Conflict of Interest and Medicine

In the context of a growing criticism on the influence of the pharmaceutical industry on physicians, scientists, or politicians, *Conflict of Interest and Medicine* offers a comprehensive analysis of the conflict of interest in medicine anchored in the social sciences, with perspectives from sociology, history, political science, and law.

Based on in-depth empirical investigations conducted within different territories (France, the European Union, and the United States) the contributions analyze the development of conflict of interest as a social issue and how it impacts the production of medical knowledge and expertise, physicians' work and their prescriptions, and also the framing of health crises and controversies. In doing so, they bring a new understanding of the transformations in the political economy of pharmaceutical knowledge, the politicization of public health risks, and the promotion of transparency in science and public life.

Complementing the more normative and quantitative understandings of conflict of interest issues that dominate today, this book will be of interest to researchers in a broad range of areas including social studies of sciences and technology, sociology of health and illness, and political sociology and ethics. It will be also a valuable resource for health professionals, medical scientists, or regulators facing the question of corporate influence.

Boris Hauray is a sociologist at Inserm (French National Institute for Health and Medical Research) and a member of the Institute for Interdisciplinary Research on Social Issues (IRIS). He was the scientific coordinator of the project MEDICI on conflict of interest in the field of medicines (French National Research Agency, 2017–2021).

Henri Boullier is a sociologist at CNRS (National Center for Scientific Research) and a member of the Interdisciplinary Research Institute in Social Sciences (IRISSO). His research focuses on the power relationships at play in health and environmental policies, in particular concerning industrial chemicals and pharmaceuticals.

Jean-Paul Gaudillière is historian of science, Senior Researcher at Inserm (French National Institute for Health and Medical Research) and Professor at EHESS (School of Advanced Studies in the Social Sciences). His recent work focuses on the history of pharmaceutical innovation and the dynamics of health globalization.

Hélène Michel is a political scientist, Professor at the University of Strasbourg, a member of the Institut Universitaire de France, and of the SAGE laboratory (Societies, Actors and Government in Europe). She has worked on interest groups, lobbying, and transparency policies in the European Union.

Routledge Studies in the Sociology of Health and Illness

'Ending AIDS' in the Age of Biopharmaceuticals
The Individual, the State, and the Politics of Prevention
Tony Sandset

HIV in the UK
Voices from the Pandemic
Jose Catalan, Barbara Hedge and Damien Ridge

The Rise of Autism
Risk and Resistance in the Age of Diagnosis
Ginny Russell

Performance Comparison and Organizational Service Provision
U.S. Hospitals and the Quest for Performance Control
Christopher Dorn

Survivorship: A Sociology of Cancer in Everyday Life
Alex Broom and Katherine Kenny

Living Pharmaceutical Lives
Peri Ballantyne and Kath Ryan

Conflict of Interest and Medicine
Knowledge, Practices, and Mobilizations
Edited by Boris Hauray, Henri Boullier, Jean-Paul Gaudillière and Hélène Michel

For more information about this series, please visit: https://www.routledge.com/Routledge-Studies-in-the-Sociology-of-Health-and-Illness/book-series/RSSHI

Conflict of Interest and Medicine

Knowledge, Practices, and Mobilizations

Edited by
Boris Hauray, Henri Boullier,
Jean-Paul Gaudillière and Hélène Michel

Routledge
Taylor & Francis Group

LONDON AND NEW YORK

First published 2022
by Routledge
2 Park Square, Milton Park, Abingdon, Oxon OX14 4RN

and by Routledge
605 Third Avenue, New York, NY 10158

Routledge is an imprint of the Taylor & Francis Group, an informa business

British Library Cataloguing-in-Publication Data
A catalogue record for this book is available from the British Library

Library of Congress Cataloging-in-Publication Data
A catalog record has been requested for this book

ISBN: 978-0-367-75115-9 (hbk)
ISBN: 978-0-367-75117-3 (pbk)
ISBN: 978-1-003-16103-5 (ebk)

DOI: 10.4324/9781003161035

Typeset in Times New Roman
by Knowledge Works Global Ltd.

Contents

List of figures   ix
List of tables   x
List of boxes   xi
List of contributors   xii
Acknowledgements   xvi

Introduction: Conflict of interest and the politics of biomedicine   1
BORIS HAURAY, HENRI BOULLIER, JEAN-PAUL GAUDILLIÈRE
AND HÉLÈNE MICHEL

PART I
Knowledge and expertise   **29**

1   **A genealogy of conflict of interest**   31
    BORIS HAURAY

2   **"Conflict of interest" or simply "interest"?**
    Shifting values in translational medicine   49
    MELANIE JESKE

3   **Managing conflicts of interest at the European Medicines**
    Agency: Success or weakness of the soft law tools?   69
    ANNIE MARTIN

4   **From the management of conflicts of interest to the**
    transformation of medical experts' profiles: The members
    of the transparency committee in France (2000–2020)   87
    JÉRÔME GREFFION AND HÉLÈNE MICHEL

PART II
Physicians and the framing of prescription practices   107

5 Conflicts of interest in medical practice: Causes and cures   109
   MARC ANDRÉ RODWIN

6 In whose best interest? Framing pharmacists' and physicians'
   (conflicts of) interest in the French market for generic drugs   129
   ETIENNE NOUGUEZ

7 The politics of industrial transparency: Constructing a database
   on the pharmaceutical funding of the health sector   147
   HENRI BOULLIER AND JÉRÔME GREFFION

8 Scientific marketing and conflict of interest: Lessons from
   the hormone replacement therapies (HRT) crisis   165
   JEAN-PAUL GAUDILLIÈRE

PART III
Mobilizations and controversies   179

9 "This Corporation Has 'Anesthetized' the Actors in the
   Drug Chain". Influence peddling and the normality
   of conflicts of interest in the Mediator® scandal   181
   SOLÈNE LELLINGER AND CHRISTIAN BONAH

10 For science, by science: The emergence and circulation of conflict
   of interest as a protest repertoire to fight against pesticides   201
   GIOVANNI PRETE, JEAN-NOËL JOUZEL AND FRANÇOIS DEDIEU

11 Conflict of interest, capture, production of ignorance, and
   hegemony: Conceptualizing the influence of corporate interests
   on public health   219
   HENRI BOULLIER, JEAN-PAUL GAUDILLIÈRE, BORIS HAURAY
   AND EMMANUEL HENRY

Postface: Conflict of interest, industry hegemony and key
opinion leader management   239
   SERGIO SISMONDO

   Index   245

Lists of figures

4.1 Graph showing total amounts received (in euros), in the form of benefits or payments between 2013 and mid-2019 by people who were TC members from 2000 to 2020. 92

4.2 Average amount received per member, between 2013 and mid-2019, according to year of entry into the TC. 93

4.3 Changes in average amounts received over the period 2013–2019, according to date on which members joined the TC (amounts normalized). 97

4.4 Average amount received per member, between 2013 and mid-2019, according to the date they left the TC. 98

4.5 Age of the TC members by period of entry into the TC. 99

4.6 Graphic representation of the *h*-index of TC members since 2000, measured in 2019. 101

4.7 Average *h*-index in 2019 and average *h*-index on joining the TC, for members since 2000, according to the period during which they joined the TC. 102

7.1 Number of articles focusing on the transparence santé website and published in the french press, by year of publication. 158

9.1 Chronology of benfluorex, 1974–2021. 183

9.2 Number of packets of Mediator® sold in France by Laboratoires Servier (September 1976 to November 2009). 183

9.3 Countries in which benfluorex was being sold in 2009. 184

9.4 Evolution of the concept of COI. 189

9.5 Cardiologists' overall perception of the pharmaceutical industry. 192

List of tables

2.1 COIs reported in major biomedical journals in 2019   65
4.1 Average age of the members in 2016 and at their entry into the
    TC and proportion of women, by period of entry into in the TC   91
4.2 Multiple linear regressions on the amount received per month
    between 2013 and mid-2019 (amounts normalized)   94
4.3 Multiple linear regressions on the h-index and number of
    publications by TC members since 2000, in 2019 and at the date
    they joined the TC   103
5.1 COIs of public servants: Intervention points   114
11.1 Four categories to explore influence, their analytical framing,
    and their uses   234

List of boxes

5.1 Analyzing COIs: a checklist 116
5.2 Sources of COIs of public employees 118
9.1 List of charges filed against the accused in the act of indictment
for the Mediator® trial opened on September 23, 2019 197
10.1 List of French books criticizing industry influence on pesticide
regulation 208

List of contributors

Christian Bonah is Professor for the History of Health and Life Sciences at the University of Strasbourg and a member of the Institut Universitaire de France. He has worked on the comparative history of medical education, the history of medicaments, as well as the history of human experimentation. Recent work includes research on risk perception and management in drug scandals as well as studies on medical films. He is currently the Principal Investigator of the ERC Advanced Grant *The Healthy Self as Body Capital: Individuals, Market-based Societies and Body Politics in Visual Twentieth Century Europe*.

Henri Boullier is Research Fellow in Sociology at CNRS (French National Center for Scientific Research) and a member of the Interdisciplinary Research Institute in Social Sciences (IRISSO). Trained in sociology and STS, his research focuses on the power relationships at play in health and environmental policies (industrial chemicals, pesticides, drugs, and veterinary medicines) and the role of companies in the production of scientific and regulatory knowledge. His book, *Toxiques légaux* (2019), analyzes how complex bureaucratic procedures and dominant toxicological protocols contribute to maintaining mass-produced toxic chemicals on the market. He is currently investigating the global circulation of pesticides and veterinary antimicrobials.

François Dedieu is Research Fellow in Sociology at INRAE (French National Institute for Agricultural Research and the Environment). His research focuses on the relationship between organizations and knowledge production in the domain of health and environmental risks. He has worked on the construction of ignorance in public policies, with the objective to study how the dangers of pesticides are recognized or left in the shadows. Recent publications include *Covid-19, une crise organisationnelle* (2020) and "Organized denial at work: The difficult search for consistencies in French pesticide regulation", in *Regulation and Governance* (2021).

Jean-Paul Gaudillière is Senior Researcher in History of Science at the Institut National de la Santé et de la Recherche Médicale. His research explores the history of the life sciences and medicine during the 20th century. His recent work focuses on the history of pharmaceutical innovation and the construction of drug markets since World War II on the one hand, and the dynamics of health globalization after WWII on the other hand. Between 2014 and 2019, he was coordinator of the European Research Council project *From International to Global: Knowledge, Diseases, and the Postwar Government of Health.*

Jérôme Greffion is Associate Professor of Sociology at Paris Nanterre University and a member of the Institutions and Historical Dynamics of Economics and Society (IDHES) laboratory. His research focuses on the economics of pharmaceuticals and the commercial strategies of pharmaceutical companies. He has extensively studied the relations between the pharmaceutical industry and doctors as well as the work of pharmaceutical sales representatives. More recently, he has also been interested in the process of setting and negotiating drug prices in hospitals.

Boris Hauray is Research Fellow in Sociology at Inserm (French National Institute of Health and Medical Research) and a member of the Institute for Interdisciplinary Research on Social Issues. He has been working on public health issues for 20 years, and more particularly on pharmaceutical knowledge, practices, and policies. He was recently the scientific coordinator of the project MEDICI on conflict of interest in the field of medicines (ANR, 2017–2021). His publications include *Santé publique, l'état des savoirs,* (co-edited with Didier Fassin, 2010) and a special issue of the journal *Sciences sociales et santé* on *Conflits d'intérêts et santé publique* (2020).

Emmanuel Henry is Professor of Sociology at Université Paris-Dauphine, PSL University and researcher at IRISSO. In 2020–2021, he was a member of the School of Social Science at *Institute for Advanced Study.* His research seeks to gain insight into how scientific knowledge and ignorance, particularly as structured by power dynamics, contribute to shaping social problems, as well as the ways in which those problems are addressed in the public sphere and managed within the framework of public policy. He is particularly interested in showing how the structuring of scientific knowledge and ignorance contributes to the construction of non-issues, that is, issues that are socially invisible and insufficiently addressed by public authorities.

Melanie Jeske is a Doctoral Candidate in Sociology in the Department of Social and Behavioral Sciences at the University of California, San Francisco. A sociologist of science and medicine, Melanie's research has focused on how developments in science, medicine, and technology shape the ways we come to know and understand our social identities, beliefs about human difference, and experiences of health and illness. Her research critically examines the social, political, and economic drivers of emergent technologies and knowledge systems.

Jean-Noël Jouzel is Senior Researcher in Sociology at CNRS and a member of the Center for the Sociology of Organizations. He is interested in controversies surrounding environmental health issues. His research looks specifically at why so little is known about occupational diseases induced by worker exposure to toxic substances. His approach combines sciences studies, the sociology of public action, and the sociology of social movements, and contributes to the growing body of work on the social construction of ignorance. He has recently published *Pesticides. Comment ignorer ce que l'on sait* (2019).

Solène Lellinger is Lecturer in History and Philosophy of Health at the University of Paris. Her research has focused on the socio-history of therapeutic agents, which she studies through their production, their regulation, and their use in care relationships. In particuler, she has tried to understand the origins and consequences of the Mediator® (benfluorex) scandal in France. She has analyzed the process of non-recognition of a serious adverse side effect of the drug for over 30 years and, above all, the effects of this non-recognition on those directly affected: the patients.

Annie Martin is Research Fellow in Law at CNRS (French National Center for Scientific Research) and a member of the SAGE laboratory (Societies, Actors and Government in Europe). She has worked on international space law, private international law, and more recently on European and international law related to pesticides. Her research focuses on the circulation of norms between international organizations as well as between private and public entities.

Hélène Michel is Professor of Political Science at the University of Strasbourg, a member of the Institut Universitaire de France, and affiliated to the CNRS and University of Strasbourg's SAGE laboratory (Societies, Actors and Governement in Europe). She has worked on interest groups, lobbying, and transparency policies in the European Union. As a political sociologist, she focuses on the sociology of actors, their trajectories, and their practices in order to figure out the logics of the influence.

Etienne Nouguez is Research Fellow at CNRS, a member of the Center for the Sociology of Organisations (Sciences Po/CNRS), and Assistant Professor of Sociology at Sciences Po, Paris, France. Specialized in economic and health sociology, his research has focused on the institutionalization of markets for health (drugs, marijuana, and food with health claims). These markets are approached as complex social organizations combining regulatory agencies, experts, companies, healthcare professionals, and consumers. But they are also analyzed as spaces for valuation in which health, social, political, and economic values are both conflicting and articulated.

Giovanni Prete is Associate Professor at the Université Paris Nord and a researcher in Sociology at the Institut de Recherche Interdisciplinaire sur les enjeux Sociaux (IRIS). His research focuses on the social and political issues of occupational health. He is particularly interested in understanding the interplay of social movements, law, science, and public regulations. In his most recent work, he has analyzed the controversies and mobilizations around the risks of agricultural pesticides for workers and the general population.

Marc Rodwin is Professor of Law at Suffolk University Law School. His research has focused on diverse facets of health law, policy, and ethics including health care consumer voice and representation; accountability in managed care; consumer protection in health care; medical malpractice; and ownership of patient health data. He has provided training on conflicts of interest related to pharmaceutical good governance for various nations under the aegis of the World Health Organization. He is the author of *Conflicts of Interest and the Future of Medicine: The United States, France and Japan* (2011); and *Medicine, Money & Morals: Physicians' Conflicts of Interest* (1993).

Sergio Sismondo is Professor in the Department of Philosophy at Queen's University. He works in the field of Science and Technology Studies, in which he has written one of the standard textbooks, *An Introduction to Science and Technology Studies* (2nd ed. 2010) and is editor of *Social Studies of Science*, one of the field's flagship journals. His empirical work for the past decade has mostly been about intersections of pharmaceutical research and marketing, focused on political economies of pharmaceutical knowledge; see his *Ghost-Managed Medicine: Big Pharma's Invisible Hands* (2018).

Acknowledgements

This book is the result of a four-year research project on conflicts of interest in the field of medicines (nicknamed MEDICI), funded by the French National Agency for Research (ANR). It brings together a selection of papers presented and discussed during its final conference, held in Paris in December 2019. We are very grateful for the support and help of many people in the ANR and Inserm (French National Institute for Health and Medical Research), but also in our respective laboratories (IRIS, Cermes3, and SAGE), who have participated in the elaboration and daily functioning of this project, and in the organization of its numerous scientific events. We would like to especially thank Carmen Mata and Issa Cissé for their joyful efficacy. We are of course particularly indebted to Estelle Girard, for her lightening and warm influence throughout the MEDICI project, from the handling of day-to-day problems to her participation in strategic decision-making.

As this research would not have been possible without them, we owe a great deal to all the physicians and scientists, administrative or elected officials, members of NGOs, and journalists, who have accepted to meet us, sometimes several times. They not only accepted to respond to our questions, but they also have, more often than once, offered us generous encouragements to undertake this social sciences inquiry into the thorny issue of corporate influence. We are also very grateful to all the colleagues and health professionals who engaged in stimulating and thought-provoking discussions during their participation in the conferences and seminars organized throughout the project, most notably the three-year-long seminar *'Conflits d'intérêts et santé publique'* organized at EHESS (School of Advanced Studies in the Social Sciences); the conference *'Intérêts agro-industriels et santé publique'* held in May 2018; the conference *'Des influences toxiques? Industrie chimique et santé publique'* held in November 2018; the conference *'Conflits d'intérêts et médicaments'* held in May 2019; and the panels on *'Corporate Influence on Science and Regulation'* we organized in the context of the annual meeting of the Society for the Social Studies of

Science held in New Orleans in September 2019. In these regards, we would like to thank Patrick Castel, Anne Chailleu, Pierre Chirac, Lisa Cosgrove, David Demortain, Marc-Oliver Déplaude, Joséphine Eberhart, Irène Frachon, Stéphane Horel, Catherine Lemorton, Paul Scheffer, Philippe Schilliger, and Frédéric Séval. The contribution of Sébastien Dalgalarrondo to this book is incommensurable, as he participated from day one to the writing of the MEDICI project, co-lead the EHESS seminar on conflict of interest for three years, and because his analyses and knowledge on corporate influence and the pharmaceutical sector have been a compass during the journey of this project.

In the last part of this adventure, we were very fortunate to benefit from the careful and supportive feedback of Emily Briggs and Lakshita Joshi, respectively editor and editorial assistant at Routledge, during the preparation of this volume. Chapter 1 and 10 were translated by Cadenza Academic Translations, Chapters 3, 4, and 9 by Adam Foulkes-Roberts & Sarah Bichot, Chapter 7 by Lucy Garnier and Chapter 8 by Liz Libbrecht. The manuscript was much improved by the careful, precise, and thorough copy editing by Cadenza.

Last but most definitely not least, we would like to thank our friends and loved ones, particularly Ingrid, Lili, and Salomé, for their constant support, patience, and love throughout this project.

Introduction
Conflict of interest and the politics of biomedicine

Boris Hauray, Henri Boullier,
Jean-Paul Gaudillière and Hélène Michel

Over the last few decades, the influence of corporate interests – particularly from the tobacco, chemical, pharmaceutical, and food industries – on public health has attracted growing concern and public attention. In medicine, this criticism has been particularly virulent as several scandals and health crises since the 2000s (such as those relating to the anti-inflammatory drug Vioxx®, antidepressants, vaccines or opioids) have shed light on the pharmaceutical industry's financial relationships with scientists, experts, physicians, and politicians, and on their potential consequences for public health. These discourses and mobilizations draw on different conceptualizations of corporate influence: some evoke the capture of regulatory agencies; others focus on the lobbying of corporate actors; while, more recently, the "production of ignorance" (Frickel and Moore, 2006) has gained increasing currency in the social sciences, echoing pioneering research on the strategies of the tobacco industry.

However, another notion, that of "conflict of interest" (COI), has been particularly successful in the discourse produced by professionals, watchdog organizations, and the media on corporate influence, with far-reaching consequences on the framing of many political and scientific dynamics. The debates triggered by the COVID-19 pandemic, from the arguments surrounding the benefits/risks of the different potential treatments to the negotiation of contracts with the vaccine producers, have once again brought this situation to light. For example, the publication by a team led by French researcher Didier Raoult of a study defending the efficacy of hydroxychloroquine in treating patients affected by COVID-19 was attacked from the day of its publication not only because of its methodological weaknesses, but also (by researchers focusing on questions of scientific integrity) because it had been published in a journal with which Raoult had close links, creating a strong suspicion of COI.[1] In return, the proponents of this therapy have repeatedly claimed that their opponents were in fact biased by their financial links with firms developing competing treatments, in particular the firm Gilead,

10.4324/9781003161035

producer of remdesivir®. Raoult even published an article claiming to demonstrate the correlation between these COIs and the public positions taken by physicians against hydroxychloroquine in France (Roussel and Raoult, 2020). More generally, and owing to the existence of a public database disclosing the financial relationships between companies and healthcare professionals in France since 2014, physicians who have gained visibility as part of COVID controversies have been attacked on social media or in the press for their links with pharmaceutical firms. Members of France's Scientific Council on COVID-19, which was established by President Macron and played a central role in the definition of the country's response to the pandemic, were also criticized for the same reason. And when the public debate switched from hydroxychloroquine to vaccines, the same controversies arose. Observers drew attention to the high price the European Union (EU) had paid for vaccines, and it was revealed that one of the EU negotiators was a fellow lobbyist for the pharmaceutical industry. To this accusation, the European Commission simply responded that this negotiator had, along with all the other negotiators, signed a disclosure form attesting that he had no COI.

This importance of the issue of corporate influence, understood through the lens of COI, in the political dynamics of COVID-19, was of course not specific to France or Europe. In the United States (US), President Trump's support for hydroxychloroquine, along with the Food and Drug Administration's (FDA) emergency authorization to prescribe it, has led journalists and politicians to point out the links of interest between Trump or people from his close circle and certain producers of the treatment. A group of US senators more widely and officially requested explanations on the COIs tainting the US's management of the pandemic, drawing attention to "recent reports that raise significant ethics and conflict of interest concerns about the White House Coronavirus Task Force and the roles and influence of Jared Kushner, President Trump, and other individuals with financial conflicts of interest".[2] A few weeks later, when Moderna announced that it had developed its first vaccine against the virus, the *New York Times* headlined 'Trump's Vaccine Chief Has Vast Ties to Drug Industry, Posing Possible Conflicts'[3], referring to Moncef Slaoui (co-leader of Trump's Operation Warp Speed): the value of his shares in Moderna had increased by $2.4 million following the announcement. The fact that COI is so widely used in the context of public or scientific controversies must be understood in the context of an increasing institutionalization of this category within many organizations in the health sector and in the law over several decades. Regulatory agencies and expert committees, scientific journals, universities, and research institutes have established increasingly precise mechanisms for documenting and controlling COIs, and in particular procedures for disclosing the financial relationships between industries and health professionals. As a consequence, in 2009, an influential report by the American Institute of Medicine stated: "Hardly a week goes by without a news story about conflicts of interest in medicine" (Lo and Field, 2009, p. xi).

Despite this centrality of COI in health controversies and in the regulation of health professions and organizations, the social sciences, unlike the fields of ethics and the biomedical sciences, have paid little attention to this issue. Focusing on medicine and the pharmaceutical industry, this book aims to fill this gap. In the context of an evolving moral and political economy of biomedicine, it proposes to explore 1) how COI has become the main category used to consider and regulate corporate influence, and 2) the effects of this problematization on the ways in which the various actors of the health sector perform and organize their activities. To do so, it gathers contributions from sociologists, historians, and political and legal scholars, who study COI within different territories (France, the European Union (EU), or the US) and various social spaces (the media, scientific organizations, public agencies, medical practices). They adopt multiple analytical perspectives, looking at professional arrangements, the construction and circulation of ideas and discourses, the definition and implementation of laws and procedures, and the dynamics of health controversies, among other aspects.

A neglected subject in the social sciences

The dominant definition of COI points to situations that create a risk that a professional's judgment or action concerning his or her primary interest will be unduly influenced by a secondary interest (Lo and Field, 2009). In the health sector, this primary interest may involve actions such as producing valid knowledge, treating a patient, and making public health decisions, while the secondary interest tends to be financial links or benefits. Behind this apparent simplicity, the category is used to account for, question, or regulate quite diverse phenomena: hidden connections or cases of scientific fraud; the role acquired by industrial actors in science and medicine (definition and conduct of clinical research, presence in the initial and continuing medical education of physicians); direct financial transfers to health professionals and health organizations (such as meals, speaking fees paid to key opinion leaders, or funding of learned societies, patient associations, or parliamentary clubs); or phenomena such as revolving door processes. Moreover, public and professional debates on the matter seem to be caught in a rut between, on the one hand, those who describe medicine as being corrupted by industry interests (Angell, 2004; Goldacre, 2012; Gøtzsche, 2013) and, on the other hand, those who denounce the systematic suspicion of health professionals and scientists collaborating with industrial actors (Stossel, 2015). The former highlight the limits and pitfalls of transparency as the main solution given to COI problems and ask for more structural reforms of the health care sector. The latter claim that the prevailing crusade against COI endangers valuable interactions between industry and academics or physicians, leads to witch hunts, and imposes an unnecessary bureaucratic burden on the sector.

From the 1980s onwards, COI became the subject of conceptual and normative debates in law and bioethics (Luebke, 1987; Thompson, 1993; Davis and Stark, 2001; Brody, 2011). These debates attempted to specify this notion by asking questions such as: Is COI primarily a risk of poor judgment or a breach of trust in a social system? And why should we focus on financial COI? They also tried to assess the normative implications of COI, i.e., is having COIs in itself morally wrong? From the late 1990s, the increasingly widespread use of disclosure statements in scientific articles and the analysis of documents obtained through litigations fostered the development in medical journals of a quasi-subfield of research on COI. These articles aimed to *demonstrate* the hypothesis underlying COI regulations: the contradictions between financial relationships with industry and the production of proper health knowledge/practices. Studies have tried to statistically prove the link between the source of funding (private/academic) and the claims made about the risks or benefits of products (Bekelman, Li, and Gross, 2003) or the impact of gifts on prescription practices (DeJong et al., 2016). Most of these studies were conducted on pharmaceuticals (Lundh et al., 2017), but some also looked at tobacco (Barnes and Bero, 1998) or food products (Lesser et al., 2007). Others have more directly exposed *misconducts* that have been interpreted as mechanisms explaining these statistical "biases": commercially driven study designs (Lathyris et al., 2010); misrepresentation of research results (Hrachovec and Mora, 2001); withholding of negative data (Whittington et al., 2004); and strong industrial control of scientific publishing through ghost- and guest-writing (Wislar et al., 2011). Some analysts have regularly criticized a focus on *financial* COI (Rothman, 1993; Rosenbaum, 2015); others have responded that because non-financial COIs (i.e., personal beliefs, academic competition, etc.) are unavoidable and impossible to regulate, highlighting their importance only serves to muddy the waters on the necessity of enforcing COI policies (Bero, 2017).

In contrast, partly because of the perception that COI is mainly an "insider category", infused with idealized professional norms of purity (see chapter 11), social science researchers have been reluctant to consider COI as a fruitful subject through which to study science and medicine. Scholars analyzing the role of corporate interests in medicine have favored other perspectives. On the one side, they have focused on more specific and tangible forms of social phenomena, such as the ghost management of science (Sismondo, 2018), corporate bias in regulation (Abraham, 1995), and scientific marketing (Gaudillière and Thoms, 2015). On the other side, they have adopted alternative frameworks of analysis, such as neoliberalism (Davis and Abraham, 2013), hegemony (Sismondo, 2018; Rajan, 2017), regulatory capture (Carpenter and Moss, 2013), and institutional corruption (Rodwin, 2013). Exceptions include the work of Sheldon Krimsky, trained in the philosophy of science, who since the 1980s has published several works on the subject. In his writings, COI points to all forms of corporate financing of science, science being considered as a public-interest-driven institution, which fundamentally raises problems of scientific integrity. Alongside works of a more philosophical nature, Krimsky (with his colleagues) has concentrated on measuring the importance of the financial links between corporations and the academic sphere (universities, experts), their disclosure (or not) in publications, and their effect on the results of research (Krimsky, 2019). Concerning this last issue, he has focused on the direct funding of research by corporations – the "funding effect" (Krimsky, 2013). The publications of Marc Rodwin (1995; 2011) have also been landmarks in the social study of COI. Rodwin has adopted a broad conception of physicians' COIs (to include all tensions between physicians' economic self-interest and their commitment to treating patients) tracing the constitution of a medical market in the US back over more than a century, examining the policies aimed at limiting its perverse effects, and comparing these to French and Japanese histories and policies.

Alongside these pioneering pieces of research, some work has described the rise of COI disclosure policies in medical journals (Hendrick, 2016) or regulatory agencies (Glode, 2002; Hauray, 2006). On this last point, Joel Lexchin and Orla O'Donovan (2010) have studied the policies implemented in three European agencies. They found that the European Medicines Agency (EMA) itself considers a quarter of the experts in its database to be "high risk", and thus criticize the agency's logic of COI management, as opposed to a logic of prohibition, which the two authors themselves advocate. Very little work has focused on the implications of this growing problematization of COI within the health sector. This lack is all the more regrettable since, as Frederic W. Hafferty and Brian Castellani (2011) have pointed out, this is probably one of the major issues through which medicine as a profession thinks about itself today. Sarah Wadmann has suggested that focusing on the problems of COIs with regard to relations between industries and physicians leads to blame games, which distract attention from the real stakes of this cooperation, i.e., the definition of research priorities (Wadmann, 2014). Kathryn Jones has studied the financial relations between pharmaceutical firms and patient groups, the management and perception of these relations by the actors involved, and has rejected the idea that they could lead to capture by economic interests (Jones, 2008). Based on solid empirical work that focuses on the actors involved, their practices, and the social dynamics at play, the very aim of this book is to make up for this lack of social studies on COI in relation to public health.

A social study of COI

A central hypothesis underlying the book is that COI is not just a new way of naming old problems of corporate influence: for more than two decades, the mounting visibility of the category has profoundly affected the world of medicine and the knowledge about financial relationships within it, along with the consequences of these relationships, the ethical experience of individuals, and the political struggle inside the field. As such, there is a need for empirical work that focuses on the actors, their practices, and the social dynamics at play. These analyses are needed to document and explain the development of COI as a central issue; to explain what this category *brings to light*, but also what it *leaves in the dark*; and to understand the materiality and social impact of the implementation of COI regulation. Based on this hypothesis, this book draws on the collective research conducted over the course of four years by a dozen French scholars on COI in medicine, and on the analyses of international scholars who have been studying corporate influence on science and medicine for years.

Using a large range of empirical data (including interviews, observations, archives, biographical and career-path studies, and statistical and content analysis of scientific publications), the book proposes an innovative analytical strategy, combining two lines of investigation. The first analyzes the socio-historical construction of COI as a social category; the heterogeneous mobilizations it triggered in the medical field or in the public sphere (as a moral judgment, a protest repertoire, a naturalized object of measurement, or a regulatory tool); and examines the different kinds of laws, rules, and procedures built in the name of COI, along with their consequences. The second line of investigation looks at the changing nature of the arrangements between corporate interests and health actors (and not just the financial transfers involved) and the way health professionals and scientists perceive them, in a contradictory landscape where private–public relationships are at the same time widely encouraged – in the name of biomedical innovation – and stigmatized. Some contributions focus more on the first line of investigation, others on the second, but they all connect these two complementary ways of developing a social study of COI. In adopting these two analytical strategies, this book will (re)place COI-related debates and processes within larger social dynamics that have affected the world of public health for several decades, the main ones being the transformations of the political economy of pharmaceutical knowledge, the politicization and scandalization of public health risks, and the development of a transparency movement in science and politics.

The transformations of the political economy of pharmaceutical knowledge

For the past two decades, a rapidly growing body of literature has regarded the pervading presence of COIs in the drug sector as a systemic rather than an idiosyncratic phenomenon. Originating in the social sciences in general and in the studies of science more specifically, inquiries about the forms of knowledge production in the pharmaceutical world reveal structural features that result in repeated and multiple situations of COI. The direct and large-scale role of the industry in both financing and designing the majority of research projects, ranging from the synthesis of new molecules to the completion of phase III clinical trials, is thus the central idea grounding the argument that situations of COI originate in the mere political economy of pharmaceutical knowledge. This section introduces this argument by recounting the dominant post-Second World War regime of industrial knowledge production, explaining how the tensions grounding this regime had turned into a crisis by the turn of the century, and detailing how both the reorganization associated with an increasing reliance on a finance-based biotech sector and the outsourcing of in-house research and development (R&D) have increased the instances of COI and made them more visible.

It is interesting to discuss this perspective on COI in relation to the analysis of the recent historiography of pharmacy, which has proposed to account for the radical transformation of the domain after the Second World War. What historians such as Chauveau (1999), Quirke (2008), Greene (2007), Tobbell (2011), Carpenter (2010), and many others have taught us over the past 15 years in this respect is that the post-war reorganization of the Northern world of drug-making was characterized by five main features:

- the changing scale of a market increasingly supported by new forms of benefits provided by health insurance (national or private), which thus turned into aggregated, collective spending
- the mergers or disappearance of vast numbers of small family-run firms that had originated in pharmacies established by university-educated professionals
- the introduction into the market of whole new classes of drugs, opening the door to chemotherapy in areas that had either not been working with therapeutic substances at all (cancer) or had not been doing so very successfully (tuberculosis)
- the rising importance of administrative rather than professional or industrial regulations, with the consequence of a significant drop in the number of products sold on the market in all major industrial countries
- the increasingly widespread use of chemical–biological–clinical screening as the dominant path to drug invention, which in the eyes of most firms gave them the possibility of finding radically new active substances

rather than copying, modifying, and combining those already included in the pharmacopoeia, therefore legitimizing large-scale investment in internal research infrastructures

The combination of these five features radically altered the construction of drug markets, placing the search for "innovations" center stage. The advent of particular structures of pharmaceutical capitalism that brought together innovations in pharmaceutical marketing (Greene, 2007; Dumit, 2012; Gaudillière, 2013) and models of drug development based on screening and randomized clinical trials (RCTs) changed the nature of market operations and led to the development of bio-capitalist economies with very specific ways of envisaging how biomedical utility and circuits of drug/commodity exchange should be connected. Rather than anticipating development and growth on the basis of competition through prices and short-term management, large post-war pharmaceutical companies increasingly turned to monopolistic practices rooted in patent protection, competition for entire therapeutic classes, and the long-term planning of launches and mass marketing – all strategies that strongly connected with, depended upon, and further fed into the in-house screening model of drug invention.

One reason for this pattern was of course the in-house dynamics of laboratory growth, which resulted in a radical increase in the chemical workforce in all large companies and consequently in the sheer number of molecules at their disposal. The other reason was the increasingly widespread use and *internalization* of controlled clinical trials. It is not that pharmaceutical firms did not engage in the evaluation of efficacy before the Second World War, but they did it through long-term collaborations with a small group of elite clinicians who were free to experiment in many directions. The mounting reference in the 1960s–1970s to controlled clinical trials, double-blind procedures, randomization, standard protocols, the statistical control of significance, and collaborative studies led by the industry was therefore a significant change of practice.

The industrialization of clinical trials brought a new coupling with scientific marketing. Scientific marketing is not publicity, but rather a different way of constructing drug markets that mobilizes science in two different ways (Gaudillière, 2013; Gaudillière and Thoms, 2015). First, it develops marketing as a research activity based not only on sales data but also, for instance, on sophisticated surveys of prescription practices and motivations. Second, it uses laboratory or clinical research for promotion. Scientific marketing was not a new concept in the 1960s, but its scale and nature radically changed when, after the Second World War, prescribing physicians became the exclusive targets of marketing departments. A key sign of this change was the growth in the 1950s–1970s of the drug representative system, which became the core instrument of scientific marketing. The hundreds and later thousands of pharmaceutical representatives employed in large firms were not only sales agents; they were given special technical training, and eventually even completed short stays in laboratories and clinical services. Clinical research and marketing were thus coupled in new ways with regular exchanges of information.

This political economy of drug knowledge production was of course not without its tensions, which were both epistemic and organizational. It was however not until the 1980s that these tensions escalated into a crisis overtly discussed in the specialized literature from the early 2000s onward under the motto of the "crisis of productivity" in drug research and development (for an overview, see Gaudillière, 2021). This idea of a crisis is exemplified with three kinds of indicators: the decrease in the number of new molecular entity (NME) approvals; the rising costs of drug R&D; and the growing rates of attrition (the probability of failure) when a molecular drug candidate moves along the screening pipeline from preclinical studies to phase I, II, and III trials, and finally to market launch.

The discussion about the crisis has also shed light on a variety of "responses" in the industry: from the most simple – putting more money in the pipeline – to attempts to diversify the knowledge (and target) basis with biotech acquisition, and finally to more recent and more fundamental changes of the organizational and economic model, with tendencies toward externalized R&D or the more radical exploration of an open source model that would limit the domination of patents as the key mode of appropriation. Though less discussed, other responses exist and include internal tinkering with the organization of research (such as increasing the number of candidates in the early stages of screening, followed by more stringent selection in the latter – more costly – clinical stages) or lobbying in favor of regulatory reforms (for example, extending the duration of intellectual property rights, or creating accelerated evaluation processes and access to the market, such as the 1983 Orphan Drug Act). What characterizes this repertoire of responses is a deep inscription in three large transformations: the rise of biotechnology, an increasingly financial economy of knowledge, and the outsourcing of many activities.

Sociologists and economists of innovation have looked at the "biotechnology turn" as an example of the creation of a "knowledge economy" (Kahin and Foray, 2006), i.e., the commodification of research through the conjunction of three elements: 1) the emergence of new forms of knowledge; 2) the creation of startups valorizing research results in a more or less straightforward way through patenting; and 3) the financing of these startups through venture capital and innovation markets. This transformation would not have taken place without major political and institutional changes (for an overview, see Gaudillière, 2015). In the US context, the 1980s thus saw the conjunction of three initiatives: 1) the transformation of Nasdaq into a speculative market for financing innovative firms not (yet) involved in the production of goods or services; 2) the passage of the Bayh-Dole Act to foster technology transfers from academia; and 3) the enlarged practices of patent approval at the US Patent and Trademark Office, which culminated in the normalization of property rights over genes, cells, and entire organisms.

This rise of an economy focusing on the early appropriation and financial valorization of biomedical research outputs has been reinforced by a general trend toward the demise of the "research factory", i.e., the reduction in *in-house* research capabilities (Buderi, 2002). A good example is provided by the rise in contract research organizations (CROs) (Mirowski and Van Horn, 2005; Sismondo, 2009), which fulfill many functions, including preparing articles and following the process of publication (ghostwriting), organizing clinical trials through networks of physicians distributed across the globe, and preparing marketing permit applications and lobbying for their approval. In the case of clinical trials, for instance, the costs of maintaining a relationship with qualified physicians, recruiting patients, and collecting and analyzing data are transferred to CROs, which – in contrast to previous contractors (clinical services, hospitals) – share the same managerial culture and efficacy criteria as the contracting firm. More broadly, outsourcing may be viewed as a new type of value formation, breaking with the Chandlerian structure of large corporations. As such, it comes with an increasing emphasis on the flexibility of tasks, delocalized production, and the search for rapidly rotating market niches.

This conjunction of crisis and reorganization of the pharmaceutical sector has in many ways strengthened the influence of companies over the production of knowledge, increasing and making more visible the links that scientists and physicians have with the industry. Sergio Sismondo (2018) has for instance powerfully argued that the phenomenon of ghostwriting – which involves key opinion leaders in a medical field of interest putting their name to articles they have not written and for which may not even have done significant research – has recently acquired novel dimensions with the expansion of dedicated contractors. One hypothesis the book engages with is therefore that the new visibility of COI in public controversies about the value of drugs, along with its mounting legal and regulatory functions, is rooted in these very processes of crisis, financialization, and outsourcing.

The politicization and scandalization of public health risks

The transformation of the political economy of pharmaceutical knowledge has created new links between corporate actors and the world of health. The consideration of these links in terms of threats to the population, and the success of the category of COI as a tool to denounce and regulate them, has taken place within a movement characterized by a growing politicization and scandalization of public health risks. This movement, enshrined in a broader reconsideration of the status of science and technology in society, has been particularly influential in the pharmaceutical sector, and "Big

Pharma" has come to embody the unscrupulous and dangerous research of profits of global companies. As chapter 1 details, although COI emerged during the 1970s in public health debates through criticisms of the composition of regulatory committees, it was really from the 1980s, and following highly visible controversies on fraud and newfound fortunes in the biomedical sector, that it was progressively institutionalized in science and medicine. It gained prominence from the early 2000s onwards, when the media, NGOs, politicians, but also many professionals, began to intensively accuse the pharmaceutical industry (and its pervasive influence, from general practitioners to ministers) of endangering the population. More generally speaking, the general moral and political landscape on public health risks has greatly evolved over the last decades, giving rise to a "crisis of trust" in the pharmaceutical sector's products and actors. This has paved the way for the mobilization of the category of COI.

The risks generated by medical practices or therapeutics have long been acknowledged, and since at least the end of the 19th century, scandals and controversies have fostered the development of a growing professional and public regulation (Daemmrich, 2004; Horowitz, 2012; Gaudillière and Hess, 2013). However, the political context in which these controversies and regulation take place evolved significantly from the 1950s onwards. While the status of science and technology had been little questioned until then, late modernity caused cracks in the idea of a natural alliance between the progress of science and technology and the improvement of the well-being of the population. Despite the withdrawal from the market of thalidomide in the early 1960s and DES in the early 1970s (see chapter 8) attracting significant public and political attention (and, in the case of thalidomide fostering crucial political reforms; see Carpenter, 2010), trust in the pharmaceutical sector's actors and products remained strong until the late 1980s. The social mobilizations on public health risks that emerged in the 1960s primarily concerned pollution and environmental contamination, notably linked to the widespread use of pesticides developed by chemical multinationals such as Dow Chemical and Monsanto (Boudia and Jas, 2014; Boullier, 2019). From the 1970s, they participated to a more general and growing criticism of the political nature of scientific knowledge and the composition of expert committees regulating science and technologies (drugs, food products, chemicals, nuclear plants). This new politicization of public health knowledge, technologies, and political bodies has been well captured by a nascent field of science and technology studies (STS). Sheila Jasanoff's work on the Environmental Protection Agency (EPA) and the FDA has notably analyzed the forms of knowledge produced and used by the regulatory agencies, and has proposed using the term "regulatory science" to designate the knowledge mobilized to assess products before they are put on the market (or, very rarely, to withdraw them), which is generally based on complex bureaucratic procedures and standardized testing protocols (Jasanoff, 1990). In this context, in the US, COI began to be occasionally denounced and procedures of COI disclosure were formalized in public agencies. In parallel, from the 1960s, focusing firstly on psychiatry, the criticism of medicine as an institution of social control (Zola, 1972), led by the specific interest of its professionals, developed through the notion of "medicalization". In 1975, Ivan Illich, in his high-profile book on the fundamental iatrogeny of medicine, *Medical Nemesis: The Expropriation of Health*, firmly denounced the power of the medical professions with a more general condemnation of industrial society, giving global visibility to these issues. However, even though the crucial role of drugs in medicalization processes was sometimes highlighted (Conrad, 1975), the role of industry "remained a somewhat muted or neglected theme in the medicalisation literature" (Williams, Gabe, and Davis, 2008, p. 813).

From the 1980s, the social reconsideration of biomedical science increased with the development of scientific entrepreneurship and a scandalization of scientific fraud and misconduct (LaFolette, 1994). In this context, COI represented a way of naming the problem and, for scientific institutions (universities, medical journal, research organizations), of responding to it by establishing disclosure procedures. This reconsideration took place within a broader tendency to question the negative impact of science and technology on society. In 1986, the German sociologist Ulrich Beck formulated his general theory on the development of a "risk society" (Beck, 1992), underlining that modern societies are exposed to risks that result from "manufactured risks" (diseases, pollution, side effects of drugs, etc.) directly attributable to human activities, a theory that resonated with the Chernobyl nuclear accident that occurred in the same year. Concerning pharmaceutical drugs and knowledge, the late 1980s and the development of patient activism in response to the AIDS epidemic marked an important turning point (Epstein, 1996; Dodier, 2003; Dalgalarrondo, 2004). It produced a new politicization of science, expertise, and medicine, and gave media visibility to the denunciation of pharmaceutical firms' strategies.

From the early 2000s, criticism of the "tightening grip of big pharma" (The Lancet, 2001) became more widespread and severe. The increased number of drug scandals (cerivastatin in 2001, hormone replacement therapy (HRT) in 2002, Vioxx® and antidepressants in 2004) pushed media, professional, and political actors to investigate and denounce the influence of pharmaceutical firms in the health sector (House of Commons, 2005; Angell, 2004). Drugs were increasingly reframed as health risk producers and pharmaceutical firms as profit-obsessed dangerous actors (Gøtzsche, 2013) who downplayed risks and created diseases to promote their products (Moynihan, Heath, and Henry, 2002). A visible consequence of this increasingly negative status of pharmaceutical corporations in society and of the acknowledgment of their problematic dominant position in the health sector was the reconsideration of the notion of medicalization in the social sciences, in which they were then given a central role (Conrad, 2005) and even the rise a field of study focusing on "the pharmaceuticalization of society" (Williams, Martin, and Gabe, 2011). This politicization of drugs and their risks was favored by a more general questioning of the impact of corporations' strategies on health, following the mad cow disease "scandal" in the late 1990s and the long-running controversies over GMOs and pesticides. In this context, the denunciation of COI gained momentum as a way of capturing the problems raised by the link between scientists, experts, politicians, and economic interests. These dynamics triggered procedural reforms from professionals, medical journals, and public agencies aiming to restore and/or consolidate their legitimacy (Carpenter, 2010; Demortain, 2020; Krimsky, 2019). These reforms were nevertheless generally conducted so as to leave out the fundamental political (pro-corporate) stances incorporated in these same structures (Hauray, 2017; Boullier, 2019; Dedieu, 2021) and left the functioning of the medical sector fundamentally unchanged (Sismondo, 2018). The strengthening of procedures aimed at controlling COI through transparency thus paradoxically fueled more than it cured the "crisis of trust" in medicine (Hauray, 2019).

The promotion of transparency in science and public life

For several decades, the expansion and success of the category of COI has been directly linked to the promotion of a transparency apparatus – the disclosure of the financial links of scientists, experts, and administrative and political officials – conceived as a remedy to corporate influence issues. As such, it has actively participated in the installation and reinforcement of transparency as a central democratic ideal. Since the late 1990s, a "transparency movement" (Lessig, 2009) has taken shape in both the political and scientific fields, driven by the mobilization of various actors (NGOs, public institutions, politicians, scholars, and so on) and new technological capacities in the production and circulation of information. This movement, which promotes both expanded access to documents/data of public interest and the unveiling of hidden relationships of officials or experts with private interests, has in return legitimized COI (and its regulations) as an appropriate solution to the increased power of corporate actors in general, and as concerns public health in particular. Over the last decade, this promotion of transparency has been increasingly criticized for its depoliticization effects and its incapacity to tackle systemic dynamics.

Transparency has an ancient history as a political norm, and "sunshine" mechanisms have long been presented in the US as a solution to the problematic domination or influence of corporate actors. Louis Brandeis – advisor to President Woodrow Wilson and future member of the Supreme Court of the United States – famously stated as early as 1913 in a series of articles devoted to the problems posed by the growing powers of the big banks: "Publicity is justly commended as a remedy for social and industrial diseases. Sunlight is said to be the best of disinfectants; electric light the most efficient policeman" (Brandeis, 1913, p. 10). In 1946, the Administrative Procedure Act recognized the right of US citizens to have access to technical and regulatory information used in regulation and policymaking, a right that was reinforced by several public decisions, most notably the Freedom of Information Act of 1966 (Jasanoff, 2006; Schudson, 2015). Even more directly connected to our subject is the passing of the Bribery, Graft and Conflicts of Interest Act in 1962, which enshrined the notion of COI in federal law for the very first time. As explained in chapter 1 of this book, this law centrally created a disclosure procedure to regulate (and above all facilitate) the mobilization of consultants or outside experts in the administration. The prevailing idea among its promoters was that transparency was sufficient to manage a desired development of the circulation of professionals between the private and the public sector. In the context marked by the rise of the consumerist movement (with the founding of the non-profit organization Public Citizen by Ralph Nader in 1971) and after the adoption of the Federal Advisory Committee Act in 1972 (which aimed to ensure that the advice produced by the increasingly numerous advisory committees is "objective and accessible to the public"), the 1970s saw transparency and disclosure procedures acquire a more central place in the democratic control of the executive branch. From the 1980s onward, disclosure procedures were also progressively established in US universities, research institutions, and academic journals (Krimsky, 2019). This norm of transparency took hold more firmly in Europe from the early 1990s, in close connection, in terms of public life, with European integration and the rise of the regulatory state (Majone, 1996). The will to modernize public governance has resulted in the implementation of COI disclosure and "freedom of information" procedures in European public administrations, particularly in newly created national and European drug regulatory agencies (Abraham and Lewis, 2000; Hauray, 2006).

In recent years, the ideals of transparency have become even more visible and the measures designed in response have proliferated, both in the political and public health spheres. In the 1990s, transparency progressively became the battle horse of a whole series of non-profit organizations and NGOs fighting against corruption and COIs in the public and political sectors at large. The objective of the Center for Responsive Politics, for instance, is to investigate the "dark money" in electoral campaigns and politics; that of Transparency International is to promote transparency and integrity in public and economic affairs; while ALTER-EU (Alliance for Lobbying Transparency and Ethics Regulation), a coalition of over 200 public interest groups, denounces the influence of corporate interests on European politics (Balanyá et al., 2000; Dinan and Miller, 2008; ALTER-EU, 2010). Corporate Europe Observatory (CEO), a European research and campaign group founded in 1997 and a member of ALTER-EU, is one of the more representative examples of the growing demand for transparency over potential COI. In recent years, CEO has been denouncing the influence of large corporations in public decision-making and the "capture" of European regulatory agencies, most notably the European Food Safety Agency (CEO, 2017; Robinson et al., 2013). To promote more stringent transparency policies, their researchers have partnered with investigative journalists and developed advanced skills in the study of COI (Horel and CEO, 2013; 2015). On the other hand, public institutions were starting to promote transparency policies during the same period, in response to those mobilizations and in an effort to fight against fraud and corruption in public life. At an international level, the IMF and the World Bank called for rigorous transparency policies as far as countries' budget and debt were concerned, arguing that the public (i.e., creditors, donors, analysts, and rating agencies rather than citizens) needed to be informed in order to hold governments accountable (e.g., World Bank, 2002). Beyond the narrow problem of public corruption, the Organisation for Economic Co-operation and Development started to draw up recommendations for "good governance" and to promote "good practice" for states and public administration, on public integrity, lobbying, and revolving doors (OECD, 2004; 2007; 2010). In these transparency initiatives promoted by NGOs and public institutions, digital tools and large databases have gradually taken on a more prominent role. In 1996, the Center for Responsive Politics launched its website, OpenSecrets. org, which inventories and analyzes large sets of data related to money in politics including donations, federal lobbying, or the personal finances of members of Congress and other officials. Using similar means of disclosure on a global scale, journalist organizations and collaborations, like ProPublica and the International Consortium of Investigative Journalists (ICIJ), organized "leaks" of large collections of documents and often disclosed them through databases aimed at citizens and journalists. For instance, the ICIJ shared the Panama and the Paradise Papers, the millions of documents that revealed offshore investments and money laundering in tax havens. In these different projects, transparency is the key driver of data journalists and open government activists alike (Parasie and Dagiral, 2013; Lathrop and Ruma, 2010). Ambitious initiatives were also launched by public institutions in an effort to increase transparency. The creation of data. gov under the Obama administration may very well embody one of the most visible instances of open government, which some have called "institutional transparency" (Coglianese, 2009; Moore, 2018). Although more strictly limited to the political sphere, similar projects were launched in the EU with the European Transparency Initiative (Michel, 2012) and the Transparency Register, a publicly accessible database that inventories all the organizations representing particular interests at the European level (professional consultancies, in-house lobbyists, NGOs, think-tanks, and so on), which currently contains more than 12,000 registrants. These digital devices and the open publication of data make it easier for citizens to monitor the relations between firms and the political and regulatory sphere. They encourage whistleblowers to take action and rely on public opinion, particularly when legal protections are lacking.

On the public health side, a turning point in the mobilization around transparency, directly linked to corporate influence, was the Tobacco Master Settlement Agreement of 1998. Tobacco companies were in fact ordered to release the internal documents produced for the case, and these "Tobacco papers" were made easily accessible to the public owing to the involvement of the University of California at San Francisco. After the inclusion of documents from cases involving pharmaceutical firms (in 2006) and food industries (in 2018), it became the Industry Documents Library. What was defined as a "portal to aid investigation about cross-industry corporate practices that are detrimental to public health" has since its creation revealed with great detail the intensity of corporate ghost management of science and expertise (Sismondo, 2018, chapter 8) and demonstrated the need to fight against secrecy. For over ten years, and in the context of acute worries about research integrity, reproducibility (Elliott, 2020), and about the influence of corporate actors on secrecy and biased knowledge (Michaels, 2008; Mirowski, 2011), the issue of transparency also gained new prominence in science, most notably through the "open data/science" banner. This dynamic has been particularly strong as concerns clinical trials: the capacity to consult initial research protocols and to access raw data (so as to assess the sincerity of the published results and to produce "independent" statistical analysis) is presented as a way of compensating for the corporate bias in knowledge and expertise on drugs. For example, in 2004, in a new attempt to respond to the dominant role of the pharmaceutical industry in clinical research, the editors of the major medical journals collectively decided that trial protocols should be publicly registered (before they began) if their investigators were to publish their results in their journals. Nowadays, a deepening of the access to individual-level clinical data used by regulatory agencies or by the authors of articles is strongly advocated (Gøtzsche, 2013). In recent years, large databases have also been set up to inventory all the financial transactions between pharmaceutical companies and physicians. The most famous is probably Open Payments, a US disclosure program "that promotes a more transparent and accountable health care system" by making the financial relationships between manufacturers and health care providers available to the public. It was adopted alongside the 2010 Patient Protection and Affordable Care Act ("Obamacare") and officially launched in 2014. This idea quickly crossed the Atlantic and inspired the creation of a French counterpart, the Transparence Santé (Transparency in Healthcare) website, which was launched the same year (see chapter 7).

This larger context of promotion of transparency has been highly suitable for disseminating the category of COI. At first sight, COI appears as an additional problem to be dealt with, in addition, in the political field, to corruption, covert financing, influence peddling or lobbying or, in the scientific field, to fabrication of data, falsification, or plagiarism. Like these issues, it is seen as endangering trust in fundamental institutions and their capacity to fulfill their public-driven "raison d'être". Moreover, COI is a problem to which transparency can be seen to constitute an adequate answer. The underlying principle behind COI is that the "secondary interest" is not in itself illegitimate, it is only the coexistence of two partly contradictory interests that is at stake and, above all, numerous observers often stress that the existence of a COI does not imply that there is or will indeed be a problematic bias in the decision, expertise, or knowledge produced. In this context, one can think or claim that, in order to discourage illegitimate behavior and enable the citizens or interest parties to fully appreciate the decisions taken or knowledge/expertise produced, it is enough to know who is involved in professional or personal relationships with whom, and to objectify (usually through the value of money transfers) and publicize these relationships.

However, COI seems to be increasingly considered as more than just an additional problem. It is also progressively constituted as the origin and/or the visible indices of the other problems fought against, like corruption or falsification of data. The advantage of COI over these faults is that, given the importance of available information on the activities or financial links of officials, experts, or scientists, COIs (or undeclared COIs) are relatively easy to spot and to expose to the public. The transparency devices feed the scandals' production and enable NGOs or investigative journalists to intervene publicly: they turn COI into a public problem and urge public institutions to take measures to tackle it. Transparency tools have thus contributed to an autonomization of COI as a political issue and contributed to very specific forms of intervention on influence with the various instruments of soft law (ethical recommendations, disclosure, online registers, strategies of shaming, etc.) – making it possible to avoid other categories, along with binding means of intervention (see chapter 3).

Some conclude from that situation that the current importance given to COI constitutes a moral crusade and/or results from a search for buzz from the media or activists, or even point to its negative effects on the well-being of populations. More generally, transparency is mocked as a buzzword, and some observers deplore the tyranny of transparency and the exaggeration of discourses and injunctions in that domain (Fung, Graham, and Weil, 2007). Others think that transparency, as promoted through the category of COI, will never be a strong enough solution to respond to the systemic influence of corporate actors on policies and knowledge (see in particular chapters 3, 5, 8, and 9). For several years, this critical appraisal of transparency has been becoming increasingly influential, as illustrated by the stimulating emerging field of critical transparency studies (Alloa and Thomä, 2018; Birchall, 2011; 2015). For them, the availability of large collections of data and the increase in the number of transparency tools are not a simple response to controversies or social mobilization: they mark the advent of an "info-capitalist-democracy" where subjects must take the place of governments in retreat, by becoming auditors of the disclosed data (Birchall, 2015). Despite its omnipresence in public debates and in institutional communications, it is not certain that the focus on COI has led to a reduction in risk and an improvement of ethics in politics or science. On the other hand, it has made individual behaviors the cause of COI, thus avoiding thinking about this issue in structural terms, that is to say by taking into account the social, political, legal, and scientific dimensions of COI (Sismondo, 2008, chapter 11).

Taking into account these three broad socio-historical dynamics, the contributions gathered in this book will provide us with a comprehensive social science analysis of COI in relation to public health, which will complement the more normative and quantitative understandings of this issue that dominate today. In doing so, they open up possibilities of comparison with other fields affected by the large-scale presence of COI, including those of chemical products, nuclear technology, air pollution, and occupational health.

Contents of the book

This book combines two lines of investigation: the first consists in analyzing the socio-historical construction of COI, while the second focuses on examining the arrangements between corporate interests and health actors, and their transformations. The different contributions in this book examine these two lines of investigation in various social spaces. They are delimited by the activity of different organizations or professions (committees, physicians, the media, etc.), in relation to specific products (anorectics, hormone treatments, etc.) or domains (biotechnology, translational medicine, general medical practice, social sciences, etc.). Three main territories of the world of public health are successively examined and form the base of the structure of the book: the production of scientific knowledge and expertise, prescription practices, and mobilizations and controversies.

Part one of the book focuses on the production of scientific knowledge and expertise, and consequently on tensions between processes and regimes of "veridiction" (Foucault, 2004) and corporate interest. The key actors whose relationships with industry are centrally examined are researchers, experts, and regulators.

In the first chapter, Boris Hauray retraces the genealogy of COI as a social category and its trajectory in biomedical sciences and drug regulatory agencies. He explores both the continuities and discontinuities in how this category has been used. In particular, he draws attention to the long-lasting contradictory motives explaining the success of this category, but also the evolution of the social issues that it has served to discuss. As a consequence, he claims that this category goes well beyond revealing a specific profession-al's COIs, playing a central role in questions about industry influences and more widely in the debate about the role of drugs in medical care.

Focused on the more recent period and on biomedical actors, chapter 2, by Melanie Jeske, discusses the ways in which the reorganization of biomedical research exemplified by the institutionalization of "translational medicine" in the US has created a climate in which activities that once might have been categorized as controversial COIs are increasingly supported, encouraged, and rewarded in academic communities. Jeske's chapter examines the tensions created in traditional academic structures, such as publishing outlets, where new debates about COI reporting and its consequences proliferate.

Chapter 3, written by Annie Martin, adopts a legal perspective in its focus on the handling of COI issues by regulatory agencies. It analyzes in particu-lar how the European Medicines Agency (EMA), which is responsible for producing scientific advice on the benefit/risk evaluation of pharmaceuti-cals in the EU, manages the COIs of its experts. Martin questions the use of soft laws, such as regularly revised internal codes of conduct, instead of the existing binding texts of EU law. In particular, she wonders if this strat-egy fundamentally aims at addressing the risk generated by the COI of its experts or if it is to be understood as a way of limiting outside interventions and criticism on the functioning of the EMA.

In the last chapter of this first part, Hélène Michel and Jérôme Greffion extend this reflection and assess the effects that the different policies intro-duced to prevent the COI of experts have had on the composition of advisory committees. Their sociological analysis draws on a statistical examination of the profiles and financial links of the members of a French committee producing scientific evaluations of products, and looks at their evolution over the last two decades, during which time many measures to tackle COI have been put in place. The two authors show that not only do the members of this committee have structurally fewer links with industry, but also that their "scientific expertise" – as assessed through several bibliometric indi-cators – has apparently improved. This result challenges the idea that "an expert who has no interest is an expert of no interest".

Part two of the book focuses on drug prescription, i.e., on how knowledge and expertise are transformed into concrete daily practices in the health sector. The central actors whose relationships with industry are examined are physicians and, in one chapter, pharmacists.

In chapter 5, Marc Rodwin paints a general picture of how the COIs of physicians have been defined and managed. He examines the definitions of COIs, presents their causes, and discusses the means that can be used to "cure" COIs. He underlines that COI can be controlled by different means: by removing the financial interests, by transforming the physician's activi-ties, or by overseeing them. These solutions have some limits and Rodwin shows that COI disclosure is a "quick fix" and a necessary step in the fight against corporate influence, but insufficient in itself.

The next chapter, by Etienne Nouguez, focuses on the mounting importance of generic medicines in the French pharmaceutical market and includes an analysis of the COI of actors often neglected, pharmacists. It shows that – in contrast to what one might expect of manufacturers challenging the patent-based economy of the sector – the competition between original and generic medicines is not so much a price competition as a struggle to "frame" the choices made by health professionals. Generic companies have interacted with France's national health insurance system in order to influence prescribers and increase the prescription of their products, playing on the particular interests of these health professionals (be they remuneration, professional status, or autonomy) and developing patterns of influence including public health objectives rather than typical situations of COI.

In chapter 7, Henri Boullier and Jérôme Greffion examine the transparency apparatus recently created in numerous countries to regulate the COIs of physicians. These publicly accessible databases promise to prevent undue influence of pharmaceutical firms through the inventory, classification, and disclosure of millions of transactions between the industry and physicians. Focusing on the case of France's Transparence Santé (*Transparency in Healthcare*) website, officially launched in 2014, their investigation looks back over the highly complex and chaotic construction of the database. They show how open data activists have endeavored to compensate for the resulting flaws in this public database and to deliver on the promise of transparency. Drawing on this example, the chapter emphasizes that these recent disclosure projects embody a new form of transparency that the authors call "industrial transparency", targeted at – and operated by – economic actors, and constitute a way for the liberal state to regulate the private sector at only at a marginal level by externalizing the interpretation and monitoring of the disclosed data.

In the last chapter of this part, Jean-Paul Gaudillière investigates the history of hormone replacement therapy (HRT) during the menopause and analyzes the strategies adopted by Wyeth, one of the main US producers of HRT, to influence prescription practices. HRT was linked to issues of COI in 2003 when the Women's Health Initiative, a very large US cohort study of its effects, demonstrated its link with a higher risk of cancer and cardiovascular disorders. As a consequence, numerous female users and patients filed court cases against Wyeth. The resulting legal documentation opens a window onto the firm's activities of scientific marketing. It shows that Wyeth's main communication partner, DesignWrite, was a full-fledged "scientific marketing organization". Gaudillière believes that COI is a category that makes it difficult to understand the systemic nature of the problems originating in this kind of industrial production of expertise. The chapter therefore concludes that we need to supplement COI with other notions, for instance with hegemony.

Part three of the book analyzes how COI is used in mobilizations, controversies, and social science debates. The central actors analyzed are the media, political actors, lawyers, and social scientists.

In chapter 9, Solène Lellinger and Christian Bonah study the roots and the political consequences of the benfluorex (Mediator®) scandal in France, a drug that was withdrawn from the market in 2009 due to the morbidity and mortality assessment of its cardiopulmonary side effects. The Mediator® scandal has come to be recognized as the key event that pushed COI to the top of the agenda of France's pharmaceutical sector and beyond. Examining parliamentary and administrative inquiries that followed this scandal, they investigate how the category of COI became central to its framing and analysis. They then study how COI issues were perceived by ordinary actors in the drug chain, specifically prescribing physicians. They demonstrate that these professionals often see COI as a problem that affects other people but not their own practice, and conclude that this denial is reinforced by the justice system's treatment of legal transgressions, which leave behind the systemic nature of the problem.

The next chapter expands the analysis of the use of COI in controversies and public debate and examines the development of COI as a "protest repertoire". Focusing on environmental health, it shows that the denunciation of corporate influence in terms of COI goes far beyond the medical sector. Giovanni Prete, Jean-Noël Jouzel, and François Dedieu argue that three major changes in the institutional and social context of activism contributed to its success: the institutionalization of risk assessment, the development of investigative environmental journalism, and the professionalization of environmental health advocacy organizations. More broadly, their chapter questions the political effects of this framing in terms of COI. It suggests that it has enabled activist organizations to give public visibility to the issue of industry influence on pesticide regulation, and that it also tends to promote a rather narrow critique of pesticides as a technology.

The concluding chapter of the book looks further into a question raised by most of the other chapters: the analytical validity, for the social sciences and their participation in the public debate, of COI as a tool to conceptualize corporate influence. To do so, it compares this notion to three dominant conceptualizations of corporate influence in the public health sector: capture, production of ignorance, and hegemony. After having presented the foundations of these four notions, the main studies attached to them, and their benefits and drawbacks, the chapter's authors advocate that a comprehensive analysis of influence requires an articulation of COI, ignorance, and hegemony: COI both as a reflection of the multiple channels of influence the industry has developed and as a powerful means of making visible the double-bind of scientists, experts, and regulators; ignorance as a way of exploring the asymmetries and power gradients at stake in the production and non-production of knowledge and their effects in regulation; and hegemony as a reminder of the key role processes of market construction and diverse political economies play in the logic of influence.

Finally, in the postface, Sergio Sismondo starts on discourses of key opinion leaders (KOL) and on the management of these professionals by the pharmaceutical industry to consider the pervasive influence of corporate actors in the medical sector. He underlines that COI is part of accounts focused on individual human agency in which many of the actors of this domain are enormously invested. For him, this conception of influence tends to put too much of an emphasis on psychology, which leads many people to think in terms of actual biases, while the hegemonic position of the pharmaceutical firms is more fundamentally at stake.

Notes

1. https://scienceintegritydigest.com/2020/03/24/thoughts-on-the-gautret-et-al-paper-about-hydroxychloroquine-and-azithromycin-treatment-of-covid-19-infections/ (Accessed: February 27, 2021).
2. https://www.warren.senate.gov/imo/media/doc/2020.04.15%20Letter%20to%20WH%20DAEO%20re.%20ethics%20compliance.pdf?fbclid=IwAR1JjJRCsfg-ahdDCIdEe-7LbHkXyreW-CFV8Ld1Cf3TJji5csZLFkHcWQI (Accessed: February 26, 2021)
3. https://www.nytimes.com/2020/05/20/health/coronavirus-vaccine-czar.html (Accessed: February 15, 2021).

References

Abraham, J (1995) *Science, politics and the pharmaceutical industry: controversy and bias in drug regulation*. London: UCL Press.

Abraham, J and Lewis, G (2000) *Regulating Medicines in Europe: competition, expertise and public health*. London; New York: Routledge.

Alloa, E and Thomä, D (2018) *Transparency, society and subjectivity: critical perspectives*. London: Palgrave MacMillan.

ALTER-EU (2010) *Bursting the Brussels bubble. The battle to expose corporate lobbying at The heart of The EU*. Brussels.

Angell, M (2004) *The truth about the drug companies: how they deceive us and what to do about it*. New York: Random House.

Balanyá, B, Doherty, A, Hoedeman, O, Ma'anit, A, and Wesselius, E (2000) *Europe inc. Regional & global restructuring and the rise of corporate power*. London: Pluto.

Barnes, DE and Bero, LA (1998) 'Why review articles on the health effects of passive smoking reach different conclusions', *JAMA*, 279(19), pp. 1566–1570.

Beck, U (1992) *Risk Society: Towards a New Modernity*. London: Sage.

Bekelman, JE, Li, Y, and Gross, CP (2003) 'Scope and impact of financial conflicts of interest in biomedical research: a systematic review', *JAMA*, 289(4), pp. 454–465.

Bero, L (2017) 'Addressing bias and conflict of interest among biomedical researchers', *JAMA*, 317(17), pp. 1723–1724.

Birchall, C (2011) 'Introduction to "secrecy and transparency": the politics of opacity and openness', *Theory, Culture & Society*, 28(7–8), pp. 7–25.

Birchall, C (2015) 'Data.gov-in-a-box': delimiting transparency', *European Journal of Social Theory*, 18(2), pp. 185–202 [online]. Available at: https://doi.org/10.1177/1368431014555259 (Accessed: January 25, 2021).

Boudia, S and Jas, N (2014) *Powerless science? Science and politics in a toxic world.* New York: Berghahn Books.

Boullier, H (2019). *Toxiques légaux. Comment les firmes chimiques ont mis la main sur le contrôle de leurs produits.* Paris: La Découverte.

Brandeis, LD (1913) 'What publicity can do', *Harper's Weekly*, December 20, pp. 10–13.

Brody, H (2011) 'Clarifying Conflict of Interest', *The American Journal of Bioethics* 11(1), pp. 23–28.

Buderi, R (2002) 'The once and future industrial research'in Teich, AH, Nelson, SD, McEnaney, C, and Lita, SJ (eds.) *AAAS Science and Technology Policy Yearbook.* Washington: Committee on Science, Engineering, and Public Policy, AAAS, pp. 245–251.

Carpenter, D (2010) *Reputation and power: organizational image and pharmaceutical regulation at the FDA.* Princeton: Princeton University Press.

Carpenter, D and Moss, DA (2013) *Preventing regulatory capture: special interest influence and how to limit it.* New York: Cambridge University Press.

CEO (2017) *Recruitment errors The European Food Safety Authority (EFSA) will probably fail, again, to become independent from The Food industry.* Corporate Europe Observatory, June 16.

Chauveau, S (1999) *L'invention Pharmaceutique. La pharmacie française entre l'État et la société au XXe siècle.* Paris: Les empêcheurs de penser en rond.

Coglianese, C (2009) 'The transparency president? The Obama administration and open government', *Governance: An International Journal of Policy, Administration, and Institutions*, 22(4), pp. 529–544 [online]. Available at: https://doi.org/10.1111/j.1468-0491.2009.01451.x (Accessed: January 25, 2021).

Conrad, P (1975) 'The discovery of hyperkinesis: notes on the medicalization of deviant behavior', *Social Problems*, 23(1), pp. 12–21.

Conrad, P (2005) 'The shifting engines of medicalization', *Journal of Health and Social Behavior*, 46(1), pp. 3–14.

Daemmrich, AA (2004) *Pharmacopolitics. Drug regulation in The United States and Germany.* Chapel Hill: The University of North Carolina Press.

Dalgalarrondo, S (2004) *Sida: la course aux molécules.* Paris: Editions de l'EHESS.

Davis, C and Abraham, J (2013) *Unhealthy pharmaceutical regulation: innovation, politics and promissory science.* Basingstoke: Palgrave Macmillan.

Davis, M and Stark, A (eds.) (2001) *Conflict of interest in the professions.* Oxford: Oxford University Press.

Dedieu, F (2021) Organized denial at work: The difficult search for consistencies in French pesticide regulation. *Regulation & Governance (in print).*

Demortain, D (2020) *The science of bureaucracy: risk decision-making and the US environmental protection agency.* London: MIT Press

DeJong, C, Aguilar, T, Tseng, C-W, Lin, GA, Boscardin, WJ, and Dudley, RA (2016) 'Pharmaceutical industry–sponsored meals and physician prescribing patterns for Medicare beneficiaries', *JAMA Internal Medicine*, 176(8), pp. 1114–1122.

Dinan, W and Miller, D (2008) '*Transparency in EU decision making, holding* corporations to account: why the ETI needs mandatory lobbying disclosure' in Serger, A (ed.) *Corruption and democracy: political finances, conflicts of interest, lobbying, justice*. Strasbourg: Council of Europe Publishing, pp. 155–160.

Dodier, N (2003) *Leçons politiques de l'épidémie de sida*. Paris: Editions de l'EHESS.

Dumit, J (2012) *Drugs for life: how pharmaceutical companies define our health*. Durham: Duke University Press.

Elliott, K (2020) 'A taxonomy of transparency in science', *Canadian Journal of Philosophy*, pp. 1–14.

Epstein, S (1996) *Impure science: AIDS, activism, and the politics of knowledge*. Berkeley: University of California Press.

Foucault, M (2004) *Naissance de la biopolitique*. Paris: Gallimard/Le Seuil.

Frickel, S and Moore, K (2006) *The new political sociology of science: institutions, networks, and power*. Madison: University of Wisconsin Press.

Fung, A, Graham, M, and Weil, D (2007) *Full disclosure: the perils and promise of transparency*. Cambridge: Cambridge University Press.

Gaudillière, J-P and Hess, V (eds.) (2013) *Ways of regulating drugs in the 19th and 20th centuries*. Basinkstokes: Routledge-Palgrave.

Gaudillière, J-P (2013) 'From *Propaganda* to scientific marketing: Schering, cortisone, and the construction of drugs markets', *History and Technology*, 29(2), pp. 188–209.

Gaudilliere, J-P (2015), "Une manière industrielle de savoir" in Bonneuil, C. and pester, D. (eds), *Histoire des sciences et des saviors. 3 Le siècle des technosciences*, Paris: Seuil, p. 85–106.

Gaudillière, J-P and Thoms, U (eds.) (2015) *The development of scientific marketing in the twentieth century*. New York: Pickering & Chatto.

Gaudillière, J-P (2021) 'Pharmaceutical innovation and its crisis: Drug markets, screening the dialectics of value', *Biosocieties*.

Glode, ER (2002) 'Advising under the influence? Conflicts of Interest among FDA advisory committee members', *Food and Drug Law Journal*, 57(2), pp. 293–322.

Greene, J (2007) *Prescribing by numbers: drugs and the definition of disease*. Baltimore: Johns Hopkins University Press.

Goldacre, B (2012) *Bad Pharma: how drug companies mislead doctors and harm patients*. London: Fourth Estate.

Gøtzsche, PC (2013) *Deadly medicines and organised crime. How big pharma has corrupted healthcare*. London: Radcliffe.

Hafferty, FW and Castellani, B (2011) 'Two cultures, two ships: the rise of a professionalism movement within modern medicine and medical sociology's disappearance from the professionalism debate' in Pescosolido, BA, Martin, JK, McLeod, JD, and Rogers, A (eds.) *Handbook of the sociology of health, illness, and healing*. New York: Springer, pp. 201–219.

House of Commons (2005) *The influence of the pharmaceutical industry*. London: House of Commons.

Hauray, B (2006) *L'Europe du médicament. Politique - expertise - intérêts privés*. Paris: Presses de Sciences Po.

Hauray, B (2017) 'From regulatory knowledge to regulatory decisions: the European evaluation of medicines', *Minerva*, 55(2), pp. 187–208.

Hauray, B (2019) 'Une médecine détournée? Influences industrielles et crise de confiance dans le domaine du médicament', *Mouvements*, 98(2), pp. 53–66.

Hendrick, RA (2016) *Managing or maintaining bias? Examining the conceptualis-ation of conflicts of interest in medical journal publishing*. Edinburgh: University of Edinburgh.

Horel, S and CEO (2013) *Unhappy meal. The European Food Safety Authority's inde-pendence problem.*

Horel, S and CEO (2015) *A toxic affair. How the chemical lobby blocked action on hormone disrupting chemicals.*

Horowitz, R (2012) *In the public interest: medical licensing and the disciplinary process.* New Brunswick: Rutgers University Press.

Hrachovec, JB and Mora, M (2001) 'Reporting of 6-month vs 12-month data in a clinical trial of celecoxib', *JAMA*, 286(19), pp. 2398–2400.

Illich, I (1975) *Medical nemesis: the expropriation of health.* London: Calder & Boyars.

Jasanoff, S (1990) *The fifth branch. Science adviser as policymakers.* Cambridge: Harvard University Press.

Jasanoff, S (2006) 'Transparency in public science: purposes, reasons, limits', *Law & Contemporary Problems*, 69, pp. 21–45.

Jones, K (2008) 'In whose interest? Relationships between health consumer groups and the pharmaceutical industry in the UK', *Sociology of Health & Illness*, 30(6), pp. 929–943.

Kahin, B and Foray, D (eds.) (2006) *Advancing knowledge and the knowledge economy.* Cambridge: MIT Press.

Krimsky, S (2013) 'Do financial conflicts of interest bias research? An inquiry into the "funding effect" hypothesis', *Science, Technology & Human Values*, 38(4), pp. 566–587.

Krimsky, S (2019) *Conflicts of interest in science: how corporate-funded academic research can threaten public health.* New York: Hot Books.

LaFolette, MC (1994) 'The politics of research misconduct: congressional oversight, universities, and science' *The Journal of Higher Education*, 65(3), pp. 261–285.

Lathyris, DN, Patsopoulos, NA, Salanti, G, and Ioannidis, JPA (2010) 'Industry sponsorship and selection of comparators in randomized clinical trials', *European Journal of Clinical Investigation*, 40(2), pp. 172–182.

Lathrop, D and Ruma, L (2010) *Open government: collaboration, transparency, and participation in practice.* Sebastopol: O'Reilly Media.

Lesser, LI, Ebbeling, CB, Goozner, M, Wypij, D, and Ludwig, DS (2007) 'Relationship between funding source and conclusion among nutrition-related scientific arti-cles', *PLoS Med*, 4(1), e5.

Lessig, L (2009) 'Against transparency', *New Republic,* October 9.

Lexchin, J and O'Donovan, O (2010) 'Prohibiting or "managing" conflict of interest? A review of policies and procedures in three European drug regulation agencies', *Social Science & Medicine*, 70(5), pp. 643–647.

Lo, B and Field, MJ (2009) *Conflict of interest in medical research, education, and prac-tice.* Washington: National Academies Press.

Luebke, NR (1987) 'Conflict of interest as a moral category', *Business and Professional Ethics Journal*, 6(1), pp. 66–81.

Lundh, A, Lexchin, J, Mintzes, B, Schroll, JB, and Bero, L (2017) 'Industry sponsor-ship and research outcome', *Cochrane Database of Systematic Reviews.*

Majone, G (1996) *Regulating Europe.* London: Routledge.

Michaels, D (2008) *Doubt is their product. How industry's assault on science threatens your health*. Oxford: Oxford University Press.

Michel, H (2012) 'EU lobbying and the European Transparency Initiative: sociological approach to interest groups'in Kauppi, N (ed.) *A political sociology of transnational Europe*. Colchester: ECPR Press, pp. 53–78.

Mirowski, P (2011) *Science-Mart: privatizing American science*. Cambridge: Harvard University Press.

Mirowski, P and Van Horn, R (2005) 'The contract research organization and the commercialization of scientific research', *Social Studies of Science*, 35(4), pp. 503–548.

Moore, S (2018) 'Towards a sociology of institutional transparency: openness, deception and the problem of public trust', *Sociology*, 52(2), pp. 416–430 [online]. Available at: https://doi.org/10.1177/0038038516686530 (Accessed: January 25, 2021).

Moynihan, R, Heath, I, and Henry, D (2002) 'Selling sickness: the pharmaceutical industry and disease mongering', *BMJ: British Medical Journal*, 324(7342), pp. 886–891.

OECD (2004) *Managing conflict of interest in the Public Service. OECD guidelines and country experiences*. Paris: OECD Publishing.

OECD (2007) *Building a framework for enhancing transparency and accountability in lobbying*. Paris: OECD Publishing.

OECD (2010) *Post-public employment: good practices for preventing conflict of interest*. Paris: OECD Publishing.

Parasie, S and Dagiral, E (2013) 'Data-driven journalism and the public good: "computer-assisted-reporters" and "programmer-journalists" in Chicago', *New media & society*, 15(6), pp. 853–871.

Quirke, V (2008) *Collaboration in the pharmaceutical industry: changing relationships in Britain and France, 1935–1965*. New York: Routledge.

Rajan, KS (2017) *Pharmocracy: value, politics, and knowledge in global biomedicine*. Durham: Duke University Press.

Robinson, C, Holland, N, Leloup, D, and Muilerman, H (2013) 'Conflicts of interest at the European Food Safety Authority erode public confidence', *Journal of Epidemiology & Community Health*, 67(9), pp. 717–720.

Rodwin, MA (1995) *Medicine, money, and morals: physicians' conflicts of interest*. New York: Oxford University Press.

Rodwin, MA (2011) *Conflicts of interest and the future of medicine: the United States, France, and Japan*. Oxford: Oxford University Press.

Rodwin, MA (2013) 'Institutional corruption and the pharmaceutical policy', *Journal of Law, Medicine, Ethics* 14(3), pp. 544–552.

Rosenbaum, L (2015) 'Reconnecting the dots — reinterpreting industry–physician relations', *New England Journal of Medicine*, 372(19), pp. 1860–1864.

Rothman, KJ (1993) 'Conflict of interest. The new McCarthyism in science', *JAMA*, 269(21), pp. 2782–2784.

Roussel, Y and Raoult, D (2020) 'Influence of conflicts of interest on public positions in the COVID-19 era, the case of Gilead Sciences', *New Microbes and New Infections*, 38.

Schudson, M (2015) *The rise of the right to know. Politics and the culture of transparency, 1945–1975*. Cambridge: Harvard University Press.

Sismondo, S (2008) 'How pharmaceutical industry funding affects trial outcomes: causal structures and responses', *Social Science & Medicine*, 66(9), pp. 1909–1914.

Sismondo, S (2009) 'Ghosts in the machine: publication planning in the medical sciences', *Social Studies of Science*, 39(2), pp. 171–198.

Sismondo, S (2018) *Ghost-managed medicine: Big Pharma's invisible hands*. Manchester: Mattering Press.

Stossel, TP (2015) *Pharmaphobia: how the conflict of interest myth undermines American medical innovation*. Lanham: Rowman & Littlefield.

Tobbell, DA (2011) *Pills, power and policy: the struggle for drug reform in Cold War America and its consequences*. Berkeley: University of California Press.

The Lancet (2001) 'The tightening grip of big pharma', *The Lancet*, 357(9263), p. 1141.

Thompson, DF (1993) 'Understanding financial conflicts of interest', *New England Journal of Medicine*, 329, pp. 573–576.

Wadmann, S (2014) 'Physician–industry collaboration: conflicts of interest and the imputation of motive', *Social Studies of Science*, 44(4), pp. 531–554.

Williams, SJ, Gabe, J, and Davis, P (2008) 'The sociology of pharmaceuticals: progress and prospects', *Sociology of Health & Illness*, 30(6), pp. 813–824.

Williams, SJ, Martin, P, and Gabe, J (2011) 'The pharmaceuticalisation of society? A framework for analysis', *Sociology of Health & Illness*, 33(5), pp. 710–725.

Wislar, JS, Flanagin, A, Fontanarosa, B, and DeAngelis, C (2011) 'Honorary and ghost authorship in high impact biomedical journals: a cross sectional survey', *BMJ*, 343, d6128.

Whittington, CJ, Kendall, T, Fonagy, P, Cottrell, D, Cotgrove, A, and Boddington, E (2004) 'Selective serotonin reuptake inhibitors in childhood depression: systematic review of published versus unpublished data', *The Lancet*, 363(9418) pp. 1341–1345.

World Bank (2002) *Strengthening public debt transparency: the role of the IMF and the World Bank*. Washington: World Bank.

Zola, IK (1972) 'Medicine as an institution of social control', *The Sociological Review*, 20(4), pp. 487–504.

Part I

Knowledge and expertise

Chapter 1

A genealogy of conflict of interest

Boris Hauray

Over the last few decades, the category of "conflict of interest" (COI) has gained importance in the medical world, both in the way its organizations operate and in the controversies that have affected it. It is extensively used by whistleblowers, groups involved in denouncing "health scandals", scientists challenging the promotion of certain therapeutic options, or journalists investigating public decisions. But it is also institutionalized in the functioning of many scientific and health organizations (universities, research centers, academic journals, regulatory agencies, and so on). Given how familiar we all are with the concept of COI, it might be easy to assume that this idea has always been present in medicine, and that it is a "neutral" way to examine and regulate the influence of industry interests. The term "conflict of interest" itself evokes an image of contradictory psychological forces shaping our behavior, something that seems quite obvious. The reality is something different: the category of COI only really became common in the medical world from the 1980s onward, and has only been a part of public discourse since the post-war period. That said, the underlying ethical uncertainties and legal principles behind COI date back much further. Marc Rodwin traces their origins to the concept of *fiducia* (trust, confidence) in Roman law, which was used in the context of property transfers (Rodwin, 2011). More specifically, in the Middle Ages, lawyers constructed a set of professional regulations that condemned "ambidexterity", meaning receiving money from both parties involved in a conflict or sharing confidential information with opposing parties (Rose, 1999). In the realm of politics, one might cite the prohibition on members of the British Parliament practicing certain professions ("offices of profit"), starting in the 16th century, because they might easily find themselves in a situation where they were both judge and defendant (Cranston, 1979). The use of the expression "conflict of interest", with its current meaning, can also be found in the early 20th century. Examples can be found in discussions of trust funds (Hadsall, 1936) and in the similar expression "conflicting interests" in codes of ethics for lawyers (McMunigal, 1992). At this time, however, COI

10.4324/9781003161035-1

had not yet become a specific idea or category that needed to be defined or demarcated (McMunigal, 1992). The philosopher Neil Luebke (1987) notes that the term's first appearance in a court decision dates to 1949, its first inclusion in an English-language dictionary to 1971, and its first entry in a legal dictionary to 1979. These definitions primarily relate to issues of public officials placing their private gain over the public interest. Legal scholar Michael Davis (2001) also points out that this term is barely half a century old and that it only began to be used in legal practice in the 1960s, entering into codes of ethics from the 1970s. What then might explain how central the category of COI has become in only a few decades?

As Paul Starr has explained (1992), social categories are a "political reduction of social complexity", one of many ways to understand reality, not all of which come to be recognized as legitimate, institutionalized in laws and procedures, or used in official statistics. Since its emergence, the category of COI has been closely tied with a specific apparatus, the declaration of interests, which has spread to different contexts (public agencies, universities and research organizations, medical journals). This has produced data that has not only been used to generate statistics, but that has also spurred media revelations. A category like COI shapes the way people in a certain field see the world. It influences their moral judgments and can influence politics as well, insofar as it drives action or serves as a tool for moral entrepreneurs (Gusfield, 1986). The aim of this chapter is therefore to trace the genealogy of this category (and that of the declaration of interest procedures accompanying it). Starting with the current state of affairs of COI, this chapter will attempt to understand its centrality, focusing on a series of instances where contradictions between private and public interests have been seen through the lens of this category. In so doing, it will of course highlight continuities, but it will also, perhaps to an even greater degree, examine the discontinuities in the historical dynamics that have led to the acceptance of this category (Foucault, 1984).

By using a documentary research approach (looking at official documents, press reviews, publications in medical journals), as well as interviews for the more recent period, this first chapter will attempt to fill in the broad strokes of how the category of COI emerged and spread. It will focus on two areas, biomedical research and regulatory authorities,[1] and on the different dynamics in the United States and France. This will enable four distinct phases in the history of COIs to be identified. The first is the emergence of this category in government circles in reference to the closeness between government and private entities. The second is its adoption by the world of biomedical research during the rise of biotech entrepreneurship. The third is its international expansion and the new use of this category to criticize the influence of large pharmaceutical groups. The fourth and final phase is marked by an increasing politicization of COIs and by an accretion of new procedures targeting them. The conclusion will discuss the social effects of these dynamics.

The emergence of COIs: Between the military–industrial complex and the regulatory state

The term "conflict of interest" entered into public discourse in the 1950s in the United States, as part of the debate around reforming what were referred to informally as "conflict of interest statutes/laws". COI emerged as a catch-all category for several laws governing the relationships between private entities and public officials, especially in terms of shareholdings and the revolving door between the public and private sectors (industry, but also law firms and lobby groups). At that time, there were two contradictory dynamics that shaped their impact on media and political spaces: (1) public distrust of important politicians' personal interests and connections, and (2) a desire to create a more appropriate space for exchanges between the private and public spheres. In the 1970s, the issue of properly applying these COI regulations continued to develop against the background of consumer mobilization and criticism of the role played by regulatory agencies and expert committees (Jasanoff, 1990).

During the Truman and Eisenhower administrations, a series of political scandals drew attention to the influence of private industries in Washington. In 1951, for example, a commission on ethical standards in government was created.[2] Its report asserted that the recurring controversies were due to the spread of influence peddling. According to the report, as the state became more involved in the economy, it expanded the "dangerous area" where selling influence could be lucrative. It, therefore, called for procedures that would make the financial interests of elected officials and civil servants public information. What President Eisenhower himself termed in 1961 the "military-industrial complex" was at the heart of public concerns. Several of Eisenhower's political appointees were attacked for their links with this domain (Davis, 1954). According to commentators at the time, the controversy that surrounded General Motors CEO Charles Erwin Wilson's nomination as Secretary of Defense in 1953 played a central role in bringing COIs into public discourse and the world of political machinations (Manning, 1964). While he ultimately gave in, Wilson initially refused to sell his large volume of General Motors shares, despite the company being a leading Department of Defense supplier. This category then developed quickly. When the Supreme Court issued its 1961 decision on the Tennessee Valley Authority, an issue that had divided Democrats and Republicans, it found the contract signed by the government to be "infected by an illegal conflict of interest".[3]

The second dynamic, conversely, arose from the idea that these "conflict of interest laws" were too rigid: written for full-time government employees, they were poorly suited to the specific situation of temporary employees. The first use of the expression "conflict of interest" in its current meaning in the *New York Times* refers to the Nimitz Commission, which was formed by President Truman in 1951 to investigate government employee loyalty, in a context marked by fears of communist espionage activities. Because the Senate resoundingly refused to grant exemptions from these rules for some of its members (notably military veterans and lawyers), the commission decided to disband, ending its investigation. This was a symbolic moment for those (mostly in the legal profession, with some from the sciences) that were advocating, more broadly, amendments that would allow the existing regulations to meet the state's growing need for expertise as it became more involved in regulating society and the economy (McElwain and Vorenberg, 1952). Those who held this view considered COIs to be unavoidable in a modern pluralistic society, which allows individuals to belong to multiple groups, without owing any total or eternal allegiance to the state (Braucher, 1961). In 1955, the New York City Bar Association created a special commission under the leadership of Professor Bayless Manning, whose 1960 report marks a turning point (Special Committee on the Federal Conflict of Interest Laws, 1960). This report asserted that, insofar as COIs are potential risks and not punishable acts, the cost of the preventive approach taken by the current regulations was too high in terms of expertise and the circulation of information between the public and private sectors, and that this approach only led to more informal kinds of consultation. In late 1960, John F. Kennedy was elected after making promises of integrity and enlightened modernity. With advice from Professor Manning, he sent a "Special Message on Conflicts of Interest" to Congress in 1961, opening the way for the legislation to be reformed. The Bribery, Graft and Conflicts of Interest Act was then passed in 1962. This law, however, did not define what a COI was, nor did it use the term beyond its title. It expanded and specified the kinds of financial interest that should bar someone from participating in public decision-making (including those of their spouses and children), and also created the separate status of "Special Government Employee" for people who were only employed by the government part-time or temporarily. It created a system of waivers for these individuals, as long as they had declared their interests to a superior, who has judged "that the interest is not so substantial as to be deemed likely to affect the integrity of the services".

These new regulations did not put a stop to controversies about politicians' private interests and connections. These controversies even spread to the executive branch, impacting regulatory agencies and expert advisers. In the United States, the 1970s saw the rise of social movements to protect the interests of consumers and the environment, putting an end to the idea that science and social progress were natural allies. In 1971, Peter Hutt's nomination as Chief Counsel of the Food and Drug Administration (FDA) was opposed in debate by some members of Congress because he had previously worked as a food industry lawyer.[4] In 1972, the Federal Advisory Committee Act was adopted – which defined a legal framework to govern the creation and operation of federal advisory committees and integrated the 1962 provisions on COI. Members of the FDA and the National Academy of Sciences (NAS) expert committees were targeted for having COIs (Boffey, 1975). In the late 1960s and throughout the 1970s, Congress criticized the cost, ineffectiveness, excessive power, and lack of democratic oversight of regulatory authorities' advisory committees. The specific issue of COIs and how to manage them within such authorities was also raised in this context. In 1976, an internal investigation within the administration revealed that 150 FDA employees were in violation of the COI laws passed in 1962. In response, the agency moved to formalize the way it applied the 1962 law to its actual practices. Previously, it had followed the guiding principle of trusting experts, both in their expertise and in their ability to manage their own COIs, removing themselves from any deliberations that might involve their personal interests (Glode, 2002). The FDA's internal policy for handling COIs was once again the target of a congressional investigation in 1977–1978. The report resulting from this investigation cited trends within the FDA that privileged cooperative relationships with industry firms, and the possible consequences this could have for decision-making (Dorsen, 1977). COIs, however, were seen as inevitable: "Because most candidates for committee service will have had some contact with regulated industry, few prospective candidates will be entirely free from conflicts of interest" (ibid., pp. 9–10). Making deliberations more transparent and enforcing declaration procedures were the main solutions proposed for this problem.

COIs enter medical science: Between biotech entrepreneurship and scientific fraud

From the late 1970s, the use of the category of COI, which had become common in the political sphere and within expert bodies, spread to scientific knowledge production through universities and medical journals. This importation may be seen as the result of a collision between two social dynamics: scientific entrepreneurship and the criticism of scientific fraud or malpractice. Politicians and the media played an important role in defining the kinds of issues discussed in terms of COIs, but biomedical professionals were also actively involved: the category of COI provided an essential tool for self-regulation, one that would not threaten the relationships between scientists and industry, protecting their autonomy.

During this period, federal regulations were put into place to strengthen the connections between academic scientists and industry firms (Blumenthal, 1994). The Bayh-Dole Act of 1980, for example, allowed universities and research centers to patent discoveries they had made using federal funds and to exploit these patents with industrial partners. Although universities have always had ties with the economic sector, these decisions marked the beginning of economic development becoming one of their core purposes (Etzkowitz, 2002). The entrepreneurial and financial ambitions of universities and of some of their researchers were particularly strong in the emerging field of biotechnology. In 1980, University of California professor Herbert Boyer, a recombinant DNA pioneer who co-founded Genentech with a young financier in 1976, became a multi-millionaire overnight after his company's IPO, nearly two years *before* it sold its first product (human insulin) in 1982. For universities, making connections with industry partners was an opportunity to re-balance their financial structure. In 1980, Harvard University was planning to create its own company to market the work of its DNA researchers, financed by venture capital, but with Harvard retaining 10–15 percent of the shares.[5] This plan was met with strong criticism in the press[6] – with suggestions that Harvard change the "veritas" in its motto to "cupiditas" – but also with public rebukes from its own professors. The project was abandoned, but this controversy revealed that Harvard already had significant indirect investments in Biogen Inc., a company co-founded by a professor, Walter Gilbert (recipient of the 1980 Nobel Prize in Chemistry), who went on to become its CEO in 1981. The category of COI, which came from the world of government – the most obvious expression of the collective interest – began to be used in scientific journals (Gingras and Gosselin, 2008) and in the press by professors who were opposed to this blurring of lines, to describe the threats that these new arrangements posed to science's public character. These critiques were joined by others after a series of scandals revealed breaches in scientists' integrity. In 1980, there were four instances of scientific fraud, all connected to the biomedical field, that received widespread media coverage. These cases were at the heart of both journalistic investigations (*Betrayers of the Truth: Fraud and Deceit in the Halls of Science* by journalists Nicholas Wade and William Broad, published in 1982) as well as political ones, with congressional hearings held on misconduct in science. These hearings began in 1981, and continued throughout the rest of the decade (LaFollette, 1994). From the beginning, they drew a clear line between fraud and the new way that research was funded, ceding more influence to commercial interests. The biotech sector was a prime example of this new way of doing things.

Both universities and medical journals were worried about protecting their reputation and about the government intervening in their affairs. Promoting declaration of interest procedures based on the administrative model, therefore, seemed like a low-cost defensive solution. In 1981, Harvard's Faculty of Arts and Sciences decided to adopt new guidelines for COIs, presented as the first of their kind in the country. These guidelines asked that professors report any work that seemed "likely to present an unacceptable conflict of interest or commitment" to a "special faculty committee".[7] Similar policies were put in place in several other US universities, notably at Yale and across the University of California system the following year. In March 1982, a conference was held that has been compared to the Asilomar Conference on Recombinant DNA. For three days, representatives from top US universities and biotech companies met behind closed doors at a hotel in Pajaro Dunes, trying to establish guidelines that would legitimize their collaboration. The final declaration notably called for new rules to govern COIs, but these were understood in a limited sense, i.e., owning shares or serving on the board of a company.[8] In 1984, the *New England Journal of Medicine* (NEJM), the most prestigious general medicine publication, decided to institute its own disclosure policy, announced in an editorial by Arnold Relman entitled "Dealing with Conflicts of Interest". This editorial is rightly seen as the starting point for this issue being taken seriously by scientific publications. It should, however, be noted to avoid any misunderstanding that this editorial was focused on new scientific entrepreneurs, and not on the existing relationships between researchers and the pharmaceutical industry, which were not seen as problematic at the time (Relman, 1980). The editorial is a clear extension of what the universities had already done, directly referencing the positions taken by the presidents of Harvard and Yale. The result was that only strong and direct financial ties, such as patents, shares, or consultancy positions related to a given article had to be declared. No time period was given for these COIs, implying that only relationships that existed the moment the article was submitted were covered. Declarations were also strictly voluntary and were not intended to interfere with the article approval process. A similar policy was adopted the next year by the *Journal of the American Medical Association* (JAMA).

At the end of the 1980s, a new scientific fraud scandal around an eye treatment that had been tested at Harvard was seen as the product of COIs. It was also revealed that several researchers had conducted trials using NIH (National Institutes of Health) financing for a heart treatment developed by the biotech firm Genentech while holding shares in that company. Some had even purchased shares just before the results were published. This led to a new round of congressional hearings and media investigation. For example, a hearing was held on September 29, 1988, entitled "Federal Response to Misconduct in Science: Are Conflicts of Interest Hazardous to our Health?" and another in June 1989, "Is Science for Sale? Conflicts of Interest vs. The Public Interest". This interaction between the political world, which was used to thinking about influence and morality through the lens of COIs, and the scientific world, which was just getting to grips with them, had a concrete effect on the gradual expansion of what constitutes a COI. For example, during one hearing, a representative expressed his surprise to the editor of the JAMA that honoraria were not included in journals' COI disclosure policies, as they were in policies for elected officials. The editor was unable to justify this lack, and later changed the journal's policy. In September 1989, the NIH unveiled its draft guidelines for COIs: NIH-funded researchers would need to make any financial relationships public and would be prohibited (along with their families) from owning shares in companies related to their research: "What we're basically saying is let's get rid of any conflicts of interest" one of the NIH directors said at the time.[9] This document faced fierce opposition from some in academia and was ultimately abandoned by the administration of President George H. W. Bush that December, because it could "jeopardize the United States' pre-eminence in biomedical research".[10] It took until 1995 for another, less strict set of guidelines to be adopted. It should also be noted that given the still vague nature of the procedures and criteria for declarations of interest, their actual use remained limited. In 1988, a report published after an internal investigation led by a student organization at Harvard and written by the future president of the NGO Public Citizen showed that there were no concrete practices behind the policy the university had adopted in 1981.[11] Also, although medical journals had adopted COI disclosure policies, declarations of interest remained rare, and reviewing them was a small part of an editor's work. A former senior editor for both the NJEM and the JAMA recalled that "in the 70s and even in the 80s, pretty well no one in the editorial board meeting would ever have brought up questions of conflict of interest" (Interview, October 2018). British journals (*The Lancet*, the *British Medical Journal*, *Nature*), meanwhile, remained outside of this debate.

Big pharma and the expansion of COIs

The 1990s saw the category of COI expand to cover new ground, both in terms of the behaviors it included and in terms of its geographic spread. As for the latter, declaration of interest procedures were imported into European administrative and public spheres as part of the movement toward "agencification". This geographic expansion went hand-in-hand with a general redefinition of the category's primary targets: it was no longer biotech entrepreneurs, but rather the structural influence of large pharmaceutical groups on research that was the subject of debate. The edges of what constituted a COI became blurred as they also became a tool for describing and criticizing the new relationships between researchers and industry firms (Sismondo, 2018).

COI and declarations of interest had been mainly seen as products of US legal and political culture. In the early 1990s, the European administrative and academic spheres were reflecting more and more on governance, discussing and promoting the rise of a regulatory state, conceived of in opposition to the traditional European interventionist state (Majone, 1996). This movement, which looked to the United States as an originating example, led to the creation of regulatory agencies in various sectors, meant to lend procedural legitimacy to political decision-making. More specifically, in the pharmaceutical sector, the European Medicines Agency (EMA) was created in 1993 to counterbalance the FDA, an agency whose credibility gave it the power to set global standards. In this context, the architects of the EMA imported the FDA's transparency "best practices", in particular its procedures for declaring COIs (Interview with a former European Commission member, April 2000). At the national level as well, COIs were a part of the formalization of expert groups' independence. For example, it was only after France launched its own "independent" agency for regulating medicines, which replaced a former Department of Health service, that declarations of interest were first used. These declarations were made public starting in 1996, and this innovation has been described by the press as innovative and courageous.[12] By the end of the 1990s, the mere existence of these declarations led more and more observers to question industry influence on experts in Europe. In the United Kingdom, for example, a 2000 article in the *Sunday Express* noted that "more than two thirds of the doctors and academics who serve on committees of the Medicines Control Agency [MCA] have investments in the pharmaceutical industry or benefit from drug company cash".[13] A few months later, *The Guardian* reported on the possible COIs arising from a former pharmaceutical industry executive being named as director of drugs licensing at the MCA,[14] while only ten years earlier, no such accusations had been made when a former Merck executive was tapped to head the same agency.

The phenomena targeted by the category of COI as concerns knowledge production gradually evolved between the 1980s and 1990s. In the 1980s, biotech entrepreneurs were seen as a source of COIs because they mixed scientific objectives with capitalistic growth strategies. By extension, researchers who owned shares in the companies whose drugs they were testing also came to be included. In the 1990s, the scope of COIs became much wider: the concept was used to discuss and categorize the various financial relationships that pharmaceutical firms had with researchers and physicians (paying for them to attend conferences, speaking fees, financing research or new equipment), as well as the balance of power between these groups. Large pharmaceutical groups thus became the primary target of the discourse around COIs. The research landscape underwent rapid changes during this period: while only 32 percent of research funding in the United States came from industry sources in 1980, this figure had risen to as high as 62 percent by 2000, giving industry players more influence over how clinical trials were designed, how data was processed, and how the results were published. The issue of bias in scientific publications was discussed in statistical studies starting in the mid-1990s, legitimizing those voices in the biomedical community that had been denouncing the problematic effects of COIs, especially because these studies were published in scientific journals. When asked about when he had first become aware of COIs, a former editor-in-chief of a major medical journal pointed to an article he had read in 1994 (Rochon, Gurwitz, and Simms, 1994):

> I remember being taken aback when I saw a study [...] that looked at the series of studies on NSAIDs [non-steroidal anti-inflammatory drugs] funded by the pharma industry, they didn't find one paper where the results went against the interest of the pharmaceutical company. Although I kind of knew that, reading this paper really hit very hard.
>
> (Interview, November 2017)

When the NEJM published an article by Henry Thomas Stelfox and his colleagues on the highly controversial topic of calcium-channel antagonists in 1998, it marked the real beginning of a period when publications' objectivity was called into question due to the COIs of their authors (Stelfox et al., 1998). This article showed that the authors in favor of using calcium-channel antagonists had significantly more financial ties to the pharmaceutical industry than those who were neutral or against their use (96 percent vs. 60 percent and 37 percent, respectively), and that these COIs were only declared in a vanishingly small minority of cases. At the beginning of the 2000s, meta-analyses would confirm these suspected biases (Bekelman, Li, and Gross, 2003). Other detailed accounts of the power relationships between researchers and industries were also published, each adding more weight to the idea that the pharmaceutical industry's influence on research had become a central issue. In 1997, for example, there was a scandal around the work of Dr. Betty Dong, a pharmacologist at a public university (the University of California): it was revealed that a pharmaceutical company had (by threatening a lawsuit) been able to prevent the publication in the JAMA of one of Dr. Dong's articles on its thyroid treatment. The company had moreover commissioned another article that used the same data to reach opposite conclusions.

The threat that industry influence posed to journals' credibility as the gatekeepers of knowledge production transformed COIs throughout the 1990s from a fringe issue into one of the medical publishing sector's primary concerns. Led by US journals, medical journals around the world, as represented by the ICMJE (International Committee of Medical Journal Editors), issued a joint declaration on COIs in 1993. The actual implementation of these principles, however, remained uneven and overall rather weak. Professionals also had a hard time thinking of their "normal" ties with industry players as COIs. One author criticized for an incomplete declaration in the JAMA defended himself in *The Boston Globe* in these words:

> It is true I did not disclose financial ties to Johnson and Johnson, but it is also true it never occurred to me. My situation is very similar to that of most experts in medical investigations – that is, I have consulted for every major and most minor companies that work in my area of interest.[15]

The idea that scientists' interests should be taken into account when judging their results remained a subject of debate until the mid-1990s, and differences in policies led to "blame games" between journals. Still, the growing evidence about COIs and their impact, as well as periodic denunciations of various articles, gradually led medical journal editors to align their positions (Krimsky and Rothenberg, 2001). This was solidified in 2001, with a joint declaration from the ICMJE entitled "Sponsorship, Authorship, and

Accountability". This declaration decried the new political economy of biomedical research and issued some new rules for acceptable divisions of tasks and responsibilities between investigators and sponsors. It described what types of contracts it considered to be unfair and called on authors to declare "all relationships that could be viewed as presenting a potential conflict of interest". All these rules were added to the organization's regulations under the heading "Conflicts of Interest". Unlike what happened in 1993, the editors announced them publicly and formally, stating that any failure to comply with these rules would result in the rejection of the article in question. These rules drew the ire of the pharmaceutical industry, which called them "patently absurd".[16] The British journal *The Lancet* can be seen as an example of how these changes occurred throughout the 1990s. At the beginning of the decade, the journal remained somewhat guarded on the issue of COIs: its COI policy simply asked authors to declare any issues that might be embarrassing should they come to light, and as late as 1997, its editor-in-chief published an editorial criticizing the growing obsession with COIs. In the early 2000s, the journal's tone changed and it published an editorial entitled "The Tightening Grip of Big Pharma" (The Lancet, 2001), with the journal finally requiring that all authors sign a COI declaration in 2002.

Politicizing and proceduralizing COIs

At the beginning of the 2000s, the category of COI was therefore solidly embedded in professional sub-fields of biomedicine, having been adopted by pharmaceutical regulatory agencies, universities and medical journals in particular. While the media and the wider public had periodically also engaged in this debate, the mid-2000s saw a fundamental shift in the category's visibility. When the anti-inflammatory drug Vioxx® was withdrawn, it unleashed a series of strong criticisms of the influence of pharmaceutical firms, especially the limited added therapeutic value of pharmaceutical "innovations", and the serious risks they can create. Revealing COIs, and undeclared interests and relationships in particular, was therefore seen as an especially effective "action repertoire". In response, the biomedical field once again tightened its procedures, to avoid scandals without really changing the sector's internal configuration.

There was a general increase in articles connecting medicine or pharmaceuticals to issues of COI in the press starting in the mid-2000s that, despite some ups and downs, has never since faded. The Vioxx® scandal played an important role in this process. Vioxx® was a recent blockbuster drug from the Merck laboratories that was withdrawn from the market in 2004 after accusations that it had killed tens of thousands of patients. The political, journalistic, legal, and professional investigations that followed in the United States, the United Kingdom, and France examined the COIs not only of regulatory agency experts and doctors but also of scientists and medical journals. The Vioxx Gastrointestinal Outcomes Research (VIGOR) study, whose manipulated results had been published in the NEJM, became the symbol of the harmful effects of connections between academic researchers and the pharmaceutical industry, but it also implicated the NEJM itself, which received almost $700,000 for reprints of the article ordered by the company. This scandal became even more consequential because it occurred in the wake of controversies surrounding cerivastatin in 2001 and hormone replacement therapy in 2002. In 2004, the industry's strategies to increase the off-label use of antidepressants for children and adolescents also came to light, especially the fact that they had succeeded in downplaying the increased risk of suicide in published articles, and in hiding the results of clinical trials that showed no more effectiveness compared to a placebo.[17] COIs, which were the most tangible form of the pharmaceutical industry's pervasive presence in this sector, became a common thread, being discussed and denounced with each new health crisis. For example, after the H1N1 flu pandemic in 2010, World Health Organization (WHO) experts were criticized for their ties with anti-retroviral drug manufacturers. Bias in the trials that had shown Tamiflu® to be effective against the virus was explained by COIs arising from Roche's involvement in setting them up. The Mediator® scandal that erupted in France and across Europe in 2010 was also quickly reanalyzed in terms of COIs, leading to resignations and legal proceedings against regulatory agency members.[18]

In this political context, where many institutions produce declarations of interest and where, thanks to the growth of the internet, it is often quite easy to consult and cross-reference them, revealing errors in declarations of interest has become a particularly effective "action repertoire" for criticizing treatment options or for denouncing the permissive attitude toward the influence of laboratories more generally. For example, in 1998, *The Lancet* published an article linking autism to MMR (measles, mumps, and rubella) vaccines that has become highly controversial, since it is widely used by anti-vaccination groups. Controversy over the results remained over the years, and *The Lancet* continued to defend the article. In 2004, however, a journalistic investigation revealed an undeclared COI by the lead author, Dr. Andrew Wakefield, that radically changed the situation. It was revealed that Dr. Wakefield had received £55,000 from a group of lawyers defending children in lawsuits against vaccine manufacturers. The editor of *The Lancet* asserted: "If we had known the conflict of interest Dr. Wakefield had in his work, it would have been rejected".[19] His co-authors also withdrew their names from the article, which was finally retracted, with Wakefield discredited. Of course, it is those working against the influence of the industry who turn most often to this "action repertoire". In the United States, after the Vioxx® investigation, Senator Chuck Grassley advocated greater transparency of the financial ties between scientists, doctors, and the pharmaceutical industry. After an initial failure to pass a "Sunshine Act" (which would publish all such financial transfer information on a public website), he went after highly influential psychiatric researchers for only reporting a fraction of their financial ties to their home universities. In particular, he targeted Harvard Medical School's Joseph Biederman, whose work had played a central role in the diagnosis and treatment of bipolar disorder in children. He used his investigatory powers as chairman of the Senate Finance Committee to look into universities and industrial firms. One of his main advisers during this time recalled:

> No one goes out into the intersection and says, you know, we should put a traffic light out there [...] laws always happen because someone's killed or, you know, something happened [...] so what I did was I put together a list of like 12 to 15 doctors who we thought were taking money from the companies [...] and we wrote letters and we sent letters to all of those universities for those doctors, saying how much money these guys, you know, are taking from the industry [...] and then we sent letters also to the companies saying how much money have you paid these doctors.
>
> (Interview, September 2018)

The articles published in US newspapers about these "hidden" payments in 2008 created an uproar. They led to further investigations and revelations (especially in the field of psychiatry), increasing support for a Sunshine Act in Congress (which was finally passed in 2010 as part of Obamacare). In France, the association Formindep was created in 2004 to fight to protect doctors' autonomy from industry firms, critiquing the relationships between these firms and opinion leaders or experts. In 2009, it secured the withdrawal of two official recommendations for treating diabetes and Alzheimer's disease because some expert committees had not followed the Haute Autorité de Santé's (HAS) (French National Authority for Health) COI rules (Dalgalarrondo and Hauray, 2020). While the EMA was criticized for its close ties with industry firms, an NGO revealed in 2010 that some patient association members who were members of its committees had not declared their financial ties to industry firms. Then, in 2011, NGOs revealed that former director of the EMA Thomas Lönngren went straight from the agency to working at a pharmaceutical industry consulting firm, in violation of the agency's COI regulations.[20] More recently in 2018, as an increasing number of voices in the oncology community were rising up against the low effectiveness and exorbitant prices of new cancer treatments, the *New York Times* and *ProPublica* revealed that José Baselga, a world-renowned cancer researcher, had failed to disclose millions of dollars in payments from drug and health care companies in dozens of research articles. He was later forced to step down from his position as chief medical officer of the Memorial Sloan Kettering Cancer Center.

The politicization of COIs led, in turn, to more formalized rules to govern them in drug regulatory agencies, starting in 2007 with the FDA and in 2010 for the EMA. As for scientific publications, in 2009, the ICMJE adopted a standard form for declaring interests in order to avoid any errors. This form went into greater detail about the different kinds of personal and non-personal relationships that should be included, stipulating a time frame of three years within which such relationships must be reported. After the Baselga scandal, the ICMJE added "the purposeful failure" to disclose COIs as the fourth type of scientific misconduct (alongside fabrication, falsification, and plagiarism). Still, this did not mean that relationships with pharmaceutical firms were called into question structurally: over the last few years, false declarations have become the primary target of professional and media attention, more than the existence of the relationships of interest themselves. An editor of a prominent medical journal summarized the situation:

> I think, you know, we always felt quite strongly that researchers need to be funded by [the] pharmaceutical industry to do their research [...] So we have no rules that we can't publish research if there's conflict of interest. We publish it but it has to be transparently declared.
>
> (Interview, May 2019)

This politicization and increasing proceduralization of COIs even resulted in the re-emergence of a certain discourse in the medical world, and sometimes even on medical journal editorial teams, that claimed that being overly strict in controlling COIs has a negative effect on medicine and on innovation. According to them, it prevents or limits beneficial cooperation between industry firms and researchers and constitutes a harmful bureaucratic burden (Stossel, 2015). Some voices in administrative circles also denounced the reduced expertise capacity resulting from the rules in place for managing COIs.[21]

Conclusion

Starting with the situation as it stands currently, this chapter has attempted to retrace the genealogy of COI as a social category, that is to say, to explore both the continuities and discontinuities in how this category has been used and how it has become a part of the field of biomedicine. The history that it has outlined enables the highlighting of a characteristic common to all the successive contexts that helped to propagate this category. Each of these episodes involved new, unfamiliar practices developing within a social space (blurring the lines between civil servants and economic interests, between knowledge production and entrepreneurship, reshaping the power balance between pharmaceutical firms and clinicians, ultimately casting doubt on the benefits of innovation), leading to a kind of moral uncertainty. In such contexts, the category of COI made it possible to both flag and denounce practices (Luebke, 1987), without invoking well legally defined categories like fraud or corruption.[22] The second major continuity is the defensive aspect of COI: this category has been able to successfully circulate between social spaces because the implementation/ reinforcement of declaration of interest procedures represented a way of responding to political or media criticism, or even of trying to prevent this criticism, without fundamentally challenging the functioning of the sector or new practices. This defensive response has had paradoxical effects. In fact, it has made the problem that it is meant to solve more visible and "objective", a phenomenon that has been largely reinforced by the growth of the internet and databases from the 2000s onward. The formalization of rules for managing COIs has not only led to a more negative moral view of the relationships with firms, but it has also produced more failures to disclose COI, of varying intentionality, which have been denounced and have led to some "second order" scandals.

Above all, rather than presenting an a-historical view that might see the trajectory of COI as a simple, gradual taking into account of one single reality, this chapter has made it possible to highlight the evolution of the social issues that this category has mostly served to discuss. It has shown that this way of thinking about corporate influence originates from the world of government, a world where the tension between the interests of private individuals and the protection of the public interest is well established. It was only taken up in scientific circles when the public became aware of certain researchers whose entrepreneurial goals were inseparable from their work of knowledge production. Later, when industry firms' strategies to control and use clinical research for their own purposes intensified, the category came to be used more widely in biomedicine. It covered a wider range of financial relationships (speaking fees, grants, and so on), some of them less direct in nature (with time frames of up to several years for reportable interests), as part of a more structural and global critique of the influence of large pharmaceutical groups. The major shift in the mid-2000s was that COIs became more than just a concern for biomedical professionals. By connecting health risks to the pharmaceutical innovation process, the issue became the subject of public scandals. Reporting omissions in COI declarations became a particularly effective "action repertoire", especially for NGOs and investigative journalists, for questioning the stubborn tolerance of the pervasive power of pharmaceutical laboratories. This chapter has also underlined that the focus of COI has, across several decades, swung between individuals and organizations. Criticism was aimed at individuals in the 1980s before becoming more focused on organizations from the late 1990s, and since the 2010s it can be seen as mixed: it is aimed at organizations, but individuals are those on the receiving end of attacks.

The limits of the category of COI as a tool for analyzing influence have been discussed frequently,[23] as have the limits of the COI regulations put into place in its name. By retracing the genealogy of COI as a social category, this chapter has attempted to demonstrate that this category does not simply designate or control certain phenomena: in just a few decades, it has become an "organizing concept", to use the terminology of Ian Hacking (2004). It is a social category that, in all of its diverse uses, has impacted the biomedical field through its combined effects on knowledge (making it possible to produce data on the concrete manifestation of the pharmaceutical industry's financial omnipresence), norms (leading to moral re-evaluations of the practices of scientists, experts or doctors), and politics. Today, this category goes well beyond revealing a specific professional's COIs, playing a central role in questions about industry influences and more widely in the debate about the role of drugs in medical care.

Notes

1. For the issue of physicians' referrals and more generally, for questions about doctors' practices, see Rodwin (2011), as well as Chapter 5 of this book.
2. The Senate Committee on Labor and Public Welfare. See Senate Committee on Labor and Public Welfare (1951).
3. U.S. vs. Mississippi Valley Generating Co., 364 U.S. 520 (1961).
4. "Peter Hutt Assures Congress He Will Avoid Conflicts of Interest", *New York Times,* September 12, 1971, p. 59.
5. "Harvard Considers Commercial Role in DNA Research", *New York Times,* October 27, 1980, p. 1.
6. "Ivy-Covered Capitalism", *Washington Post*, November 11, 1980.
7. "Colleges are uneasy over faculties' outside jobs", *New York Times*, November 16, 1981.
8. Draft statement of the Pajaro Dunes Conference, March 25–27, 1982.
9. "NIH Moves to Curb Industry-Science Ties", *Boston Globe*, October 6, 1989, p. 1.
10. "U.S. Scraps Rules on Conflicts in Health Research", *New York Times,* December 30, 1989.
11. Robert Weissman Scholars, Inc.: Harvard Academics in Service of Industry and Government, Harvard Watch, Cambridge, MA, 1988.
12. Sophie Coignard, "Les prodiges de l'effet placebo", *Le Point,* June 29, 1996.
13. Jonathan Calvert and Lucy Johnston, "Scandal of Drug Doctors' Shares", *Sunday Express*, August 6, 2000. The MCA was charged with regulating medicines in the United Kingdom at the time.
14. Sarah Boseley, "Alarm as drug company chief joins watchdog", *The Guardian,* December 28, 2000.
15. Judy Foreman, "Drawing the fine line on Retin A US panel slaps doctors for allegedly touting it as a wrinkle smoother", *Boston Globe*, November 23, 1992.
16. "A Stand for Scientific Independence", *The Washington Post*, August 5, 2001.
17. See Chapter 11.
18. See Chapter 9.
19. "MMR – the truth behind the crisis", *The Sunday Times*, February 22, 2004.
20. https://www.beuc.eu/publications/2011-00156-01-e.pdf.
21. See Chapter 4.
22. See Chapter 11.
23. See Chapter 11.

References

Bekelman, JE, Li, Y and Gross, CP (2003) 'Scope and impact of financial conflicts of interest in biomedical research: a systematic review', *JAMA*, 289(4), pp. 454–465.

Blumenthal, D (1994) 'Growing pains for new academic/industry relationships', *Health Affairs*, 13(3), pp. 176–193.

Boffey, PM (1975) *The brain bank of America: an inquiry into the politics of science.* New York: McGraw-Hill.

Braucher, R (1961) 'Conflict of interest and federal service', *Harvard Law Review*, 74(8), pp. 189–192.

Cranston, RF (1979) 'Regulating conflict of interest of public officials: a comparative analysis', *Vanderbilt Journal of Transnational Law*, 12(2), pp. 215–255.

Dalgalarrondo, S and Hauray, B (2020) 'Conflit d'intérêts et traitements anti-Alzheimer: de la construction à la contestation d'une promesse médicale', *Sciences Sociales et santé*, 38(3), pp. 77–104.

Davis, M (2001) 'Introduction' in Davis, M and Stark, A (eds.) *Conflict of interest in the professions.* New York: Oxford University Press, pp. 3–19.

Davis, RD (1954) 'The federal conflict of interest laws', *Columbia Law Review*, 54(6), pp. 893–915.

Dorsen, N (1977) 'Interim report – conflicts of interest on standing advisory committees of the bureau of drugs, FDA' in *United States Department of Health, Education, and Welfare, Review panel on new drug regulation: interim reports.* Volume 3. Washington: United States Department of Health, Education, and Welfare.

Etzkowitz, H (2002) *MIT and the rise of entrepreneurial science.* London: Routledge.

Foucault, M (1984) 'What is enlightenment?' in Rabinow, P (ed.) *The Foucault reader.* New York: Pantheon Books, pp. 32–50.

Gingras, Y and Gosselin, P-M (2008) 'The emergence and evolution of the expression "conflict of interests" in *science*: a historical overview, 1880–2006', *Science and Engineering Ethics*, 14(3), pp. 337–343.

Glode, ER (2002) 'Advising under the influence? Conflicts of interest among FDA advisory committee members', *Food and Drug Law Journal*, 57(2), pp. 293–322.

Gusfield, JR (1986) *Symbolic crusade: status politics and the American Temperance movement.* Champaign: University of Illinois Press.

Hacking, I (2004) *Historical ontology.* Cambridge: Harvard University Press.

Hadsall, JM (1936) 'Conflict of interest when a trustee invests trust funds', *Chicago-Kent Review*, 14(4), pp. 329–350.

Jasanoff, S (1990) *The fifth branch. Science advisers as policymakers.* Cambridge: Harvard University Press.

Krimsky, S and Rothenberg, LS (2001) 'Conflict of interest policies in science and medical journals: editorial practices and author disclosures', *Science and Engineering Ethics*, 7(2), pp. 205–218.

LaFollette, MC (1994) 'The politics of research misconduct: congressional oversight, universities, and science', *The Journal of Higher Education*, 65(3), pp. 261–285.

Luebke, NR (1987) 'Conflict of interest as a moral category', *Business & Professional Ethics Journal*, 6(1), pp. 66–81.

Majone, G (1996) *Regulating Europe.* London: Routledge.

Manning, B (1964) 'The purity potlatch: an essay on conflicts of interest, American government, and moral escalation', *The Federal Bar Journal*, 24, pp. 239–256.

McElwain, E and Vorenberg, J (1952) 'The federal conflict of interest statutes', *Harvard Law Review*, 65(6), pp. 955–983.

McMunigal, KC (1992) 'Rethinking attorney conflict of interest doctrine', *Georgetown Journal of Legal Ethics*, 5(4), pp. 823–877.

Relman, AS (1980) 'The new medical-industrial complex', *New England Journal of Medicine*, 303(17), pp. 963–970.

Rochon, PA, Gurwitz, JH, Simms, RW, et al. (1994) 'A study of manufacturer-supported trials of nonsteroidal anti-inflammatory drugs in the treatment of arthritis', *Archives of Internal Medicine*, 154(2), pp. 157–163.

Rodwin, MA (2011) *Conflicts of interest and the future of medicine: the United States, France and Japan*. New York: Oxford University Press.

Rose, J (1999) 'The ambidextrous lawyer: conflict of interest and the medieval legal profession', *The University of Chicago Law School Roundtable*, 7(1) [online]. Available at: https://chicagounbound.uchicago.edu/roundtable/vol7/iss1/7 (Accessed: February 2, 2021).

Senate Committee on Labor and Public Welfare (1951) *Ethical standards in government*. Washington: United States Government Printing Office.

Sismondo, S (2018) *Ghost-managed medicine: Big Pharma's invisible hands*. Manchester: Mattering Press.

Special Committee on the Federal Conflict of Interest Laws (1960) *Conflict of interest and federal service*. Cambridge: Harvard University Press.

Starr, P (1992) 'Social categories and claims in the liberal state', *Social Research*, 59(2), pp. 263–295.

Stelfox, HT, Chua, G, O'Rourke, K and Detsky, AS (1998) 'Conflict of interest in the debate over calcium-channel Antagonists', *New England Journal of Medicine*, 338 (2), pp. 101–6.

Stossel, TP (2015) *Pharmaphobia: how the conflict of interest myth undermines American medical innovation*. 1st edn. Lanham: Rowman & Littlefield Publishers.

The Lancet (2001) 'The tightening grip of big pharma', *The Lancet*, 357(9263), p. 1141.

Chapter 2

"Conflict of interest" or simply "interest"? Shifting values in translational medicine

Melanie Jeske

In 2019, at least 70 percent of original research articles published in the *Journal of the American Medical Association*, *Science Translational Medicine*, and *Nature Biotechnology* were written by researchers with conflicts of interest (COIs) to disclose.[1] Such statistics emphasize the extent to which private interests have become enmeshed in the production of biomedical knowledge. They suggest that competing interests are no longer an obstacle for those working in academic biomedical research – certainly, conflicting interests are not a barrier to publishing in prestigious journals – and raise critical questions about how we govern the role and influence of industry and private interests in the conduct of biomedical research in the United States.

Controversies surrounding COIs and debates over the best ways to manage them are a hallmark of biomedical research. Throughout the 20th century, but particularly beginning in the 1980s, arbiters of biomedical knowledge production have become concerned with the consequences of private interests on the production of objective, scientific knowledge (Hauray, Chapter 1). In the wake of biotechnological advances in the 1970s and 1980s, and the potential of pursuing the commercialization of such advances (e.g., through the passage of the 1980 Bayh-Dole Act), we are witnessing an alignment of commercial and scientific goals under the logic of "translational medicine". In this chapter, I argue that translational medicine, as an organizing principle in biomedicine, infuses new values as a central part of what it means to do successful, efficient, and effective biomedical research. Translational medicine valorizes collaboration between government, universities, and industry, challenging previous beliefs about the dangerous role of industry in academic science. The chapter closes with a consideration of the challenges this raises for how we conceptualize and govern COIs in academic biomedical research and offers reflections on what is at stake in this new regime of biomedicine.

10.4324/9781003161035-2

Governing COIs

That biomedical research, pharmaceutical development, and biotechnology innovation are profitable endeavors is not a new revelation. Stakeholders in biomedical research communities have long pursued intellectual property rights to *potentially* lucrative biomedical advances. And although the interest that universities and their academic researchers have in securing the intellectual property rights of discoveries is by no means a recent phenomenon, many scholars would agree this was not a widespread, patterned practice until the late 20th century (Berman, 2012).[2] Coinciding with the biotech correct to "biotechnology" boom of the 1980s, universities across the United States established technology transfer offices, and career academics interfacing with industry became more widespread. Over the past several decades, the "traditional" values of academic research have become more relaxed, supporting and encouraging researchers to explore the commercial possibilities of their research.

Historically, one-way industry interests in the practice of medicine and the production of biomedical knowledge have been managed is through the disclosure of relationships that might compromise the integrity of biomedical research, creating an environment in which "transparency" about such conflicts is paramount.[3] COIs are defined as instances where producers of biomedical knowledge hold concurrent positions that may give rise to other interests that compete with their role of producing "objective" knowledge. To date, much research on COI has focused on the pharmaceutical industry as well as clinical care settings, in which health care practitioners are asked to disclose interactions with pharmaceutical and medical device companies because these relationships may negatively impact patient care (Grundy, Bero, and Malone, 2013; Grundy, Habibi, and Shnier, 2018). Increased concerns surrounding COIs in biomedical research, especially clinical trials, date to the late 1990s, when a number of high-profile clinical trial cases in which investigators held undisclosed COIs led to adverse events and sometimes patient death. Such cases resulted in increased public scrutiny over industry–clinician relationships. For instance, the Physician Payments Sunshine Act, also known as section 6002 of the Affordable Care Act, was passed in 2010, making it compulsory for medical product manufacturers to disclose any payments or gifts made to physicians and teaching hospitals, as well as physician ownership and investment in medical product companies. Reports showed that 84 percent of physicians had some form of interaction with drug, medical device, biologicals, and/or medical supplies manufacturers. And at the time, there was a growing consensus that these relationships could potentially "bias physician decision making, encourage inappropriate prescribing that drives up health care costs, and undermine the independence and rigor of clinical research" (Richardson, Saver, and Lott, 2014, p. 2).

Similarly, COI reporting has become routine in the realm of scientific publication and presentation practices. Early scientific and biomedical journal policies for COI disclosure date to 1984 in the United States, with the *New England Journal of Medicine* (NEJM), and 1994 in the United Kingdom, with *The British Medical Journal* (BMJ) adopting policies (Hauray, Chapter 1; Cosgrove, Bursztajn, and Krimsky, 2009). At this time, observing changes in relations among biomedical researchers and industry, journal editors felt it was increasingly important to institute policies. As Arnold Relman, editor-in-chief of the NEJM at the time, wrote upon instituting the journal's policy:

> It is obvious that business arrangements have an increasing role in medical research these days, and common sense suggests that readers ought to be told about those arrangements. Public support for medical research rests in no small measure on trust in the integrity of investigators. When important commercial associations are not disclosed, suspicions inevitably arise, and the public trust is jeopardized.
>
> (Relman, 1984, p. 1183)

Though Relman does not claim that such arrangements necessarily lead to the corruption of objective knowledge, he highlights that the lack of disclosure by scientific journals and researchers jeopardizes public trust in science.

Of particular interest in the social science and science and technology studies (STS) literature has been the politics surrounding COI and what such interests mean for the production and dissemination of knowledge. This scholarship underscores the notion of corporate influence as a threat to the objectivity and validity of biomedical research, for instance showing how pharmaceutical-sponsored research is associated with results favoring sponsor interests (Resnik, 1998; 2000; Sismondo, 2008; 2009). This literature has also highlighted that shifting academic–industry relations not only implicate individual researchers, but increasingly institutions. As universities and other non-profit research institutes pursue intellectual property and industry partnerships, industry partners may be perceived as having inappropriate influence over the institution's decision-making. As such, research institutions and universities have had to develop strategies to manage this, such as creating committees to independently evaluate decisions, as well as establish private institutions that operate independently in order to support and manage spin-outs and investments (Resnik, 2015). This scholarship has interrogated the practices and values at play in the local management of COIs, highlighting the interests institutions have in retaining local governance (Boyd and Bero, 2007). As COI disclosure is now requisite across many settings, scholars have examined the unintended consequences associated with the ritualization of disclosure. For instance, the public may perceive researchers with disclosed conflicts to be more trustworthy, presumably on the basis of their transparency. In effect, this literature demonstrates that disclosure might enable a moral licensing in which "anything goes" so long as it has been disclosed (Grundy et al., 2018), posing new challenges for COI governance. Against this backdrop, where COIs are recognized as something to minimize and manage, the encouragement of industry involvement in translational medicine stands in stark contrast. In this chapter, I consider how the field of translational medicine, which aligns the priorities of government funding agencies, academic researchers, and industry in new ways, renders existing COI governance inadequate.

Methods

Following qualitative traditions of constructivist grounded theory and situational analysis (Charmaz, 2014; Clarke, Friese, and Washburn, 2017) this chapter draws on a content analysis of federal health agency documents such as strategic plans, mission statements and charters, annual reports, position statements, and funding announcements, as well as published scientific journal articles and editorials on translational medicine and COI policy published between 2000 and 2020. I examined how the role of industry as a stakeholder in translational medicine efforts and programs was described, and how commercialization, relations with industry, and potential COIs were discussed. In tracing published commentary and editorials on COIs and translational priorities, I analyzed how arguments about translational value were constructed, and how discussions about the purpose and consequence of COI disclosure were framed. Using constructivist grounded theory analytic practices, I coded these documents in Dedoose, a qualitative data analysis software program. Coding procedures utilized codes developed a priori from areas of interest as well as those inductively developed from the data. After this stage, a family of codes to explore commercialization, academic–industry–government boundaries, and priorities in translational medicine were developed for focused coding. Coded data was then exported for further analysis following analytic practices of grounded theory and situational analysis.

"Translation" as a crisis in biomedicine

At the turn of the 21st century, leaders in the biomedical research community began to voice concerns over the lack of movement from bench research discoveries to patient bedsides. After decades of technological advances and "basic" biomedical discoveries, alongside increased federal funding for biomedical research, there was mounting pressure to move advancements in pre-clinical research through to patients, as tools (e.g., diagnostic devices) and treatments. Although the failure to translate basic research to applied bedside therapies and tools was not a *new* problem,[4] resounding critique of this chasm, or "valley of death" (Zerhouni, 2003), in biomedical research ignited efforts to fund "translational" research, cementing translational medicine efforts as a priority in federal health research (Robinson, 2019a; Solomon, 2015). In general, translational medicine and its allied fields are concerned with solving the problems that inhibit discoveries made in basic biomedical research from making it to the frontlines of health care delivery in the form of pharmaceutical development, diagnostic devices, as well as community health interventions and prevention programs (Solomon, 2015). "Translational medicine" has indeed become a buzzword in biomedicine, and institutionalized efforts in the name of translation have become a central organizing principle in biomedicine (Jeske, forthcoming).

In the early 2000s, both the National Institutes of Health (NIH) and the Food and Drug Administration (FDA) released strategic plans specifically to address translational problems. The NIH, the federal funding agency and main funder for biomedical research in the United States, released its "Roadmap", which set out its priorities and established the "Common Fund" in order to carry out the Roadmap's strategic plan. Similarly, the FDA, the federal regulatory agency charged with regulating pharmaceuticals and medical devices, released its 2004 report, "Innovation/Stagnation: Challenge and Opportunity on the Critical Path to New Medical Products" (hereafter referred to as the Innovation/Stagnation Report), which outlined plans to develop the "critical path" pipeline for shepherding pharmaceuticals and medical devices from pre-clinical research to the market. As the FDA explained in the Innovation/Stagnation Report:

> Many accomplished scientists in academia, government, and industry are working on these challenges, and there has been much success in recent years. But the fact remains that the pace of [product] development work has not kept up with the rapid advances in product discovery. The result is a technological disconnect between discovery and the product development process – the steps involved in turning new laboratory discoveries into treatments that are safe and effective.
>
> (2004, p. iii)

This excerpt highlights that despite the best efforts by the government, industry, and academic researchers, there is an enduring disconnect between "product" (such as pharmaceuticals and medical devices) discovery and development. As I have detailed elsewhere, the solution to this "pipeline" problem was not simply that scientists needed to deliver on bringing their discoveries and developments to the bedside. Translation has been positioned as such a fundamental problem with the very infrastructure of academic biomedical research that a whole new field and set of actors and practices have emerged to attend to remedy it (Jeske, forthcoming).

Critiquing academic biomedical research

Translational medicine advocates situate the norms and patterned practices of academic research – such as incentive structures in academic research, the slow pace of academic research and publishing standards, and the production of siloed knowledge along disciplinary and agency boundaries – as the root of translational problems (Jeske, forthcoming). Most crucially, translational medicine proponents point out that the incentive structures for professional advancement are not aligned with bringing products to market, that is, to the bedside, which is the primary goal of translational work.[5] In traditional academic science, researchers are rewarded for the quality and quantity of scientific publications; academic capital is derived from publishing research and obtaining research funding. As translational medicine proponents argue, these venues are not particularly interested in publishing translational work, which might not achieve the "pristine" quality of pre-clinical studies. Scientific journals, especially high-ranking publication outlets, typically require novel discoveries and are unwilling to publish studies that demonstrate negative findings (Marincola, 2003). Explaining "how science fails us" in the initial volume of the *Journal of Translational Medicine,* the first journal dedicated to translational medicine, Marincola argued:

> Here is where the scientific community drops the ball. Often scientists that designed new potential therapies based on fundamental scientific breakthroughs are not inclined to learn why things did not work as well in humans as they did in the pre-clinical settings because there is no room in prestige journals for negative results. Indeed, the scientific community is not generally interested in negative results. In addition, difficulty in publishing results derived from phase I studies is compounded by the fact that often data are of compromised quality and not of the pristine quality achievable in the pre-clinical setting.
>
> (2003, p. 2)

Marincola and other key proponents of translational medicine argue that negative and less-than-pristine findings offer important insights into why therapeutic compounds and strategies fail. Because journals do not typically publish this work, it can lead to redundancy in what failed experiments and strategies investigators try. When it comes to achieving translational goals, they argue, knowledge about what does not work is just as valuable, if not more, than knowledge about what does work in pre-clinical settings. As I discuss in the next section, this particular issue led to the development of dedicated translational medicine journals, providing outlets for translational research and thus aligning the incentive infrastructure of academia with the goals of translational medicine.

Due to this inefficient pipeline, high rates of failure are observed when trying to move pharmaceuticals and biomedical technologies from laboratory development, through pre-clinical research, clinical trials, and eventually to patient bedsides. Most prominently discussed in translational medicine documents as evidence of this are the many therapies that are (a) safe, as demonstrated in pre-clinical models, but then are shown to be toxic to humans, and (b) effective in pre-clinical models (non-human animals and 2D cell culture models) but are not effective in humans. The NIH estimates that 30 percent of medications shown to be effective in pre-clinical animal studies fail in human clinical trials because they are found to be toxic to humans. An additional 60 percent fail in clinical trials because they are not effective in humans (Tagle, 2019). Thus, taken together, around 90 percent of drugs effective in mice and other non-human animals are ultimately deemed unsuitable for use in humans (Marincola, 2003; Mak, Evaniew, and Ghert, 2014).[6] Put simply, "animal experiments, test tube analyses and early human trials do simply not reflect the patient situation well enough to reliably predict efficacy and safety of a novel compound or device" (Wehling, 2008).

Finally, translational medicine constructs high economic costs – in terms of financial investment and time – as the "consequence" of these high rates of failure in moving from bench-side discoveries to bedside treatments. Claims about the high costs of drug development abound in translational medicine documents. Advocates are quick to cite the billions of dollars being invested in what they consider a rather inefficient and ineffective research infrastructure (Mankoff et al., 2004; Mak et al., 2014), with estimations that it takes 10–15 years and $2.6 billion (this estimate, notably, is inclusive of the costs of failures) on average to bring new drugs to market (PhRMA, 2016).

These high costs have historically been footed by both private industry as well as the federal government. However, as Robinson (2019b) has shown, in responding to this burden, the "riskier" parts of research and development have been shifted to the government-funded side, particularly as pharmaceutical and biotechnology industries have shrunk their research and development arms. This is an open secret; advocates of translational medicine, which of course includes industry stakeholders, understand this to be a step toward achieving translational ends. As Francis Collins, current director of the NIH, remarked in 2010 in an interview on the success of the Common Fund:

> For rare and neglected diseases, economic considerations will limit private-sector interest; but NIH-funded researchers can explore the earlier stages in the drug-development pipeline to "de-risk" projects that would otherwise lie untouched. Similarly, for common diseases, many of the new molecular discoveries are of uncertain value for drug development, but NIH investigators can validate these drug targets and develop promising lead compounds, as well as carrying out process engineering on the pipeline itself. The goal will be to bring each project just far enough to become of interest to the private sector to pick up.
>
> (Wadman, 2010)

This suggests that the NIH recognizes how it can serve the needs of industry, and ultimately the public, by getting new drugs to market by "de-risking" the development pipeline. Because the NIH recognizes that industry will not invest in "risky" research and development, in the sense that return on investment may be unlikely, it positions itself – and by nature, taxpayers – to take on this burden.

In the framing of translation as a problem, industry is not seen as part of the problem; instead, its techniques and commercialization acumen are seen as valuable forms of expertise for *solving* the problem of translation. As scholars have shown, how problems are framed and discursively constructed matters because this construction opens up what are seen as potential interventions and constrains the possibilities for solving a problem (e.g., Saguy, 2012; Shostak, 2013; Jeske, 2021). As I describe in the following section, the particular framing of translational problems – namely the infrastructure of academic biomedical research – has led to the establishment of a specific infrastructure for achieving translational goals: one that prioritizes industry needs and embeds private interests more deeply in the infrastructure of biomedical research.

Establishing an infrastructure for translational medicine

In order to solve translational pipeline problems and accomplish its goals, translational medicine advocates needed to tweak the existing academic infrastructure in particular ways that would support translational endeavors. As I discuss in this section, such efforts consisted of establishing publishing outlets and funding streams that fit within the infrastructure of academic science, as well as reorganizing relations between government, academia, and industry. In doing so, translational medicine aligns the values of these three sectors in the pursuit of translation. It establishes a new organizing principle for getting biomedical research done: one that fosters more intertwined partnerships between academic researchers, industry, and government and formally engages industry needs, stakeholders, and interests throughout the research process (Jeske, forthcoming).

As discussed in the previous section, one pathway that translational medicine took in order to fit its goals within the existing infrastructure of academic science was to establish scientific, peer-reviewed journals. As scholars have shown, the establishment of professional communities and reputable journals are key to field-building and legitimation efforts (Frickel, 2004; Jeske, 2021). Such journals offer an avenue for researchers to publish work that might have otherwise not been pursued, perhaps because investigators may have thought it would be unpublishable in high-profile biomedical journals.[7] Thus, an important development for institutionalizing translational medicine was to establish high-profile scientific journals devoted to publishing translational research, journals that would provide credible alternatives for researchers working in translational spaces. These include the *Journal of Translational Medicine* (established in 2003), *Science Translational Medicine* (established in 2009), the *American Journal of Translational Research* (established in 2009), *Clinical and Translational Science* (established in 2008), and *Annals of Translational Medicine* (established in 2013), among others. These journals specifically seek to publish translational advances and aim to be widely disseminated; as such, several of them are open access publications.

Crucially, translational medicine's explicit move to bring industry into academic spaces represents a departure from past scientific practice, in which industry affiliation and involvement in academic science was something to manage and distance. Under translational medicine's logic, industry becomes a central actor in the defining of research agendas and a partner in the research process. Key here is that sectors that were previously understood to be in some ways in opposition to one another, in terms of their value systems, are now being strategically aligned. This is an important turn for translational medicine to be able to straddle the boundaries it does, but it is also where new tensions emerge.

Federal agency strategic plans like the 2003 NIH Roadmap and the 2004 FDA Innovation/Stagnation Report, two important agenda-setting documents that guide and legitimate translational efforts, explicitly call for new partnerships and collaborations with stakeholders – namely industry – throughout the research process. The programs and initiatives launched through strategic plans concretized industry partnerships and collaboration across government, academia, and the private sector and were an important part of developing an infrastructure to support translational research. For instance, the Roadmap called for "vastly different" interdisciplinary research teams, and collaborations between traditional academics and the private industry:

> To devise and use the state-of-the-art technologies developed from the roadmap effort, we will need the expertise of nontraditional teams of biological scientists, engineers, mathematicians, physical scientists, computer scientists, and others. The private sector will play an essential role in this new paradigm, and federal agencies will be required to do more collaborating with industry and each other. We recognize that the research teams of the future will look and feel vastly different from their predecessors.
>
> (Zerhouni, 2003, p. 64)

Although the Roadmap remains vague about the precise role of industry, the private sector is framed as being "essential" to successful biomedical research teams of the future. Notably, in creating the Roadmap concept, the NIH "consulted with more than 300 nationally recognized leaders in industry, government, academia and the public" (NIH, 2014, p. 3).

In 2012, the NIH established the National Center for Advancing Translational Sciences (NCATS). Unlike most institutes and centers at the NIH, NCATS does not focus on a particular disease area. Instead, it "is all about getting more treatments to more patients more quickly" (NCATS, 2020). NCATS offers a clear explanation of how it understands translation to be both a scientific and organizational problem:

> Developing a potential therapy to the point of regulatory approval can require expertise in molecular biology, medicinal chemistry, compound synthesis and formulation, pharmacology and toxicology, technology transfer, clinical science, regulatory science, and entrepreneurship, as well as the integration of patient perspectives. However, academic advancement and tenure structures and professional and cultural barriers can make teamwork difficult to navigate. For this reason, NCATS places high value on innovation in team science and partnership development, and it designs and tests novel partnership structures that cut across traditionally siloed scientific disciplines, organizations and sectors.
>
> (NCATS, 2016, p. 25)

NCATS explicitly brings industry into its organizational structure. As it states on its website, its governance includes "diverse representation, including those from disease advocacy organizations and private equity firms, along with renowned scholars in translational science and regulatory review" (NCATS, 2020). Throughout the programs it funds, NCATS partners with the FDA as well as industry in order to prevent the problems that it understands to emerge from siloing across sectors. In this way, the embedding of private interests in the governance of federal funds is foundational to the infrastructure of translational medicine.

A critical part of ensuring the success of this infrastructure comes from getting buy-in from academic researchers conducting translational research. Creating an infrastructure where commercialization is the central part of the logic is multifaceted. As I have described, one piece of this comprises engaging industry interests in the shaping of research agendas, ensuring that industry stakeholders are involved in the earliest stages of research and in the federal oversight of the translational medicine agenda. But this infrastructural change is also dependent on reframing individual academic researchers' capacity, and their definition of productivity, such that commercial and entrepreneurial pursuits are seen as desirable, worthy endeavors. These efforts are geared toward encouraging investigators to think about the commercial potential of their research and technologies and equip them with the funds, tools, and networks to pursue paths toward commercialization – and to envision themselves not only as researchers but as potential entrepreneurs. Thus, another facet to building an infrastructure for translational medicine is the creation of opportunities for academic researchers to (1) engage with potential industry partners, and (2) seek training to develop their own entrepreneurial capacities. Such opportunities stem both from federal agencies, through the creation of programs like Small Business Innovation Research (SBIR) and Small Business Technology Transfer (STTR), as well as more localized efforts that individual universities, non-profit research institutes, and their technology transfer offices initiate.

The SBIR and STTR programs were established in 1982 and 1992 respectively, across multiple federal agencies with large extramural research budgets.[8] These programs are used to fund small businesses with technologies under development that have a "strong potential for technology commercialization" (NIH, n.d.). SBIR grants are available to academic researchers as well as individuals employed by non-profit research institutions (such as research institutes established in partnership with universities). At the NIH, both of these programs move awardees through a three-phase program where they demonstrate the feasibility and proof of the concept (Phase I), moving forward to research and development (Phase II), and then commercialization (Phase III). In Phases I and II, awardees can apply for additional assistance programs such as the Niche Assessment Program, I-Corps™, and the Commercialization Accelerator Program. In each of these, investigators learn skills essential to commercializing technologies, such as how to conduct a market study and interpret the findings, and how to network with biotechnology sector experts, build commercial relationships, and identify revenue opportunities. These assistance programs effectively provide training for investigators to become entrepreneurs and foster successful start-ups. I-Corps™ at the NIH, for instance, markets its program as an "innovative program to develop and nurture a national innovation ecosystem that builds upon biomedical research to develop technologies, products and services that benefit society". As I-Corps™ puts it succinctly, it enables investigators to gain "years of entrepreneurial skills in only weeks" (NIH, n.d.).

These opportunities serve two purposes: first, they are actively pushing for an ethos of commercialization in biomedical research, and second, they are imbricating commercialization into the incentive structure of academic research. Such awards count as bringing revenue into universities, and importantly, it has become commonplace for universities to count patents toward tenure and promotion. These training avenues are critical to embedding the ethos of commercialization into traditionally academic spaces: like establishing journals where the antagonistic practices of academic publishing are minimized, these avenues shift the infrastructure to be more welcoming to commercialization efforts where it may otherwise have raised concerns.

The efforts taken to align the goals of academic researchers, funders, and industry interests in the pursuit of translation discussed in this section raise critical questions about how COIs are conceptualized in this hybrid, blurring space where once distinct value systems are increasingly congruent.

As I discuss in the next section, a critical examination of this ethos of commercialization at more meso- and micro-levels is key to how we understand and govern COIs. Within the infrastructure that translational medicine has established, the intermingling of industry interests and academic research is both supported and encouraged. Critically, it is not just about existing, external private interests that may infringe on academic research through more traditional relationships such as consulting, speaker fees, or serving on an advisory board of a pharmaceutical or biotech company. It is now inclusive of the commercial potential of academic research and researchers themselves; in other words, under the logic of translational medicine a new class of biomedical researchers are being trained to always already be thinking about the potential commercialization of their research. This marks another key success of translational medicine: these goals are understood as allied and, crucially, *in the service of* public health.

Shifting values, persistent tensions: Questioning what counts as a "conflict of interest"

> To change the reward system, one must first change the mind-set of leaders and senior faculty in academic institutions. Some faculty members believe that drug discovery and development are antithetical to academia. Intellectual curiosity and love of teaching more likely attracted them to academia than a desire to commercialize technology. Although their perspectives need to be fostered in academic institutions, the translation of research discoveries to benefit patients is also a critically important and worthy academic endeavor. Fear of corporate interests tainting academic research is unwarranted.
>
> (Parrish et al., 2019, p. 412)

In our current moment of biomedicine, in which translational priorities are in vogue, COIs and the ways they are governed have come under renewed scrutiny. As the above excerpt puts in sharp relief, advocates of translational medicine, galvanized in their effort to survive and overcome the "valley of death", have questioned the base for concern about industry involvement in academic research. As I have described in the previous sections, translational medicine calls for a deeper engagement between academic researchers and industry in order to fulfill its goals of bringing bioscience discoveries from laboratories to patient bedsides. This shift in values – from distancing industry relations to embracing them – creates a challenge for STS scholars in terms of how COIs should be conceptualized and governed, precisely because such interests are no longer seen as conflicting. Indeed, the solution translational medicine offers requires a shift in the long-held beliefs about the role of industry in academic biomedical research.

Since at least the 1980s, scientific journals have established COI disclosure policies (Hauray, Chapter 1). Over time, and in the wake of various scandals, journals have increased enforcement of these policies from being recommended to being required. Notably, alongside the rise of translational priorities that I have discussed in this chapter, journals have found themselves in a tough place. New tensions around COI reporting have surfaced: ones that question how COI reporting aligns with translational priorities and the consequences not of COIs themselves but of disclosure policies. Scientific journals, the arbiters of COI disclosure policies, toe the line between enforcing transparency but not wanting to discourage academic–industry relationships in the name of translation.

Citing revelations of COIs at the NIH and investigators' failure to disclose competing financial interests in high-profile journals, *Nature* (and other *Nature* titles) clarified and extended their reporting policy in 2004 (e.g., Nature Neuroscience, 2003; Nature, 2004). After detailing the definition of competing financial interests and its policy on reporting them, *Nature Cell Biology* offered commentary on the intended purpose of such policies:

> The aim is to add transparency to the increasingly elaborate net of financial interests that pervades not only industrial and biotechnology research, but also academia – both at the institutional and personal level. It is not our aim to castigate research with a profitable bottom line – far from it. [...] We hope it is self-evident that the aim of this policy is not to denigrate application-oriented research; rather, it is to foster transparency, particularly at this exciting time of ever-increasing and ever-more intricate affiliations between academia and industry, and the increased level of public scrutiny this has precipitated.
>
> (Nature Cell Biology, 2004, p. 67)

Implicit here is the notion that COI disclosure operates to chastise research conducted by scientists with COIs. Thus, the journal editors must toe the line between enforcing and tightening their policy around the disclosure of competing interests, while also making it clear that they are interested in publishing the very work that might be most vulnerable to such conflicts: that which is translational, or "application oriented". Indeed, because of the infrastructure translational medicine promotes and its valorization of commercialization, it is perhaps most at risk here.

Journals' disclosure policies range from vague to strict ones, with varying ramifications when rules are not followed. But even where there are clear definitions of what constitutes a COI and how to appropriately disclose one, they all rely on a common understanding of what a *conflict* is – and this is precisely where we must consider how the meaning of conflict is, in fact, shifting under the logic of translational medicine. Consider the Royal

Society of Chemistry, which manages a collection of over 40 journals in the chemical sciences, biology, biophysics, engineering, medicine, and materials science. Its policy relies on a shared understanding of what an "embarrassing" exposé could be:

> The relevant Royal Society of Chemistry journal concerned should be informed of any significant** conflict of interest that editors, authors or reviewers may have, in order to determine if any action may be appropriate (such as adding a declaration of an author's conflict of interest to a published piece, or disqualifying a reviewer). Conflicts of interest are almost inevitable and it is not intended to attempt to eliminate these.
>
> **Significance may be judged by considering whether an undeclared conflict of interest could be embarrassing were it to become publicly known after the fact.
>
> (Royal Society of Chemistry, n.d.)

This policy recognizes that COIs are pervasive in the fields of research it publishes, and explicitly states that they are not intending to disavow such relations; indeed, they are merely seeking transparency. But they also capture the essence of the problem translational medicine presents: Would these COIs necessarily be "embarrassing", if they are understood to be in alignment with the goals of the researchers and in the name of bringing laboratory discoveries to the patient bedside?

Tensions surrounding scientific publishing and translational medicine values and priorities came to the fore in an editorial series published in the NEJM in 2015. Jeffrey Drazen, then editor-in-chief, solicited a series of essays that re-examined COI policies. In both his editorial and the three subsequent pieces by Lisa Rosenbaum, national correspondent for the journal, it was posited that anti-industry bias in scientific publishing is dangerous. In his editorial that launched the series, Drazen tells the story of Selman Waksman, a soil microbiologist practicing in the 1940s. Waksman won the Nobel Prize for the discovery of streptomycin, used to treat tuberculosis. As Drazen recounts it, "Waksman realized that if his discovery was to be of value to the world, he needed a partner capable of manufacturing adequate amounts of the material under conditions that would make it suitable for use in humans" (Drazen, 2015, p. 1853). That partner happened to be Merck, a powerful pharmaceutical company.

Drazen uses this example, and draws on other institutional proponents of translational medicine who have detailed similar examples of academia–industry partnership, to emphasize the *social value* of such academia–industry relations and their ability to commercialize laboratory discoveries, turning them into clinical interventions. Rosenbaum notes that the goals of industry and academic science are in fact aligned given they "share a mission", that of fighting disease (2015, p. 1860). She argues that the "collective conscience" that has brought public and scholarly attention to COIs in biomedical research has had negative consequences (ibid.). Rosenbaum's essays suggest that public concerns over COIs are emotionally charged, as opposed to being rooted in empirical evidence; that non-financial competing interests could be just as problematic as financial ones (including an example of her own clinical care practices as a tired resident); and that charged debates about the importance of COIs are getting in the way of getting treatments to patients. Few of Rosenbaum's claims are supported by evidence – in fact, as previously discussed in this chapter there is much evidence that speaks to the contrary – and it is noteworthy that these claims were aired on such a high-profile platform.

Unsurprisingly, this series of essays was met with harsh criticism. Perhaps most scathing was the criticism from previous senior editors of the NEJM, who wrote an essay in the BMJ: "In a series of rambling articles, [...] Lisa Rosenbaum, supported by editor-in-chief, Jeffrey Drazen, tried to rationalise financial conflicts of interest in the medical profession" (Steinbrook, Kassirer, and Angell, 2015, p. 2942). They called out the "colorful" language and "fanciful" arguments, alongside the lack of empirical evidence for such claims (ibid.). Baseless or not, these claims were aired in a highly regarded venue. While the NEJM had been among the first journals to adopt a COI disclosure policy (Hauray, Chapter 1), this 2015 series of essays suggests that such a firm stance has very much eroded.[9] As the debate about the purpose of COI disclosure continues to play out, journals are adopting standardized forms of disclosure, and often removing disclosure statements from the main text of articles. A reader then must download an additional file, which may be dozens of pages long or more, in order to understand the nature of a given researcher's conflicts. Such distancing requires additional labor on the part of the reader to find and interpret potential COIs.

As values in translational medicine shift, this new regime is being met with the different perspectives of key actors and institutions. While some traditional academic outlets accept the value of commercialization as a priority and a legitimate way to achieve translational goals, others continue to question the consequences these new values hold for the production of objective, bias-free biomedical knowledge. But even the perception that the practice of COI disclosure is meant to chastise researchers for such collaborations seems to be a moot point: in the face of the statistics I opened this chapter with, it certainly does not appear that COIs – in the form of relationships with existing private companies or of a more entrepreneurial variety – are inhibiting researchers from publishing their work in highly regarded scientific journals.

Conclusion: What is at stake?

In 1984, when the NEJM was among the first journals to adopt a COI disclosure policy, editor-in-chief Arnold Relman remarked:

> Connections between industry and academic medical scientists are not new. It has long been common practice for manufacturers of pharmaceuticals and medical devices to retain the services of academic scientists as consultants or to subsidize their research studies – particularly clinical trials of marketable products in which the company is interested. But in recent years, as the commercial possibilities of new biomedical discoveries have become increasingly attractive, these connections have become more pervasive, complex, and problematic.
>
> (1984, p. 1182)

Relman recognized that relations between academic scientists and industry were becoming even more intricate in the wake of the commercial *potential* that accompanied biomedical discoveries in the late 20th century, and that scientific journals needed to take action. Nearly 40 years later, this potentiality is even more challenging to govern. COI disclosure policies have arguably been successful in encouraging transparency about who has these relationships and how commonplace they have become. But disclosure alone is not enough to understand how they shape the research agendas pursued, and, increasingly, those left undone. Even in journals where conflicts, or "competing interests", are disclosed attached to the main text of the research, authors sometimes claim that "none of these relationships impacted the work of this study" alongside their disclosure of industry affiliations, relationships, and entrepreneurial activities.

This chapter has highlighted how the values and infrastructure needed to achieve translational goals in legitimate biomedicine industry involvement in all corners of biomedical research, not only in the development of pharmaceuticals but also in the tools and technologies that become basic tools in biomedical research and in the ethos of researchers themselves. The way in which translational medicine has been constructed, it promises a social good that is difficult to critique: getting biomedical advances into the hands of the public. But *how* this is accomplished – through the embedding of industry more deeply in the infrastructure of biomedical research – is not the only and inevitable pathway. The very notion that industry is necessary to solve and save biomedical research is a particular framing. Under the logic of translational medicine, beliefs about the appropriate role of industry in biomedicine; alignment of the government, academia, and industry; and pathways to achieving broader impact all prioritize private interests in the name of public health. STS scholars have long documented the ways in which interests – of all sorts – shape scientific research agendas, those pursued and those not. This is why we must now reflect on the tools we have to make visible the power relations in this infrastructure, and to govern and potentially reclaim it. Simply disclosing COIs is no longer enough – if it ever was.

COI governance was developed when relationships that are somewhat easy to identify as an *external* influence to the research itself were the norm, such as researchers interacting with or being appointed a role (e.g., as a consultant or board member) within pre-existing corporate entities that have an interest in the outcomes of studies. But as I have shown in this chapter, industry influence and commercialization values are becoming deeply entrenched in – and inextricable from – the very infrastructure of biomedical research. As the meaning of the work biomedical researchers conduct has shifted under the logic of translational medicine, so too must the ways we conceptualize industry involvement in biomedical research, the interests that are served, and what is ultimately at stake for the public.

Notes

1. At least 70 percent of research articles published in the *Journal of the American Medical Association* (JAMA), *Science Translational Medicine* (STM), and *Nature Biotechnology* (NBT) were authored by teams comprised of researchers with COIs (Table 2.1). This estimate includes all articles where at least one member of the authorship team had one (or more) COI to disclose. For the purposes of this analysis, I defined "research" articles based on the type of content published in a given genre from each journal. This included more than just the full-length research articles; I included article types whose content offered empirical evidence in the form of analysis or development of a resource (e.g., a database). In JAMA, I included both the "original research" and "preliminary correspondence" categories. For STM publications, I included research articles and research resources, and for those in NBT, I included research articles, research letters, analysis, and resources. Descriptions of these genres can be found on the journal websites. JAMA, STM, and NBT were selected for this analysis because they are outlets in which translational medicine researchers routinely publish.

Table 2.1 COIs reported in major biomedical journals in 2019

Journal	Number of issues in sample (2019)	Number of research articles	Percentage of articles in which any author reported a COI	Percentage of articles in which the lead or senior author reported a COI
JAMA	48	158	80% (N = 127)	47% (N = 74)
STM	51	210	76% (N = 186)	63% (N = 153)
NBT	12	99	70% (N = 69)	65% (N = 64)

2. Early efforts to commercialize technologies to create revenue streams for universities from faculty inventions date to 1925, when the Wisconsin Alumni Research Foundation (WARF) was established at the University of Wisconsin following the development of a method for fortifying foods with vitamin D by one of its faculty Harry Steenbock. For more information, see: https://www.warf.org/about-us/history/history-of-warf.cmsx.

3. Although these policies have been in place for decades, there continue to be instances where prominent researchers fail to disclose potential conflicts, leading to ethics reviews and often their resignation from positions of power. For a recent example, see: https://www.nytimes.com/2018/09/08/health/jose-baselga-cancer-memorial-sloan-kettering.html.

4. I am not suggesting that conversations surrounding translating basic research findings into applications originated at the turn of the 21st century. Particularly in conversations around the use of non-human animals in biomedical research, the inefficiencies in translating findings have been well documented since at least the 1960s. However, at the national level, federal health agencies began investing in translational efforts at the turn of the century. As other scholars have discussed, I agree that translational medicine is perhaps best understood as a "reconfiguration of the structure of biomedical research" rather than a new paradigm (Robinson, 2019b, p. 4392).

5. As I discuss in detail elsewhere, evaluations of translational efforts are often discussed in terms of the number of products or therapies commercialized. In this way, translation comes to signal commercialization (Jeske, forthcoming).

6. Non-human to human safety and efficacy has proven a major hurdle in pharmaceutical development. While not within the scope of this paper, the inefficiencies of animal models have become a major motivation for developing human cell-based pre-clinical models.

7. Indeed, in in-depth interviews conducted for the broader project this chapter is part of project, biomedical researchers often spoke of the difficulties they have had getting translational work published and grants funded, especially those involving the use of novel models.

8. The US Congress created the SBIR program in 1982. The STTR program was created in 1992. Federal agencies with extramural budgets of over $100 million are required to dedicate a certain percentage of their budget to SBIR, and federal agencies with extramural budgets of over $1 billion are required to dedicate a certain percentage of their budget to STTR.

9. One might also interpret the journal's decision not to disclose COIs alongside the main text of its published material, as other journals continue to do, as a reflection of its stance on COIs.

References

Berman, EP (2012) *Creating the market university: how academic science became an economic engine.* Princeton: Princeton University Press.

Boyd, EA and Bero, LA (2007) 'Defining financial conflicts and managing research relationships: an analysis of university conflict of interest committee decisions', *Science and Engineering Ethics*, 13(4), pp. 415–435.

Charmaz, K (2014) *Constructing grounded theory.* Thousand Oaks: Sage Publishing.

Clarke, AE, Friese, C and Washburn, RS (2017) *Situational analysis: grounded theory after the interpretive turn.* Thousand Oaks: Sage Publishing.

Cosgrove, L, Bursztajn, HJ and Krimsky, S (2009) 'Developing unbiased diagnostic and treatment guidelines in psychiatry', *New England Journal of Medicine*, 360(19), pp. 2035–2036.

Drazen, JM (2015) 'Revisiting the commercial–academic interface', *New England Journal of Medicine*, 372(19), pp. 1853–1854.

FDA (2004) *Innovation or stagnation? Challenge and opportunity on the critical path to new medical products*. Washington DC: U.S. Department of Health and Human Services.

Frickel, S (2004) *Chemical consequences: environmental mutagens, scientist activism, and the rise of genetic toxicology*. New Brunswick, NJ: Rutgers University Press.

Grundy, Q, Bero, L and Malone, R (2013) 'Interactions between non-physician clinicians and industry: a systematic review', *PLOS Medicine*, 10(11), p. e1001561.

Grundy, Q, Habibi, R and Shnier, A, et al. (2018) 'Decoding disclosure: comparing conflict of interest policy among the United States, France, and Australia', *Health Policy*, 122(5), pp. 509–518.

Jeske, M (2021) 'Constructing complexity: collective action framing and rise of obesity research', *BioSocieties*, 16(1), pp. 116–141

Jeske, M (forthcoming) Crossing the valley of death: translational medicine and the commercialization of biomedical research.

Mak, IW, Evaniew, N and Ghert, M (2014) 'Lost in translation: animal models and clinical trials in cancer treatment', *American Journal of Translational Research*, 6(2), pp. 114–118.

Mankoff, SP, Brander, C and Ferrone, S, et al. (2004) 'Lost in translation: obstacles to translational medicine', *Journal of Translational Medicine*, 2(14).

Marincola, FM (2003) 'Translational medicine: a two-way road', *Journal of Translational Medicine*, 1(1).

NIH (n.d.) *What is SBIR and STTR?* National Institutions of Health [online]. Available at: https://sbir.nih.gov/about/what-is-sbir-sttr (Accessed: January 29, 2021).

Nature (2004) 'Conflicts at the NIH (cont.)', *Nature*, 430(1).

Nature Cell Biology (2004) 'Nothing to declare?' *Nature Cell Biology*, 6(6), p. 467.

NCATS (2016) *2016 Report*. National Center for Advancing Translational Sciences Improving Health Through Smarter Science. Bethseda: NCATS.

NCATS (2020) *Center Overview*. National Centre for Advancing Translational Sciences [online]. Available at: https://ncats.nih.gov/about/overview (Accessed: January 29, 2021).

Nature Neuroscience (2003) 'Financial disclosure for review authors', *Nature Neuroscience*, 6(997).

NIH (2014) *A decade of discovery: the NIH roadmap and common fund*. National Institutes of Health.

NIH (n.d.) *I-Corps at NIH* [online]. Available at: https://sbir.cancer.gov/icorps (Accessed: January 29, 2021).

Parrish, MC, Tan, YJ and Grimes, KV, et al. (2019) 'Surviving in the valley of death: opportunities and challenges in translating academic drug discoveries', *Annual Review of Pharmacology and Toxicology*, 59(1), pp. 405–421.

PhRMA [Pharmaceutical Research and Manufacturers of America] (2016) *2016 biopharmaceutical research industry profile*. Washington: PhRMA.

Relman, AS (1984) 'Dealing with conflicts of interest', *New England Journal of Medicine*, 310, pp. 1182–1183.

Resnik, DB (1998) 'Conflicts of interest in science', *Perspectives on Science*, 6(4), pp. 381–408.

Resnik, DB (2000) 'Financial interests and research bias', *Perspectives on Science*, 8(3), pp. 255–285.

Resnik, DB (2015) 'Institutional conflicts of interest in academic research', *Science and Engineering Ethics*, 25(6), pp. 1661–1669.

Richardson, E, Saver, R and Lott, R (2014) 'Health policy brief: the physician payments Sunshine Act', *Health Affairs,* October 2014. Project HOPE.

Robinson, MD (2019a) *The market in mind: how financialization is shaping neuroscience, translational medicine, and innovation in biotechnology.* Cambridge: MIT Press.

Robinson, MD (2019b) 'Financializing epistemic norms in contemporary biomedical innovation', *Synthese*, 196(11), pp. 4391–4407.

Rosenbaum, L (2015) 'Reconnecting the dots – reinterpreting industry–physician relations', *New England Journal of Medicine*, 372(19), pp. 1860–1864.

Royal Society of Chemistry (n. d.) *Author responsibilities: ethical guidelines and code of conduct for authors* [online]. Available at: https://www.rsc.org/journals-books-databases/journal-authors-reviewers/author-responsibilities/ (Accessed: January 29, 2021).

Saguy, AC (2012) *What's wrong with fat?* New York: Oxford University Press.

Shostak, S (2013) *Exposed science: genes, the environment, and the politics of population health.* Berkeley: University of California Press.

Sismondo, S (2008) 'How pharmaceutical industry funding affects trial outcomes: causal structures and responses', *Social Science & Medicine*, 66(9), pp. 1909–1914.

Sismondo, S (2009) 'Ghosts in the machine: publication planning in the medical sciences', *Social Studies of Science*, 39(2), pp. 171–198.

Solomon, M (2015) *Making medical knowledge.* New York: Oxford University Press.

Steinbrook, R, Kassirer, JP and Angell, M (2015) 'Justifying conflicts of interest in medical journals: a very bad idea', *BMJ*, 350, p. 2492.

Tagle, D (2019) 'The NIH microphysiological systems program: developing in vitro tools for safety and efficacy in drug development', *Current Opinion in Pharmacology*, 48, p. 146–154.

Wadman, M (2010) 'The bridge between lab and clinic', *Nature*, 468(877).

Wehling, M (2008) 'Translational medicine: science or wishful thinking?', *Journal of Translational Medicine*, 6(31).

Zerhouni, E (2003)'Medicine. The NIH Roadmap', *Science*, 302(5642), pp. 63–72.

Chapter 3

Managing conflicts of interest at the European Medicines Agency

Success or weakness of the soft law tools?

Annie Martin

Adopting a legal perspective, this chapter sheds light on the instruments chosen to manage conflicts of interest (COIs) in the European Union (EU), especially at the European Medicines Agency (EMA). European law has no comprehensive regulatory framework specifically dedicated to COIs. Instead, they are regulated by two categories of normative instruments.

The first category is positive law – legally binding texts. Although the expression "conflicts of interest" does not appear in any EU primary legislation, provisions of the Treaty on the Functioning of the European Union (TFEU), such as Article 245 on the Commissioners' "duty to behave with integrity and discretion", could cover COIs. In secondary legislation, texts such as EU Staff Regulations[1] are relevant even though they do not actually use the term COI. The text establishing the EMA, adopted in 2004 (EMA Regulation),[2] falls into this category. COIs are not explicitly mentioned, but Article 63.2 asserts that certain categories of persons "shall not have financial or other interests in the pharmaceutical industry which could affect their impartiality". In secondary legislation, the term COI first appeared in a 1987 directive on legal expenses insurance. Since then, around 50 regulations and directives concerning numerous sectors have used the expression, but only 2 of them give a general definition. All these texts represent COI as a "risk" that may affect "impartiality" and/or "independence" in the decision-making process, but only some of them describe the risk as "unacceptable". Some suggest a difference between "major" and "minor" COIs. The aim of the texts is always to "avoid" and "manage" COIs. This aim is to be achieved by the drafting – by Member States, various organizations, and/or agencies – of "policies", "processes", and "measures". "Rules" are rarely mentioned. These policies, processes, measures, and rules may (or may not) include transparency.

The second category of normative instruments that regulate COIs is the dense institutional documentation in which the expression COI is widely used. However, the legal status and justiciability of this documentation is highly uncertain, although it may contribute to the emergence of a future

10.4324/9781003161035-3

legal concept. Soft law such as codes of conduct and "measures" developed by institutions and agencies could be included here. For example, Article 63.2 of the EMA Regulation stipulates that the Agency's Code of Conduct "shall provide for" its "implementation". The choice of soft and flexible law instruments to name and regulate COIs is not limited to the pharmaceutical sector and the EU. It is a result of the evolution of governance in a context of globalization, and is characteristic of the development of administrative law at European level (Bertrand, 2014) and at global level (Benvenisti, 2014).

Research on global governance law has established the emergence of new global actors, such as informal, transnational, public–private institutions. In the pharmaceutical sector, the ICH[3] (Berman and Wessel, 2012), recognized for its capacity to influence public regulators (Hauray, 2006, pp. 258–263), has worked with industry on drafting guidelines since 1991. Semi-independent agencies, central to the development of neoliberal ideas (Palacios Lleras, 2017), have also emerged as global actors and now clearly assert their global regulatory role; examples include the EMA and the Food and Drug Administration (FDA) (Lumpkin et al., 2012).

The emergence of global governance has led international organizations and academic researchers to ask: what constraints should be imposed on decision-making processes within governance bodies and how can their powers be checked? In other words, COI is a global governance issue. The Organisation for Economic Co-operation and Development (OECD), a strong inspiration for the EU, points out that managing COIs (OECD, 2003) is one aspect of a more general problem: "accountability". This concept, which originated in corporate enterprise (Supiot, 2015), is now central to the theory of global administrative law. It features strongly in academic research on European agencies, and is also employed to restore public confidence in institutions. In this sense, promoting accountability in decision-making processes is one response to the democratic deficit. European institutions use the concept to express governance by numbers and legitimize a way of thinking about legal and social relations in terms of accounting rather than justice (Lavaine, 2019). Not surprisingly, from a legal point of view, the conceptualization of COIs may be perceived as a mode of managerial regulation (Taillefait, 2014), which is another register of usage for the term "accountability".

The choice of soft law as a means to incorporate the term COI into the EU's regulatory system can be partially explained by the global governance context. However, numerous questions remain. Why have existing binding texts been neglected? Has the soft law option been successful, or has it failed to improve public confidence in regulators, or in the EMA's scientific expertise? What European rationale is at work here and what are the consequences? To answer these questions, I first review the debate on COIs and the emergence of EU tools, and then examine the structure and content of measures drawn up by the EMA to "manage" COIs.

The emergence of COIs in European soft law tools

The emergence of the debate on COIs at the EMA and above all the choice of tools selected to manage them cannot be understood without explaining the struggle between the Commission and Parliament.

At institutional level: A long struggle for hard law

COI first became a topic of political contention between Parliament and the Commission in 1999 (European Parliament, 1999). Internal factors, coupled with pressure from Parliament, led to the collective resignation of the Santer Commission (Georgakakis, 2000). This had, however, been preceded by the adoption of a soft law instrument,[4] the first Code of Conduct for Commissioners (European Commission, 1999). Using an instrument of uncertain legal status was nothing new for the EU at that time (Snyder, 1994; Senden, 2004).

This regulatory option remains problematic, however, because of the existing Article 213 of the Treaty establishing the European Community (EC Treaty) (Article 245 of the TFEU), which imposes on the Commissioners "a solemn undertaking" of respect of obligations arising from their office, "in particular their duty to behave with integrity". Although certainly inspired by ethical considerations, this is more than ethics understood as individual awareness; it is primary hard law. The text of the article expresses the founding values of the EU, such as democracy and rule of law, listed in Article 2 of the Treaty on EU (TEU). Furthermore, this article gives the European Court of Justice (ECJ) the power to sanction Commissioners, but only "on application by the Council acting by a simple majority or the Commission". The Cresson case, which triggered the Santer Commission's resignation, is the sole occasion in which the Court has implemented Article 213(2) of the EC Treaty in a procedure initiated against a Commissioner.[5] In its judgment, the Court stated that "obligations arising from the office" were "to be broadly construed" (ECJ, 2006, para. 70). They could therefore cover COI situations, as the Commission suggested in its legal arguments. In this case, appointing a close acquaintance, without using the rules for their proper purpose, was considered a serious breach of the Commissioner's obligations.

How else can the adoption of the Code of Conduct – despite the existence of Article 213 of the EC Treaty – be explained? One explanation offered is the vagueness of this article. A proposal to amend the text to make it more explicit was unsuccessful, and the political sensitivity of the issue explains the final choice of a soft instrument (Cini, 2014).

I am not convinced by this argument. The TFEU contains other vague provisions, such as the precautionary principle (Article 191.2 TFEU) elaborated by the ECJ. Since Article 245 of the TFEU expressly gives competence to the Court, and given that a judicial review mechanism is crucial in the rule of law, the key question is: why is the Cresson case the only one that has been brought before the ECJ? The subsequent history of the Code supports the view that effectively combating any behavior by Commissioners that may constitute violations of obligations arising from their office comes up against political considerations.

The Code has been revised three times (European Commission, 2004; 2011; 2018), as a result of combined pressure from NGOs (Alter-EU, 2008), Parliament, and the European Ombudsman. Given the "considerable and durable" dimension of the damage to the Commission's legitimacy in the Cresson case (Geelhoed, 2006, para. 122), Parliament requested assessments of the Code specifically focusing on the effectiveness and efficiency of the COI regime (European Parliament, 2009; 2014; 2019a). Parliament pointed out that the Code was not a legal provision and therefore not "judiciable". It found many deficiencies, including the lack of definition, and denounced cases of failure to implement the Code, incremental revision, and so on. The Code, rarely criticized by academics (Bodson, 2017), consequently refers to COI under "ethical issues", and introduced the first definition of it in 2018. Cases heard by the Ombudsman, and many other cases, confirm the Code's ineffectiveness. For example, in the "Dalligate" affair, the Ombudsman noted that the President of the Ad Hoc Ethical Committee, whose role includes assessing issues relating to the post-term employment of Commissioners,[6] was in COI since he was a lawyer at a major multinational law firm.[7] In the Barroso case, the Ombudsman stated that there was a breach of duty under Article 245 of the TFEU, even though the notification period stipulated in the Code had expired.[8]

Finally, I suggest that, as in international law, one reason for the choice of soft law could be that "the impact of soft law on behavior is smaller in magnitude than the impact of hard law" (Guzman and Meyer, 2010, p. 180). De facto, the litigation has been shifted to the Ombudsman. However, she cannot impose sanctions; this right is reserved to the ECJ under Articles 245 and 247 of the TFEU. Furthermore, the Ombudsman's recommendations are not binding (ECJ, 2007, para. 44). This is why she reproached the Commission for not referring the case to the ECJ,[9] and why there may be a political explanation for the reluctance to do so. A final question emerges: is it necessary to prepare new soft rules to make existing hard law explicit if neither is being effectively enforced?

The emergence of COI as an issue is also linked to the agencification of the EU. The abundant academic literature on "agencification" and "accountability" focuses on agencies' independence from Member States and European institutions, and only scratches the surface of the question of independence from the private sector. In the social sciences, academic literature on the EU's pharmaceutical sector rarely raises the issue of the EMA's management of COIs (Lexchin and O'Donovan, 2010) and COI is a recent topic in legal research (Gabbi, 2011; Vos, 2016). In institutional discourse, COIs became topical mainly after the Commission's White Paper on European Governance, which expressly referred to "accountability" as a principle of democratic governance at European and global level, and announced the increasing use of "non-legislative instruments" (European Commission, 2001). Eager to expand regulatory agencies as actors of EU governance, the Commission has put forward proposals on agencies' accountability, including COI, since 2002 (European Commission, 2002; 2005). In 2009, the Lisbon Treaty incorporated the objective to develop "non-legislative instruments" in many of its articles, and also provided a framework for the use of soft law. However, it did not alter the situation of agencies that had been created without a constitutional basis.[10] Agencies, therefore, remain a "promised land" for soft law and a sensitive topic for the institutions, which agreed on no more than a political declaration in 2012 (Joint Statement).[11] Although not legally binding, the Joint Statement underlined the agencies' accountability and the need for a coherent policy on COI. Finally, in 2013, the Commission published another non-legally binding text, guidelines presented as a set of tools to help agencies draft their own COI policies (European Commission, 2013). In these guidelines, COI appears as a risk that can be prevented and managed through its identification, declarations of interest, and transparency of decision-making procedures.

In sum, there has been a densification of soft law, a growing use of the concept of ethics as part of a normative system conveying the idea that COI is a pertinent notion that can be used to interpret existing hard law and protect public interest. On the one hand, soft law is assumed to be the more efficient choice[12]; on the other hand, Parliament clearly promotes the inclusion of the Code of Conduct into hard law (European Parliament, 2019a) and the adoption of various hard law texts on COI, including texts on administrative rules of procedure, on the transparency register, on democracy, and on decentralized agencies (European Parliament, 2016; 2017; 2018; 2019b). This could move the litigation to the ECJ and warrant real sanctions of COIs, on the condition, however, that submission of cases to the Court are not limited to those institutions that are recalcitrant.

Under pressure: The emergence of the debate at the EMA

The choice of soft law instruments, validated by the Commission, to manage COI at the EMA, arises partly from the above-mentioned context of agencification. The EMA was set up in 1993 in a context of European harmonization, the changing role of the state, the financialization of the economy, and the harmonization of the international medicinal products market. Looking to expand its fields of competence and pursuing the objective of harmonization of the European market including medicinal products, the Commission proposed the creation of a first wave of agencies in 1989. The global harmonization objective was shared by the United States. The Bayh-Dole Act of

1980, aimed at developing the biotechnology industry, was one of several texts adopted in a context of innovation policy and technology transfer. The act allowed universities and researchers to obtain privately-owned patents on the results of federally funded research. This radically changed public research and intensified links with industry (Lemmens, 2004). Ten years later, controversy emerged surrounding the rise of COIs engendered by the text (Boumil and Berman, 2010). Despite the controversy, the OECD, exaggerating the effect of economic growth attributed to the Act (Mowery and Sampat, 2004; OECD, 2007, p. 98), advocated the diffusion of the American policy. Accordingly, and to promote "technological innovation", the patent law system was revolutionized with the World Trade Organization's adoption of the TRIPS[13] Agreement in 1994. Patent law became a global property instrument that structured the medicinal products market and propelled industry toward the blockbuster and financialized model (Abecassis and Coutinet, 2018; Tulum and Lazonick, 2018). The EMA, initially placed under the authority of DG Enterprise and Industry until 2010, was created to sustain European industry and innovation in a worldwide perspective of economic and normative competition in which the FDA had regulatory leadership.

In 1994 the Management Board (MB) adopted guidelines relating to experts' interests, and the list of experts and their declarations of interest have been available at the Agency's offices since 1995. The guidelines themselves have not been published, so we do not know who drafted them or under what circumstances.

The term COI first appears in the Agency's published documents in 1999, in internal discussions concerning the EMA's first Code of Conduct published that same year. The Code, which has been revised at least five times, refers to COI but does not define the term (EMEA, 1999).

In 2004, Article 63.2 of the EMA Regulation expressly referred to the EMA's Code, but COI has been a quasi-permanent debate at the EMA since 2009, sparked by numerous COI events in the pharmaceutical sector, such as corporate-funded patient groups at the EMA (CEO, 2009), the withdrawal of the drug Mediator® in France, and the denunciation by the Council of Europe of COIs at the World Health Organization during the H1N1 pandemic (Deshman, 2011).

In 2011, the EMA's Executive Director stepped down, announcing his intention to start a consultancy business. NGOs reacted strongly, invoking COI and the violation of Article 16 of the Staff Regulation (Alter-EU, 2011). In retrospect, considering this Regulation and the EMA's Code (EMA, 2011a),[14] the Agency considered there was no COI, but introduced a two-year restriction on post-employment activities in the private sector. Parliament had the most significant reaction, postponing the decision granting discharge for the budget for two consecutive years. Declaring itself to be "seriously concerned" by "the lack of respect to implementing procedures regarding the identification and management of conflicts of interest for [EMA's] staff and experts" (European Parliament, 2011, p. 177), Parliament considered the first decision taken in the case of the Executive Director was a breach of Article 16 of the Staff Regulations (European Parliament, 2012a, p. 382).

Under pressure from Parliament, the European Court of Auditors exposed cases of COI at the EMA, some of which were due to the Commission (European Court of Auditors, 2012, pp. 18–25). The EMA was invited to add a section to its annual reports detailing actions taken to prevent and manage COIs (European Parliament, 2012b, pp. 84–87). It subsequently revised its processes and, above all, applied them.[15]

One case dealt with by the Ombudsman illustrates the EMA's failure to enforce the Regulation and its own processes (European Ombudsman, 2014). In 2011, after Parliament's decision, the EMA required its staff members to sell any shares they held in pharmaceutical companies within six months.[16] An EMA employee, who had declared her "financial interests" to the EMA when she was recruited, refused to sell her shares before the deadline and complained to the Ombudsman. The Ombudsman considered that ownership of shares in pharmaceutical companies was problematic and said that hard law regulation applicable to EMA staff had existed since 2004. This means that the EMA had not been enforcing the law for many years.[17]

As with the Commission, the problem lies in ensuring that COI policy "is correctly implemented with particular regard to the possibility of sanctioning breaches and omissions by concerned individuals" (Gabbi, 2011, p. 225).

The EMA's processes: "to increase the level of allowable conflicts of interests"?

Since 1993, the EMA Regulation has explicitly referred to interests in the pharmaceutical industry. In essence, the current Article 63 of the Regulation contains three provisions. The first concerns the means: transparency. The names and professional qualifications of EMA committee members must be published; all MB members, committee members, rapporteurs, and experts listed on the EMA's website since 2011 (EMA, 2011b) must declare their sole "financial interests" annually; "indirect interests" potentially relating to the pharmaceutical industry must be declared in a register held by the Agency and accessible on request; and, at each meeting, the persons cited above must declare any specific interests that could be considered to be prejudicial to their independence with respect to the items on the agenda. The latter declarations are to be made available to the public. The second provision defines the aim: Article 63 states that all these persons shall "act in the public interest and in an independent manner" and "shall not have financial or other interests in the pharmaceutical industry which could affect their impartiality". The third provision makes the EMA responsible for implementing Article 63 in the Code of Conduct. The EMA must therefore guarantee the effectiveness of the independence/impartiality objective. In fact, the letter of the law is broadly clear about the objective pursued (Section 2.1) but the uncertain wording gives the EMA power of interpretation (Section 2.2).

When the means, transparency, justifies the end, impartiality

Article 63.2 of the EMA Regulation stipulates that concrete measures shall be explained in the Agency's Code of Conduct "with particular reference to the acceptance of gifts". In practice, the Code establishes a general framework and refers to other documents that the EMA calls "rules" applying to "competing interests" (EMA, 2016a, p. 5). These other documents specifically concern experts and scientific members (EMA, 2016b), MB members (EMA, 2016c), staff members, and national experts, as well as breach of trust procedure for scientific committee members, experts, and MB members. The EMA has also developed numerous other procedures.[18] This fragmentation of COI processes across several texts could be problematic in the event of litigation because of the multiplication of documents to be interpreted and enforced under the EMA Regulation. The only indication found in case law is when the ECJ referred directly to the Rules of Procedure of the EMA's Committee for Orphan Medicinal Products, without even citing the EMA Regulation, to assess an expert's impartiality (ECJ, 2010, para. 89). This is surprising, given that this committee is expressly cited by the EMA Regulation as being part of its structure.

The section of the Code concerning invitations and gifts is more precise than the EMA Regulation. It defines them and establishes a general norm: EMA staff, or other concerned persons, should not accept any direct or indirect gifts, or hospitality, and any such gifts or hospitality must be returned and declared.

The section of the Code concerning the declaration of interest adds little information to the EMA Regulation. Specifically, it indicates that rapporteurs and experts must update their declaration as soon as their interests change, and that failure to fill in the declaration of interests in a complete and/or correct manner may be considered a breach of trust toward the EMA. The principle is that each individual is responsible for his or her own declaration: it is up to declarants to assess whether their interests might affect their impartiality. This is fundamental from the point of view of the control exercised by the ECJ, which would appear to be formal. In a case related to the impartiality of an EMA expert, the Court noted that the expert's "solemn declaration" that he had no interests in the pharmaceutical industry complied with the declaration requirements of the EMA committee's Rules of Procedure. This was sufficient to exclude COI and violation of the duty of impartiality (ECJ, 2010, paras. 90–93). However, in this case, the applicant did not claim that the declaration was false or incomplete and did not contest the verification of such a declaration by the EMA, the latter being essential in a system based on individual conscience. In light of that fact, the EMA opened to external sources the possibility of alleging improprieties including the declaration of interests of scientific committee members and experts (EMA, 2017).

Article 63.2 of the EMA Regulation contains two sources of uncertainty. The first relates to the objective pursued. The text uses two terms: independence from the pharmaceutical industry and impartiality of MB and committee members, rapporteurs, and experts. Which of these is the pertinent legal concept for managing COIs? Some academics, reasoning in terms of accountability, consider that "independence is [...] not a general concept or principle". However, they prefer it to "the principle of impartiality [...] proposed by Parliament" which "seems to be inadequate" to ensure that agencies act independently "from commercially driven interest" (Vos, 2016, pp. 226–227).

"Impartiality" is a principle of European law enshrined in Article 41 of the EU Charter of Fundamental Rights (Charter), concerning the right to good administration. EU institutions and bodies such as agencies must respect this principle (ECJ, 2013, para. 154). The Court regularly recalls its two components: subjective impartiality, by virtue of which no member of the institution concerned may show bias or personal prejudice, and objective impartiality, under which there must be sufficient guarantees to exclude any legitimate doubt as to possible bias on the part of the institution (ECJ, 2017, para. 91). "Impartiality", expressly stated in Article 63.2 of the EMA Regulation, is the pertinent legal concept when it comes to dealing with COIs. Private pharmaceutical companies are starting to invoke COI to contest the Commission's decisions based on the advice of the EMA. In two cases in which the Commission followed the EMA's recommendation, the pleas concerned the "lack of impartiality" of one of the experts on the EMA committee. The ECJ recalled three points: it was an administrative procedure involving complex scientific assessments in respect of which the Commission has "broad discretion" (ECJ, 2010, para. 77); the institution had a duty to examine the case impartially according to well-established case law (ECJ, 2010, para. 87; 2019, para. 24); and it was applicable to the Commission and to the EMA's committee and experts. To put it plainly, COIs are considered as de facto situations for the assessment of possible violation of the obligation of impartiality.

The second difficulty is that Article 63.2 suggests that there is a difference between direct and indirect interests, but does not define either of these. This makes interpretation problematic and gives the EMA a margin of appreciation. The text contains two regimes of declarations of interests. The only requirement relating to "indirect interests" in the pharmaceutical industry is that they must be declared on a register that is accessible on request. "Financial interests", however, must be declared annually. At the same time, the text prohibits MB members, committee members, rapporteurs, and experts from having "financial or other interests" in this industry "which could affect their impartiality".

In the EMA's Code of Conduct, direct interests are defined as "of personal benefit to the individual [...] likely to influence or give the appearance of influencing his/her behaviour"; indirect interests are "other interests that may have some influence over the individual's behaviour"! The Code explains that according to the EMA's interpretation of Article 63.2, direct interests are "in principle incompatible" with being a member of the MB or a scientific committee, a rapporteur or expert, or an EMA staff member; but indirect interests are not prohibited. This interpretation follows the structure of Article 63.2, whose first phrase prohibits "financial or other interests" and whose second phrase introduces the expression "indirect interests", the declaration requirements for which are less stringent. We could say that Article 63.2 opposes "financial interests" and "other interests" understood as "not financial". But Article 63.2 also says the two categories "financial or other interests [...] could affect [...] impartiality". So how pertinent is the Code's distinction between direct and indirect interests?

Interestingly, the policy documents specifically relating to experts and MB members (EMA, 2016b; 2016c) begin with this problematic distinction and confirm that the point of departure of the EMA's interpretation is the regime of transparency established by Article 63.2 rather than the objective of impartiality. Both documents assert that "taking into account" Article 63.2 "in the field of declarations of interests, two categories of interests are possible, i.e., direct and indirect interests". They go on to define direct interest as employment with a company, consultancy, a strategic advisory role for a company, and financial interests. Indirect interests are "principal investigator, investigator, [or] grant or other funding to an organization/institution". Both policies define the categories that are supplemented by procedural guidance on the inclusion of declared interests in the EMA's electronic declaration of interests form (for scientific committee members and experts).

The "main objective" of the policies – "impartiality" as stated by Article 63.2 – comes in second place in the two texts, which alleges that "this has to be balanced". To achieve this "balancing" of impartiality with the need to secure the best scientific expertise and the role of MB members, a number of levels and categories of interests are introduced.

For experts, Level 1 corresponds to "no interests declared"; Level 2 concerns indirect interests declared and are subject to the balancing interpretation; and Level 3 covers direct interests declared. These levels are combined with three categories. The first category results in non-involvement in the EMA's activities during the term of the mandate, in the event of a leading role with a pharmaceutical company during previous employment. The second category results in full involvement in the EMA's activities and concerns certain direct and indirect declared interests, which are no longer present (financial interests, grant or other funding to an organization, interests related to close family members). For the remaining declared interests not included above, the interests are considered to be over, following a three-year cooling-off period. The text relating to the MB is in the same vein. Finally, one has to scrutinize the various boards listed in the annex to the documents to discover precisely where, case by case, the EMA prohibits a COI. For example, an expert who is principal investigator during the term of their EMA mandate: cannot be appointed as vice-chair of a scientific committee; must be replaced for the discussions, final deliberations, and voting as appropriate in relation to the relevant medicinal product or a rival product in a working party; cannot be involved as a member of a scientific committee with respect to procedures involving the relevant medicinal product; and cannot act as a rapporteur, take on any other leading/coordinating role, or be formally appointed as a peer reviewer for the relevant medicinal product or a rival product. Neither can they be involved as an expert on a scientific committee with respect to procedures involving the relevant medicinal product, i.e., they can take no part in discussions, final deliberations, or voting as appropriate as regards the medicinal product, and so on.

If we take the opposite perspective to that adopted by the EMA, the question is not whether the role of principal investigator, for example, is a direct or indirect interest requiring, under Article 63.2, an annual declaration or a declaration accessible on request, but whether having such a role and participating in the EMA's specific activity is compatible with the principle of impartiality in its subjective and objective components. Recently, the ECJ considered, in the case of an EMA committee's rapporteur, that it was "not necessary to prove lack of impartiality due to the specific characteristics" of his role "in the procedures conducted before" the EMA committee. The ECJ stated, "it is sufficient for a legitimate doubt to arise which cannot be dispelled" and concluded that the Committee had failed to respect the obligation of impartiality enshrined in Article 41 of the Charter (ECJ, 2019). In these circumstances, it was not necessary to examine the argument relating to the requirement of subjective impartiality.

This judgment, rendered on request of a pharmaceutical company, does not of course settle the problem of conformity of the EMA's measures with the principle of impartiality. Another aspect of the problem is illustrated by the scientific advice provided by the EMA.

The EMA Regulation puts on industry the burden of proof of quality, safety, and efficacy, required to obtain marketing authorization. However, Article 57.1.n allows the EMA to provide scientific advice to assist industry in proving these aspects. The EMA openly encourages companies to request such paying advice (Ehmann et al., 2013), invoking a correlation between the advice provided and significantly higher success in obtaining marketing authorization as well as reduced assessment turnaround (Hofer et al., 2015).

NGOs have criticized the opacity of this system and highlighted the risk of COI. They alleged that the EMA was becoming a co-developer of medicines, that it could not refuse marketing authorizations after providing paying advice, and that it encouraged these requests for financial reasons. Before the Ombudsman, the EMA admitted that some members of the Scientific Advice Working Party, which provides scientific advice, are also members of the Committee for Medicinal Products for Human Use, which is responsible for the final assessment. The EMA justifies this by arguing that experts are scarce (European Ombudsman, 2019). Stakeholders consulted by the Ombudsman had contrasting views. National authorities and industry representatives considered that the EMA's practices were adequate and transparent; NGOs and researchers in the public sector stressed the risk of bias and called for the scientific advice provided to be published, along with the names of the experts who had provided the advice, in order to check that there were no COIs.

On both points, the Ombudsman agreed with the NGOs. She asked the EMA to strictly ensure that the same persons were not involved in scientific advice and final assessment, and to publish the experts' names and scientific advice.

The spirit of interpretation by the EMA: Facilitate COI to facilitate innovation?

It has been demonstrated that "the justificatory basis for regulatory behaviour specific to medicines comes from regulators interpreting their goals as a requirement to maximise market potential" (Warren-Jones, 2016, p. 64). De facto, the EMA asserts that its goal is to "facilitate innovation" (EMA, 2005, p, 13; Ehmann et al., 2013), but the EU's action in health innovation is based mainly on an economic rationale. A health care rationale remains a potential to be exploited (Mahalatchimy, 2018). This may explain why a member of the EMA's Scientific Advice Working Party (Eichler, Kong, and Grégoire, 2006),[19] invoking "low ideological barriers", advocates collaboration between academics and industry. Above all, the EMA's public documents expressly refer to "allowable conflicts of interests", which is clearly different from "allowable links of interest". A 2008 internal audit made important recommendations on COIs,[20] but the MB nevertheless considered it was "feasible to increase the level of allowable conflicts of interests" (EMEA, 2009).[21] Responding to Parliament's reaction, the EMA set up a Scientific Coordination Board whose remit was to look at factors "putting the system under pressure" such as, for example, "the continuous strengthening of the rules on allowable conflicts of interests" (EMA, 2012). This Board coordinated the EMA's strategic reflection on regulatory science (EMA, 2020, p. 7), which explains that "top experts" with industry connections are rare, but essential to enable the EMA to fulfill its mission of fostering innovation. The EMA, therefore, recommends adopting a "proportionate approach" to COIs in order to facilitate access to "the best international expertise in key areas of regulatory science" (EMA, 2020, p. 50).

This view, clearly asserting that the problem lies in the regulation of COIs that the EMA "allows", is reflected in the latest version of its Code of Conduct (EMA, 2016a). The only section of the Code that uses the expression "conflict of interest" is that related to invitations and gifts. The EMA has replaced "terminology such as conflict, risks" with "more neutral language", in order to "address the perception issue" (EMA, 2018, p. 12). "Competing interest" is the new buzzword used to designate COIs. Underlining the different wording used in the Commission's Guidelines on COIs in EU agencies (European Commission, 2013) and the radically different opinion of NGOs (CEO, 2019), I question whether this choice of vocabulary by the EMA will contribute to the emergence of a coherent policy on COI, as requested in the Joint Statement of 2012.

Notes

1. Council Regulation 723/2004/EC of March 22, 2004 amending the Staff Regulations of officials of the European Communities and the Conditions of Employment of other servants of the European Communities, *OJ* L 124, 27.4.2004, 1.
2. Regulation 726/2004/EC of the European Parliament and of the Council of March 31, 2004 laying down Community procedures for the authorisation and supervision of medicinal products for human and veterinary use and establishing a European Medicines Agency, *OJ* L 136, 30.4.2004, 1. First text: Council Regulation 2309/93/EEC of July 22, 1993 laying down Community procedures for the authorization and supervision of medicinal products for human and veterinary use and establishing a European Agency for the Evaluation of Medicinal Products, *OJ* L 214, 24.8.1993, 1.
3. International Conference on Harmonisation of Technical Requirements for Registration of Pharmaceuticals for Human Use, renamed the International Council for Harmonisation of Technical Requirements for Pharmaceuticals for Human (ICH) Use in 2015.
4. This was Jacques Santer's choice.
5. In 1999, the Council decided to take the M. Bangemann case to the ECJ on the basis of Article 213(2) of the EC Treaty, but it was finally resolved amicably.
6. Pursuant to Article 1.2 of the 2011 Code for Commissioners, "Whenever former Commissioners intend to engage in an occupation during the eighteen months after they have ceased to hold office [...], they shall inform the Commission in good time [...]. If the planned occupation is related to the content of the portfolio of the Commissioner, the Commission shall seek the opinion of the Ad Hoc Ethical Committee. In the light of the committee's findings it shall decide whether the planned occupation is compatible with Article 245" of the TFEU.
7. This law firm had a tobacco company among its clients. Michel Petite, president of the Ad Hoc Ethical Committee and former Director General of the Commission's legal service, had a role in the Dalli case: Decision of the European Ombudsman, 297/2013/(RA), 19.12.2013.

8. In July 2016, shortly after the "cooling-off" period stipulated in the Code for Commissioners (18 months), José-Manuel Barroso was appointed to a senior position with Goldman Sachs International. The case was referred to the Ombudsman. In mid-September 2017, President Juncker announced a revision of the Code. See: Recommendations of the European Ombudsman, 194/2017/EA, 334/2017/EA, and 543/2017/EA, 6.3.2018; Decision of the European Ombudsman, 194/2017/EA, 334/2017/EA, and 543/2017/EA, 20.7.2018.

   The Ombudsman also found that the Commission had failed to take appropriate measures to avoid the risk of COI in the case of the nomination of its Secretary-General: Decision of the European Ombudsman, 488/2018/KR and 514/2018/KR, 11.2.2019.

9. Decision of the European Ombudsman, OI/2/2014/PD, 30.6.2016.

   See also: Decision of the European Ombudsman, 2077/2012/TN and 1853/2013/TN, 9.9.2016; Decision of the European Ombudsman, OI/3/2017/NF, 28.2.2019; and Report of the European Ombudsman on the publication of information on former senior staff so as to enforce the one-year lobbying and advocacy ban, SI/2/2017/NF, 28 2.2019.

10. But introduces them in many provisions, such as Article 298 TFEU.

11. Joint Statement of the European Parliament, the Council of the EU and the European Commission on decentralised agencies, 19.7.2012. https://europa.eu/european-union/sites/europaeu/files/docs/body/joint_statement_and_common_approach_2012_en.pdf.

12. The Commission ordered a study which referred to ethics and OECD guidelines on COI, entitled *Regulating Conflicts of Interest for Holders of Public Office in the European Union* (Demmke et al., 2007). The Parliament denounced the Commission for using this study "to assert its ethical 'lead' amongst the EU institutions, as grounds for not pursuing any reform of the CoC".

13. Article 7 of the Agreement on Trade-Related Aspects of Intellectual Property Rights (TRIPS) (WTO, 1994).

14. Shortly after, the EMA announced a clarification of its COI policy: EMA/451985/2011, 10.6.2011.

15. The EMA decided to publish special reports: EMA/302717/2015, 19.8.2016; EMA/175527/2016, 16.9.2016; EMA/184994/2017, 22.6.2017; EMA/463632/2017, 11.4.2018; EMA/131220/2019, 1.4.2019.

16. In its conclusions, the EMA explained this decision was taken in urgency, under the pressure of private entities and of the Parliament.

17. The Ombudsman also suggested ways for the EMA to further strengthen its rules on declarations of interests by its staff owning a patent in the area of pharmaceutics: Decision of the European Ombudsman, 1606/2016/JAS, 22.11.2017.

18. https://www.ema.europa.eu/en/about-us/how-we-work/handling-competing-interests#code-of-conduct-and-reports-section.

19. Hans-Georg Eichler, the first author of this publication, was a member of the Scientific Advice Working Party from 2005 to 2007: https://www.ema.europa.eu/en/about-us/who-we-are/task-forces. Last consulted 8.6.2020.

20. A French citizen applied to the Ombudsman for access to the audit report: Decision of the European Ombudsman, 2914/2009/DK, 14.3.2012.

21. The expression "allowable conflicts of interests" appears in the Minutes of the 67th and 72nd meetings of the MB (EMA/MB/404038/2010), (EMA/MB/465305/2011).

References

Abecassis, P and Coutinet, N (2018) *Économie du médicament*. Paris: La Découverte.

Alter-EU (2008) Critique of flawed study on regulating EU conflicts of interest. February.

Alter-EU (2011) European drug regulator challenged over revolving door case involving former Director. February 25.

Benvenisti, E (2014) 'The law of global governance', *The Pocket Books of The Hague Academy of International Law*, 24.

Berman, A and Wessel, RA (2012) 'The international legal form and status of informal international lawmaking bodies: consequences for accountability' in Pauwelyn, J, Wessel, R and Wouters, J (eds.) *Informal international lawmaking*. Oxford: Oxford University Press, pp. 35–62.

Bertrand, B (2014) 'Rapport introductif: les enjeux de la soft law dans l'Union européenne', *Revue de l'Union européenne*, 575, pp. 73–84.

Bodson, B (2017) 'Commissaires européens et conflits d'intérêts', *Journal de droit européen*, 25(237), pp. 86–97.

Boumil, M and Berman, HA (2010) 'Revisiting the physician/industry alliance: the Bayh-Dole Act and conflict of interest management at academic medical centers', *Michigan State University Journal of Medicine & Law*, 15(1), pp. 1–18.

CEO (2009) *Register fails to throw light on corporate-funded patient groups*. Corporate Europe Observatory, September 15.

CEO (2019) *High prices, poor access: what is Big Pharma fighting for in Brussels?* Corporate Europe Observatory, May 9.

Cini, M (2014) 'Institutional change and ethics management in the EU's college of commissioners', *The British Journal of Politics and International Relations*, 16(3), pp. 479–494.

Deshman, AC (2011) 'Horizontal review between international organizations: why, how, and who cares about corporate regulatory capture', *The European Journal of International Law*, 22(4), pp. 1089–1113.

Demmke, C, Bovens, M, Henökl, T, van Lierop, K, Moilanen, T, Pikker, G, Salminen, A (2017) *Regulating Conflicts of Interest for Holders of Public Office in the European Union*. Maastricht: European Institute of Public Administration.

Ehmann, F, Papaluca Amati, M, Salmonson, T, Posch, M, Vamvakas, S, Hemmings, R, Eichler, H-G and Schneider, CK (2013) 'Gatekeepers and enablers: how drug regulators respond to a challenging and changing environment by moving toward a proactive attitude', *Clinical Pharmacology & Therapeutics*, 93(5), pp. 425–432.

Eichler, H-G, Kong, SX and Grégoire, J-P (2006) Outcomes research collaborations between third-party payers, academia, and pharmaceutical manufacturers', *The European Journal of Health Economics*, 7(2), pp. 129–136.

ECJ (2006) Judgment of 11 July, Commission vs. Cresson, C-432/04, EU:C:2006:455.

ECJ (2007) Judgment of 25 October, Komninou e.a. vs. Commission, C-167/06 P, *Rec.* I, 141.

ECJ (2010) Judgment of 9 September, Now Pharm AG vs. Commission, T-74/08, *Rec.* 2010 II-4661.

ECJ (2013) Judgment of 11 July, Ziegler vs. Commission, C-439/11P, EU:C:2013:513.

ECJ (2017) Judgment of 20 December, Spain vs. Council, C-521/15, EU:C:2017:982.

ECJ (2019) Judgment of 27 March, Dr. August Wolff GmbH & Co. KG Arzneimittel and Remedia d.o.o. vs. Commission, C-680/16 P, EU:C:2019:257.

European Commission (1999) *Code of Conduct for Commissioners*, SEC(1999)1479.

European Commission (2001) *European governance: a white paper*, COM(2001) 428.

European Commission (2002) The operating framework for the European Regulatory Agencies, COM(2002)718 final.

European Commission (2004) *Code of Conduct for Commissioners*, SEC(2004)1487/2.

European Commission (2005) Draft Interinstitutional Agreement on the operating framework for the European regulatory agencies, COM(2005)59 final.

European Commission (2011) *Code of Conduct for Commissioners*, C(2011) 2904 final.

European Commission (2013) Guidelines on the prevention and management of conflicts of interest in EU decentralised agencies, December 10.

European Commission (2018) Commission decision of 31 January 2018 on a Code of Conduct for the Members of the European Commission which repeals and replaces the Code of Conduct of 20 April 2011 and the Commission decision establishing the Ad Hoc Ethical Committee of 21 October 2003, C(2018)700 final.

European Court of Auditors (2012) *Management of conflict of interest in selected EU Agencies*, Special Report no. 15. Luxembourg.

EMA (2005) The European Medicines Agency road map to 2010: preparing the ground for the future, EMEA/H/34163/03/Final, March 4.

EMA (2011a) Decision of the management board under article 16 of the staff regulations. Notification by Thomas Lönngren of activities after leaving the service, EMA/MB/218686/2011.

EMA (2011b) European Medicines Agency launches new database of European experts, EMA/794549/2011. September 30.

EMA (2012) European Medicines Agency's Scientific Coordination Board starts reflection on best cooperation between scientific committees, EMA/274306/2012. April 25.

EMA (2016a) *The European Medicines Agency Code of Conduct*, EMA/385894/2012, Revised 1. 16 June.

EMA (2016b) European Medicines Agency policy on the handling of competing interests of scientific committees' members and experts, Policy 44, EMA/626261/2014, Revised 1. October 6.

EMA (2016c) European Medicines Agency policy on the handling of competing interests of Management Board members, Policy 58, EMA/MB/715362/2015, Revised 1. October 6.

EMA (2017) EMA's handling of information from external sources disclosing alleged improprieties concerning EMA activities related to the authorisation, supervision and maintenance of human and veterinary medicinal products, Policy 72, EMA/283205/2013. March 17.

EMA (2018) 2016 and 2017 European Medicines Agency annual reports on independence, EMA/463632/2017. April 11.

EMA (2020), EMA Regulatory Science to 2025. Strategic reflection, EMA/110706/2020.

EMEA (1999) *EMEA Code of Conduct*. December 2.

EMEA (2009) Minutes of the sixty-third meeting of the Management Board, EMEA/MB/366757/2009. October 1.

European Ombudsman (2014) Decision closing the inquiry into complaint 642/2012/TN against the European Medicines Agency (EMA).

European Ombudsman (2019) Decision in strategic inquiry OI/7/2017/KR on how the European Medicines Agency engages with medicine developers in the period leading up to applications for authorisations to market new medicines in the EU, July 17.

European Parliament (1999) First report on allegations regarding fraud, mismanagement and nepotism in the European Commission, March 15.

European Parliament (2009) The Code of Conduct for Commissioners – improving effectiveness and efficiency, PE 411.268, May 12.

European Parliament (2011) Resolution of the European Parliament of 10 May 2011 with observations forming an integral part of its Decision on discharge in respect of the implementation of the budget of the European Medicines Agency for the financial year 2009, *OJ* L 250, 27.9.2011: 174–179.

European Parliament (2012a) Decision of the European Parliament of 10 May 2012 on discharge in respect of the implementation of the budget of the European Medicines Agency for the financial year 2010. Resolution of the European Parliament of 10 May 2012 with observations forming an integral part of its decision on discharge in respect of the implementation of the budget of the European Medicines Agency for the financial year 2010, *OJ* L 286, 17.10.2012: 377–386.

European Parliament (2012b) Resolution of the European Parliament of 23 October 2012 with observations forming an integral part of its decision on discharge in respect of the implementation of the budget of the European Medicines Agency for the financial year 2010, *OJ* L 350, 20.12.2012.

European Parliament (2014) Update of the study on 'The Code of Conduct for Commissioners – Improving Effectiveness and Efficiency', PE 490.697.

European Parliament (2016) Resolution of 9 June for an open, efficient and independent European Union administration, (2016/2610(RSP)), P8TA(2016)279.

European Parliament (2017) Resolution of 14 September on transparency, accountability and integrity in the EU institutions, (2015/2041(INI)), P8TA(2017)358.

European Parliament (2018) Resolution of 14 November on the need for a comprehensive EU mechanism for the protection of democracy, the rule of law and fundamental rights, 2018/2886(RSP), P8-TA(2018)456.

European Parliament (2019a) Follow up to the 2009 and 2014 studies on the Code of Conduct for Commissioners – improving effectiveness and efficiency, 15 July.

European Parliament (2019b) Resolution of 14 February on the implementation of the legal provisions and the Joint Statement ensuring parliamentary scrutiny over decentralised agencies, (2018/2114(INI)), P8TA(2019)134.

Gabbi, S (2011) 'Independent scientific advice: comparing policies on conflicts of interest in the EU and the US', *European Journal of Risk Regulation*, 2(2), pp. 213–226.

Geelhoed, LA (2006) Opinion of European Court of Justice Advocate General on case C-432/04, 23 February.

Georgakakis, D (2000) 'La démission de la Commission européenne: scandale et tournant institutionnel (octobre 1998 – mars 1999)', *Cultures & Conflits*, 38–39, pp. 39–59.

Guzman, AT and Meyer, T (2010) 'International soft law', *Journal of Legal Analysis*, 2(1), pp. 171–225.

Hauray, B (2006) *L'Europe du médicament. politique – expertise – intérêts privés*. Paris: Les Presses Science Po.

Hofer, MP, Jakobsson, C, Zafiropoulos, N, Vamvakas, S, Vetter, T, Regnstrom, J and Hemmings, RJ (2015) 'Impact of scientific advice from the European Medicines Agency', *Nature Reviews Drug Discovery*, 14, pp. 302–303.

Lavaine, M (2019) 'La circulation des concepts juridiques dans la globalisation du droit administratif: l'exemple de la "redevabilité"', *Revue française de droit administrative*, 6, pp. 1002–1010.

Lexchin, J and O'Donovan, O (2010) 'Prohibiting or "managing" conflict of interest? A review of policies and procedures in three European drug regulation agencies, *Social Science & Medicine*, 70(5), pp. 643–647.

Lemmens, T (2004) 'Leopards in the temple: restoring scientific integrity to the commercialized research scene', *The Journal of Law, Medicine & Ethics*, 32(4), pp. 641–657.

Lumpkin, M, Eichler, H-G, Breckenridge, A, Hamburg, MA, Lönngren, T and Woods, K (2012) 'Advancing the science of medicines regulation: the role of the 21st-century medicines regulator', *Clinical Pharmacology & Therapeutics*, 92(4), pp. 486–493.

Mahalatchimy, A (2018) 'La promotion de l'innovation en matière de santé: quelles logiques à l'oeuvre dans l'Union européenne?', *Revue des affaires européennes*, 4, pp. 627–636.

Mowery, DC and Sampat, BN (2004) 'The Bayh-Dole Act of 1980 and university–industry technology transfer: a model for other OECD governments? *The Journal of Technology Transfer*, 30(1), pp. 115–127.

OECD (2003) *Managing conflict of interest in the public service*. OECD Guidelines and Overview.

OECD (2007) 'Higher Education Management and Policy', *Journal of the Programme on Institutional Management in Higher Education*, 19(1).

Palacios Lleras, A (2017) 'Neoliberal law and regulation' in Brabazon, H (ed.) *Neoliberal legality: understanding the role of law in the neoliberal project*. New York: Routledge, pp. 61–76.

Senden, L (2004) *Soft law in European community law*. Oxford: Hart Publishing.

Snyder, F (1994) 'Soft law and institutional practice in the European community' in Martin, S (ed.) *The construction of Europe, essays in honour of Emile Noël*. New York: Springer, pp. 197–225.

Supiot, A (2015) *La gouvernance par les nombres. Cours au Collège de France (2012–2014)*. Paris: Fayard.

Taillefait, A (2014) 'Le développement contemporain des régimes juridiques des conflits d'intérêts: l'exemple du secteur de la santé', *Médecine & Droit*, 2014(124), pp. 3–8.

Tulum, Ö and Lazonick, W (2018) 'Financialized corporations in a national innovation system: the U.S. pharmaceutical industry', *International Journal of Political Economy*, 47(3–4), pp. 281–316.

Vos, E (2016) 'EU agencies and independence' in Ritleng, D (ed.) *Independence and legitimacy in the institutional system of the EU*. Oxford: Oxford University Press, pp. 206–228.

Warren-Jones, A (2016) 'Regulatory justifications: regulating European medicines to maximise market potential', *Law, Innovation and Technology*, 8(1), pp. 61–99.

World Trade Organization (1994) Agreement on Trade related aspects of Intellectual Property Rights. April 15.

Chapter 4

From the management of conflicts of interest to the transformation of medical experts' profiles

The members of the transparency committee in France (2000–2020)

Jérôme Greffion and Hélène Michel

Focusing on France, this chapter looks at the health agency experts whose role it is to assess medicinal products. It examines the effects that the measures taken to prevent conflicts of interest (COIs) have on the profile of the experts recruited and selected. Over the past three decades, these measures have included new legislation and the adoption of "best practices" by the agencies. Since 1994, experts working for the French Medicines Agency (today ANSM) have been required to file a declaration of interests, which is collected and examined by a special department modeled on the Division of Ethics and Integrity at the US Food and Drug Administration (FDA) (Tabuteau, 2010). In 1998, legislation made it compulsory for experts working for this agency to declare their interests and for these declarations to be disclosed. These obligations were extended in 2002 to cover all experts in France, irrespective of the agency or committee they sat on, although the implementing decree was not promulgated until 2007[1] (Hérail, 2015). More recently, in 2011, the so-called Bertrand Law[2] completed this legal arsenal by requiring all doctors to disclose any interests and benefits received (Boulier and Greffion, Chapter 7). This law was inspired by the Physician Payments Sunshine Act, adopted in the United States the previous year (Hauray, 2018).

These measures have been widely debated. Some organizations, such as Formindep, an association that calls for independent healthcare information along the lines of the No Free Lunch movement, deplore the inadequacy of measures taken against certain experts they consider complicit with an industry that is only interested in profit and has little concern for public health. Other people consider the measures excessive and argue they risk depriving the administration of good experts. Future Health Minister (2017–2020) Agnès Buzyn, for example, stated during her Senate hearing when she was a candidate for the presidency of the French National Health

10.4324/9781003161035-4

Authority (HAS), that "by seeking experts who have no industry links, we are going to run into difficulties in the highly specialized disciplines".[3] Going even further in denouncing these measures, representatives of the French pharmaceutical industry repeatedly argue that, "an expert who has no interest is an expert of no interest". However, none of these positions are based on empirical evidence. Although we know that agencies and experts have over time achieved compliance with the disclosure requirements (Cour des comptes, 2016), we do not know whether the measures have given rise to more deep-seated changes, in particular with regard to the closeness of experts' industry links and more broadly in relation to the profile of experts recruited to sit on assessment committees. This chapter aims to fill this gap.

To this end, our study looks at the members of the Transparency Committee (TC), which was part of the French Medicines Agency from 1993 and has been part of the HAS since 2004 (Le Pen, 2018). It plays an important role in the French system of health technology assessment, since its decisions have a decisive impact on the medicines market in France. The TC intervenes after a medicinal product has obtained Marketing Authorisation (MA), granted by the European Medicines Agency or, increasingly rarely, the French Medicines Agency. Following a benefit/risk assessment, the TC determines the "actual clinical benefit" (SMR) of the medicinal product – a measure of its therapeutic benefit, used to determine the level of reimbursement under the national health insurance system (Nouguez and Benoît, 2017). In addition, the TC assesses the clinical added value of medicinal products in comparison to existing products and rates the improvement in actual clinical benefit (ASMR). The SMR and the ASMR do not consider the economic aspects. Price negotiations are dealt with by a separate committee, the Economic Committee for Health Products (CEPS), which refers to the scientific assessments of the TC.

Over the last 20 years (2000–2020), 118 people have sat on the TC – either as chair, vice-chair, full member, or alternate member – 100 of them by virtue of their scientific competencies.[4] Our study of how experts' profiles have changed in the context of regulation of their interests focuses on these 100 members, whose average length of service on the TC is 5 years and 2 months. On the basis of interviews and a statistical analysis of the experts' profiles[5] focusing on their industry links, ages, and publications, we attempt to show whether and how the recruitment of experts has changed over this period.

A prestigious and regularly renewed committee

Since 2000, the TC has been renewed seven times – in 2003, 2005, 2008, 2011, 2014, 2015, and 2018 (with some occasional changes in between these key dates). The number of renewals on each occasion varies (Figure 4.2 shows the number of members renewed during each period). The committee has between 25 and 30 members, with numbers varying slightly from one term of office to another. Although there is an official call for candidates, it is often the case that the chair of the TC approaches doctors and pharmacists to ask them to submit their candidature. The chair is a university professor and hospital practitioner, appointed by the government because of his "scientific expertise".[6] It is often someone who has reached the end of his career, or may even be retired, and who has usually already sat on various committees or had a managerial role in the university such as dean or head of faculty. In recognition of their institutional career in the medical field, former chairs of the TC, as well as some experts, are now members of the French Academy of Medicine and nearly one-quarter of the experts have been awarded the Order of Merit or the Legion of Honor. The chair of the TC is expected to help shape the government's health policy with regard to the assessment of medicinal products. In collaboration with the HAS, he/she selects the TC members and makes sure that there is balance in geographical origin and that a wide range of medical specialized fields are represented. Drawing on his/her knowledge of the medical field and personal contacts, he/she approaches doctors who have achieved a certain level of recognition in their area of research. They are generally drawn from one of the top ten training hospitals in France and if they are academics have a very strong track record of publications. General practitioners (GPs) and pharmacists selected have links with the hospital sector. The chair may also ask the professional organizations to recommend personalities from different fields of specialization.

Membership of the TC is considered a mark of recognition that enhances scientific reputation. As most of the experts interviewed stated, joining the TC is "*very rewarding, it's very [...] prestigious*". One GP and university lecturer commented, "*In the eyes of the medical community, a member of the TC is [...] someone who is good at their job!*" For those who already have an established scientific and institutional reputation in the medical field, the TC is less important – it is one committee among many on which they may be invited to sit and they are more likely to decline the invitation. On the other hand, an expert lower down in the medical and academic hierarchy, such as a GP, is likely to be more enthusiastic about joining it.

Experts who sit on the TC are not paid; they can only claim expenses. Yet committee work demands time and effort – the experts examine files running to several hundred pages and attend meetings twice a month on average. In the words of more than one member, "*you need to be public service minded*". But we should not assume that the TC is devoid of interest as far as health professionals are concerned, or that the members give up their time to carry out assessments merely out of a sense of devotion to duty. Experts may emphasize the amount of work involved, but none of them complain about it. On the contrary, former members are nostalgic about their role and are disappointed when they can no longer sit on the committee – either because they have completed the maximum number of terms of office, or because their industry links are apparently too numerous to permit them to renew their term of office. They all see the assessment role as being an important one, not only because *"it's nice to be able to judge other people's work"*, but because it gives them a certain authority within the medical and scientific field.

The "public service ethic" alluded to above does not appear to prevent doctors from working in collaboration with the industry. On the contrary, such collaboration is seen as essential for any research activity, in the same way as *"carpenters have to work with wood"*, to cite a metaphor used in the interviews. However, not all hospital practitioners are courted to the same extent by the industry, even within the same specialist field, and not all of them are equally inclined to work with industrial partners. For those doing clinical research, links with industrial partners offer opportunities to work on new drugs and consequently publish articles in prestigious scientific journals, and ultimately move ahead more rapidly in their careers. In this context, the interests that experts maintain with the industry are an additional indicator of their scientific reputation.

Moves to tackle COIs have made it more difficult to combine scientific prestige resulting from obtaining private funding with institutional recognition. Several of the experts interviewed said that the rules were becoming more stringent. One university professor, a cardiologist working in a training hospital, commented, *"It used to be quite simple, if we had declared an interest link with a certain laboratory and that laboratory submitted an application, we would withdraw from the meeting so as to avoid indicating any preferences. But now, if you have a link [...] you have to withdraw from all the meetings relating to the company. Since their holdings are increasingly vast, it's becoming [...] crazy!"* Another respondent added that, given "all these new rules", he would "today no longer be able to sit on the committee". So, to what extent are the measures adopted to prevent COIs undermining relations between researchers and the industry and, as a result, the link between researchers and expertise?

A policy to tackle COIs with a measurable impact

To assess the effects of the measures introduced to prevent COIs on expert–industry links, we used data taken from the "Transparence Santé" database over the period from 2013 to mid-2019.[7] We grouped TC members together according to the date they joined the TC, and looked at the closeness of their industry links over the period. We tested the existence of a correlation between the period during which they joined the TC and the extent of their industry links between 2013 and 2019, using models that enabled us to control a set of effects likely to impact members to a different degree depending on the date on which they joined the committee (length of time since joining the TC or presence on the TC at the moment when the link was created, career advancement, etc.). By bringing to light a correlation between the date of entry into the TC and the strength of structural industry links, we aimed ultimately to be able to deduce the changes over time in the process by which members were recruited. In other words, we were looking to see whether such a change in recruitment did, in fact, take place, whether it resulted in a selection of members who had structurally weaker links with the pharmaceutical industry, and whether the change was sudden or gradual.

This synchronous comparison of the interests of experts who joined the TC over a period of more than 20 years might be open to challenge if the ages of the experts from 2013 to 2019 (and therefore their career status) were very different, since this would affect the nature and quantity of their links. However, this is not the case: the difference in terms of average age,[8] in 2016,[9] between the three groups of new members who joined the TC since 2008 is minimal (Table 4.1). The difference between the average age of these three groups and the two groups that joined prior to 2008 is greater, but is still reasonable and is less than seven years. This is due to the fact that the TC members were gradually being recruited at an older age (see below). This closeness in age between members with different entry years does therefore allow us to make a synchronous comparison between their interests without assuming that there are any significant structural effects (and we verify the age effects in our regression analyses).

The analysis of the data from the Transparence Santé database shows first of all that the 96 TC members[10] received significantly higher amounts from pharmaceutical companies than did doctors generally, estimated at approximately €6,000.[11] TC members received a little over €24,000 each on

Table 4.1 Average age of the members in 2016 and at their entry into the TC and proportion of women, by period of entry into in the TC

Period of first entry into the TC	Number of members	President of the TC	Average age of the members in 2016[a]	Average age of the members at their entry into the TC (standard deviation)	% of women
Before 2003	17	B. Dupuis	63.4	47.3 (6.5)	12%
2003–2005	25	G Bouvenot	62.2	50.0 (7.9)	20%
2008–2013	19	G. Bouvenot	57.1	50.9 (12.1)	21%
2014–2015	22	L. Guillevin	56.3	54.6 (10.9)	32%
2017–2020	17	C. Thuillez	56.8	59.2 (13.9)	6%

Field: Our selection of 100 members of the TC between 2000 and 2020.

[a]Excepting deceased members and one member too old to be included in our analysis of the links of interest.

average over the period from 2013 to mid-2019 (equivalent to €3,700 a year) in the form of benefits in kind or payments, as declared in the Transparence Santé database. However, this average figure hides significant disparities between members, as can be seen by a standard deviation of more than two and a half times the average. Twenty-seven percent of the members declared no amount received from pharmaceutical companies, and nearly 50 percent received less than €1,000 (Figure 4.1). At the opposite end of the scale, the maximum amount received was €410,000.

These disparities are also evident if we compare the groups of experts according to the date on which they joined the TC. Broadly speaking, those members who joined the TC before 2008 received significantly more than those members who joined after this date (Figure 4.2). The disparity remains, albeit lessened, if we exclude from the analysis the nine top beneficiaries (five of whom belong to the shorter, pre-2008 period). Excluding these nine top beneficiaries – those who received the highest amounts over the period from 2013 to mid-2019 and who can be clearly detached from the rest (Figure 4.1) – enables us to test whether the changes observed concern all the members or only the most extreme and relatively rare cases.

The linear regression approach enables us to verify the existence of this correlation between amounts received and date of joining the TC, controlling for certain factors such as gender and age. In our most basic models, the amount received by members per month is significantly[12] correlated to the date on which they joined the TC: compared to members who joined in 2014–2015 (period chosen as reference), members who joined in 2000

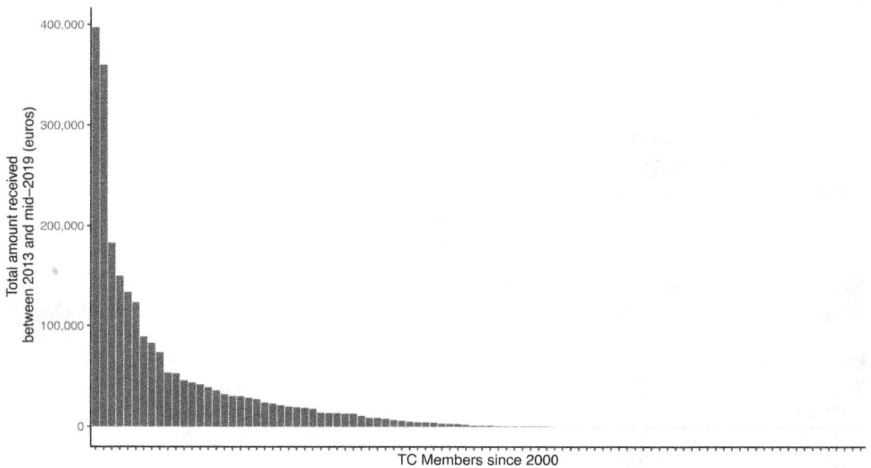

Figure 4.1 Graph showing total amounts received (in euros), in the form of benefits or payments between 2013 and mid-2019 by people who were TC members from 2000 to 2020.

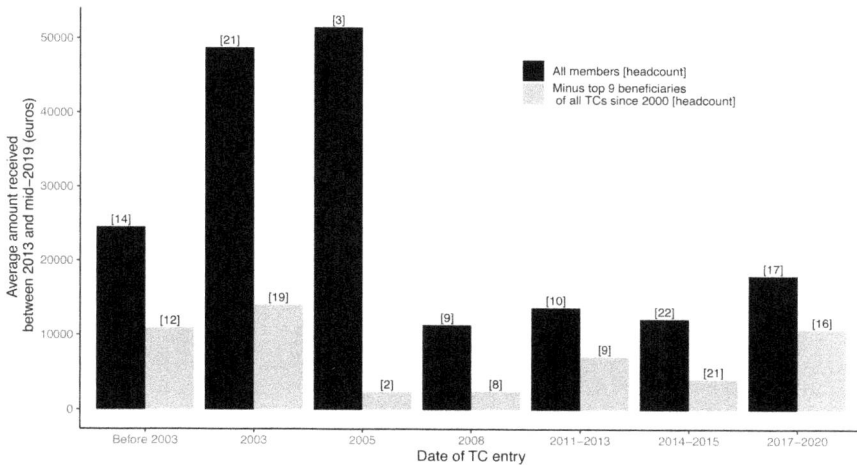

Figure 4.2 Average amount received per member, between 2013 and mid-2019, according to year of entry into the TC.

received higher amounts and those who joined in 2003–2005 received much higher amounts (Table 4.2, models 1 and 6). Women, irrespective of their date of entry, received significantly lower amounts from companies; because none of them are among the top beneficiaries (the gender gap is no longer significant for models 6 to 10).

We realized however that it would be necessary to develop more complex models than these initial ones, in order to take account of two factors that could have an impact on the extent of the interests. These are, first, the fact of being on the committee, divided into the length of time the members spent on it and the length of time elapsed since leaving (at the date they received the amount), and second, their presence on the committee on the date on which the amounts received were examined. The underlying assumption was that the members could capitalize on the experience they acquired while serving on the TC to develop links with companies once they had left the committee. We did in fact observe that although members who sat on the TC in 2003 received much higher amounts over the 2013–2019 period than those who sat on it in 2015, this was mainly because they received higher amounts in fees for consultancy services and, to a lesser extent, for speaking engagements and research contracts. In addition, the more detailed information sometimes available on payments suggests that industrial partners seek in particular former TC members' competency with regard to the drug market access process. This is confirmed in our interviews with former TC members who have retired from their medical positions but who continue to do consultancy work in the field of drugs.

Table 4.2 Multiple linear regressions on the amount received per month between 2013 and mid-2019 (amounts normalized)

	All members					Minus top 9 beneficiaries				
	Model 1	Model 2	Model 3	Model 4	Model 5	Model 6	Model 7	Model 8	Model 9	Model 10
Joined TC in 2000 or before	225.0 (97.8)*	81.7 (107.9)	115.7 (151.1)	623.7 (213.9)**	608.9 (216.0)**	189.3 (65.9)**	156.2 (73.2)*	554.8 (102.9)***	701.5 (143.6)***	710.2 (145.2)***
Joined TC in 2003 or 2005	765.3 (84.8)***	649.6 (92.4)***	664.7 (103.6)***	1017.9 (147.7)***	1002.4 (151.0)***	277.6 (56.3)***	252.1 (61.4)***	418.1 (68.3)***	520.9 (98.0)***	531.4 (101.3)***
Joined TC in 2008–2013	−7.1 (89.6)	−47.2 (90.5)	−43.4 (91.2)	90.3 (99.5)	79.2 (102.1)	12.3 (60.2)	3.0 (60.8)	41.9 (61.1)	79.1 (66.2)	87.0 (69.0)
Joined TC in 2014–2015	Ref.	Ref.	Ref.	Ref.	Ref.	Ref.	Ref.	Ref.	Ref.	Ref.
Joined TC in 2017–2020	54.7 (91.7)	−59.3 (98.6)	−64.6 (100.0)	−220.3 (110.2)*	−215.0 (110.7)+	153.5 (60.0)*	127.7 (64.9)*	72.0 (65.6)	26.0 (72.7)	23.0 (73.1)
Out of the TC when benefits/payments received		233.8 (74.5)**	242.2 (78.9)**	208.1 (79.5)**	206.0 (79.7)**	Ref.	51.2 (49.2)	141.5 (51.8)**	132.6 (52.2)*	133.4 (52.2)*
Time elapsed since final exit of TC when benefits/payments received (months)			−0.3 (1.0)	−3.4 (1.3)*	−3.8 (1.5)*			−3.5 (0.6)***	−4.4 (0.9)***	−4.2 (1.0)***
Time spent in TC (months)				−4.3 (1.3)***	−4.6 (1.4)**				−1.3 (0.9)	−1.1 (0.9)
Woman	−407.2 (72.7)***	−428.7 (73.0)***	−429.5 (73.1)***	−434.3 (73.0)***	−435.0 (73.0)***	−52.1 (47.0)	−57.5 (47.3)	−62.0 (47.2)	−65.0 (47.2)	−64.7 (47.2)
Younger than 45 when benefits/payments received	−1.1 (104.7)	11.3 (104.7)	10.7 (104.7)	3.7 (104.7)	−92.4 (222.5)	−65.7 (69.2)	−64.7 (69.3)	−70.1 (69.1)	−71.8 (69.1)	−15.1 (155.6)

(continued)

Table 4.2 Multiple linear regressions on the amount received per month between 2013 and mid-2019 (amounts normalized) (Continued)

	All members					Minus top 9 beneficiaries				
	Model 1	Model 2	Model 3	Model 4	Model 5	Model 6	Model 7	Model 8	Model 9	Model 10
Aged 45–54 when benefits/payments received	148.9 (81.1)+	122.4 (81.5)	122.6 (81.5)	90.5 (82.0)	50.5 (115.8)	46.5 (55.6)	39.7 (56.0)	46.7 (55.9)	38.0 (56.2)	59.7 (77.5)
Aged 55–66 when benefits/payments received	Ref.	Ref.	Ref.	Ref.	Ref.	Ref.	Ref.	Ref.	Ref.	Ref.
Aged 66–70 when benefits/payments received	−131.6 (79.0)+	−123.4 (79.0)	−122.0 (79.1)	−85.4 (79.8)	−58.4 (97.0)	−132.6 (53.1)*	−130.2 (53.2)*	−124.3 (53.1)*	−114.4 (53.5)*	−130.2 (66.1)*
Aged 71 and over when benefits/payments received	−491.5 (97.5)***	−481.4 (97.5)***	−482.5 (97.5)***	−493.0 (97.5)***	−439.8 (146.2)**	−191.4 (63.3)**	−189.9 (63.4)**	−199.0 (63.2)**	−203.3 (63.3)**	−234.7 (99.7)*
Age when joined TC (yrs)					−4.1 (8.4)					2.4 (5.8)

*** $p < 0.001$; ** $p < 0.01$; * $p < 0.05$; + $p < 0.1$

Source and field: See Figure 4.1.

Method: for each year between 2013 and 2019, depending on the type of declaration (benefits, contracts, payments), the amounts have been normalized by taking as a reference value the amounts attributed to all health professionals (the totals by category of beneficiary, by year and by type of declaration have been calculated on the basis of the "Transparence santé" database on the eurosfordocs.fr website). This normalization takes account of the significant and irregular increase in the amounts declared in the "Transparence santé" database, which varies depending on the type of declaration, and can be explained by the time taken by companies to adapt (in the case of benefits, the database is very incomplete prior to 2012, then significantly expands until 2014) and by the late introduction of the obligation to declare payments (hence a sharp increase in 2017 – see the chapter by Boullier and Greffion). Incidentally, this normalization also removes the effects related to the companies' changes in strategy regarding their links with health professionals. The amounts have also been adjusted for annual inflation (using figures from INSEE, the French Office for Statistics). The length of time, in months, between the date a member left the TC and their receipt of the amount was set at zero when the person had not yet joined the TC or if they were still a member.

Interpretation (model 1): among the members who sat on the TC between 2000 and 2020, women received €407 less than their male counterparts (in euros, normalized) per month between 2013 and mid-2019. For women who joined the TC between 2003 and 2005 rather than in 2014–2015 (the reference period), this amount was €765 higher.

The regression models show that while these members do exploit their experience or the legitimacy they acquired during their time with the TC to develop industry links, they do so to a decreasing extent once they have left the committee (negative correlation with the time elapsed since they left the committee, models 4–5 and 8–10). If we take the members as a whole, this effect is only noticeable for an equal length of time on the TC (compare models 3 and 4). Indeed, the length of time spent on the TC has a significant negative impact on the amounts received, which are negatively correlated. This appears to concern, above all, the members who have very close links (compare models 4–5 and 9–10). An initial interpretation could be that the members with more industry links stayed on the TC for a shorter length of time because they had to leave it sooner, precisely because of these interests. Another, perhaps less plausible, interpretation, might be that a longer time spent on the TC transformed the practices of the top beneficiaries, who no longer wished to or had the possibility to forge or renew links with the companies.

It was observed that members do indeed have a tendency to significantly reduce their industry links when they are sitting on the TC. If we look at the changes in amounts received over time (Figure 4.3), we can observe this reduction in amounts received at the beginning of the period of entry into the TC (for the members who joined the TC in 2014–2015 and in 2017–2020). For those members who were both on the TC or who had been in it during the period over which we gathered data on interests (i.e., 65 members), the amounts received in the months when they were not sitting on the committee are 39 percent higher than for the months when they were sitting on it. This "presence on the committee" effect is significant in nearly all our regression models. Thus, even though the selection of members takes into account the content of their public declaration of interest, in which candidates must declare their links for the previous five years, it would appear that the members adopt much shorter-term strategies limiting these links during the periods in which they sit on the committee.

In our complex models taking account of all these effects related to being on the TC or having been on it,[13] there is ultimately a clear distinction in terms of closeness of their links with the pharmaceutical industry between members who joined before 2008 and those who joined after 2008 (models 5 and 10). The cut-off point in the process of selection of TC members would thus be somewhere between 2005 and 2008. Since the periods before and after the cut-off point cover the terms of several chairs, and since the cut-off point occurs in the middle of the chairmanship of Professor Bouvenot, we can say that the changes observed more likely reflect structural and institutional changes than changes in practice introduced by a particular chair. This cut-off point also coincides with a change in the way COIs were managed within the HAS; on December 20, 2006, a "Guide to Declarations of Interest and the Prevention of Conflicts" was adopted (new

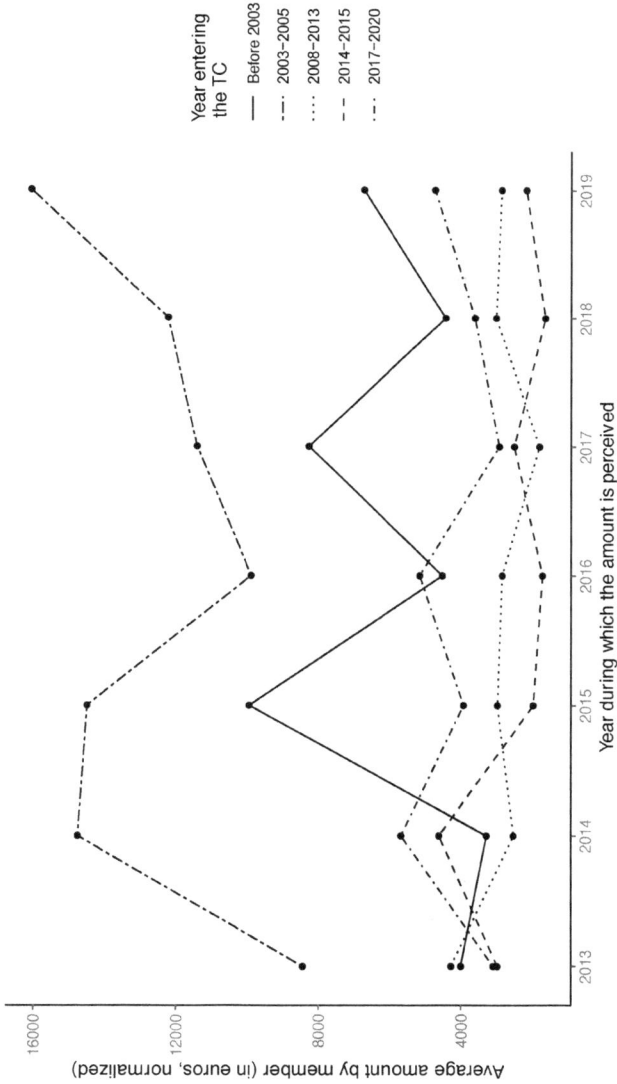

Figure 4.3 Changes in average amounts received over the period 2013–2019, according to date on which members joined the TC (amounts normalized).

versions followed in 2010 and 2013) and in 2007 orders were issued making it compulsory for experts on all advisory committees to publish their declarations of interest. The Mediator® scandal and the Bertrand Law, much later, did not really affect the process under which experts were selected, at least as far as we can see from the data declared in the Transparence Santé database. The transformation had the greatest impact on those experts who had the strongest industry links, but it affected all the other members as well.

While this change in the selection process concerned the mechanisms for selecting experts joining the committee, as studied in detail, it also undoubtedly involved the removal of certain experts who were already members of the committee and who were incited to leave. This additional aspect regarding the selection took place for the most part in 2008 and 2011 (Figure 4.4).

In the mid-2000s, the simultaneous introduction, at national level and within the HAS, of new provisions concerning the disclosure of interests and the regulation of COIs, and the very sharp reduction in the extent of the links of newly recruited experts, leads us to think that these provisions did have a real impact on the make-up of the TC. While those experts most closely linked to the industry were dismissed, the process aiming to select experts less closely linked to the industry affected all TC members. However, these transparency measures may not have fully resolved the problem of experts' partiality, related to their allegiance to the financers. On the one hand, it is possible, although this cannot be measured, that the change in the policy for managing interest links actually had the effect of encouraging

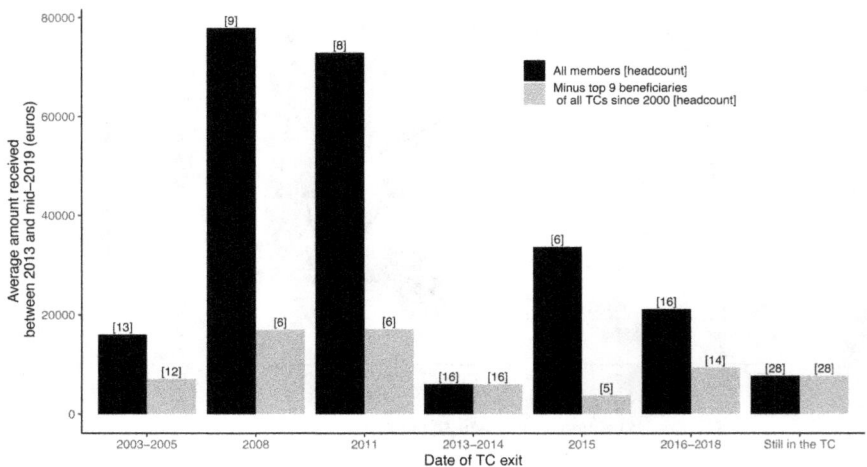

Figure 4.4 Average amount received per member, between 2013 and mid-2019, according to the date they left the TC.

the individuals in our sample to hide their links with companies to a greater extent after the period 2005–2008.[14] On the other hand, experts could put their collaborations temporarily on hold in such a way as to appear "clean" at the time of their appointment; some current members have said this is the case in interviews.

Older experts: A possible consequence of the regulation of interests

The reduction of expert–industry links over time coincides with another phenomenon that it could in fact have caused: the tendency for members to be recruited to the committee at an older age, and an increase in the age disparity between members. The average age of members rose gradually from a little over 47 for members who joined before 2003 to a little over 59 in 2017–2020. This represents an increase of 12 years, with the largest increase (a little over 8 years) occurring after 2014 (Table 4.1). At the same time, the age disparity between newly recruited members increased significantly (the standard deviation more than doubled). Age distribution thus evolved from being, for members recruited before 2003, relatively concentrated around the intermediate category of 45–54, in the majority (nearly 60 percent), to an increasingly widespread distribution for the following periods. It reached an almost bimodal distribution, either side of an almost empty 45–54 category, for the last wave of recruitment in 2017–2020, made up of 24 percent of new members in the under-45 bracket, mostly at the start of their career, and 53 percent in the over-65 bracket, who were probably retired[15] (Figure 4.5).

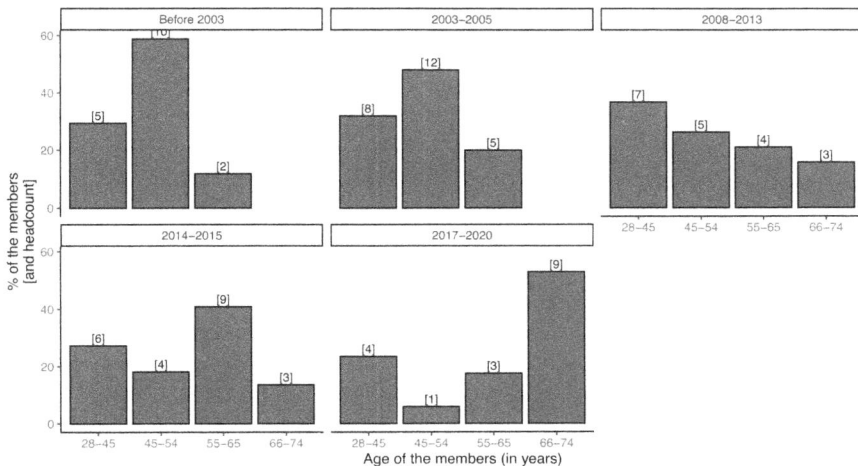

Figure 4.5 Age of the TC members by period of entry into the TC.

This change in the recruitment of members, with an increasing number of retired professionals or those at the end of their career, happened at the same time as the cut-off identified above between 2005 (last recruitment of members with very close links) and 2011 (last departure of these members). In fact, while the average age of new recruits rose sharply after 2014, the first perceptible changes appeared a little earlier with the first members over 65 recruited (Figure 4.4). This change in the age of members could be the consequence of a recruitment policy seeking to minimize new members' industry links. It is clear (Table 4.2, all models) that among former and current TC members, the over-70s receive much lower amounts and, if we look at the sub-group that excludes those with the closest industry links, the fact of being over 65 also correlates with lower amounts (models 6 to 10). This decrease with age is probably due to their career stage and the move to retirement. However, it could also reflect a number of group strategies that involve spreading out the different functions of researcher and expert at different stages in people's careers. One expert who was one of the nine top beneficiaries told us that, in one professional organization, *"they ask their oldest members to stop [...] to not maintain their links with the pharmaceutical industry for three years so that the younger ones can develop these links. In that way, it would be the more [...] experienced who could once again take on roles as experts in the institutions. [...] Since the older individuals suffered from no longer having the expertise, and in order to again find room for experts in the institutions, they asked the oldest to stop, so that the younger ones could replace them with regard to the industry, so that they, the older ones, could take up a role again in the institutions"*. This group strategy could be satisfactory for the youngest people who were keen to have access to the funding and research projects that up until then had been taken by their elder colleagues.

The marked aging of TC members could be a consequence of the new provisions introduced regarding experts' interest links: the older professionals, as a result of the career path effects, have fewer links and are more likely to be recruited. This likely effect on the profile of experts does not show up in the statements or views of the members or of the pharmaceutical industry, unlike the criticisms relating to the lower quality of experts.

Do the members have less scientific legitimacy than before?

This fairly recent tendency to disallow the selection of experts with very close industry links has been criticized by former members. Two of them, who are among the top nine beneficiaries and consequently those most affected by the new regulations, consider that the TC is depriving itself of "good" experts: *"Since conflicts of interest have become a factor in the choice of experts, those from outside who join the committee to assess and comment on applications are often not the best, because the best have been rejected"*. The other one says, *"People are recruited to the TC who do not like working with firms. Well, it's either that they don't like doing so, or that the companies don't want to take them on. They therefore have a particular profile, and are perhaps not as good as others"*. What is the value of these criticisms pointing to a poorer scientific caliber of experts?

To answer this question, we have sought to document changes in the scientific caliber of members since 2000 using a number of bibliometric indicators, in particular the number of papers and their *h*-index.[16] These indicators cannot be the sole reflection of an expert's scientific caliber and for this reason, they are often criticized in the scientific sphere. However, they are useful in that they can demonstrate a certain form of scientific legitimacy and make it possible to draw objective comparisons between experts. This scientific legitimacy varies significantly within the TC (Figure 4.6): a few members have published little or nothing (dispensing pharmacists and private practice GPs and specialists), whereas people who are at the same time practitioners, professors, and researchers within hospitals or at medical research institutes have often published and been cited extensively, and they, therefore, have a very high *h*-index.

An initial synchronous analysis examining the average *h*-index of TC members in 2019 revealed a fairly even degree of scientific legitimacy among members regrouped and examined according to the period they were recruited, aside from those recruited in 2003–2005, for whom the average *h*-index is a bit higher (Figure 4.7). This synchronous comparison of groups recruited during distinct periods has been possible because they are of a similar age (Table 4.1, age in 2016) and therefore generally at a similar stage of their career. Moreover, as they are close in generational terms, they have evolved within a field of scientific publication whose logics are fundamentally similar.

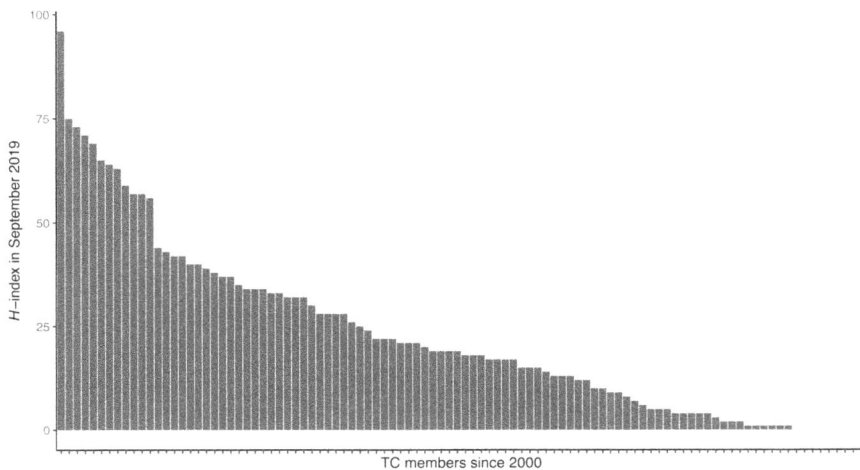

Figure 4.6 Graphic representation of the *h*-index of TC members since 2000, measured in 2019.

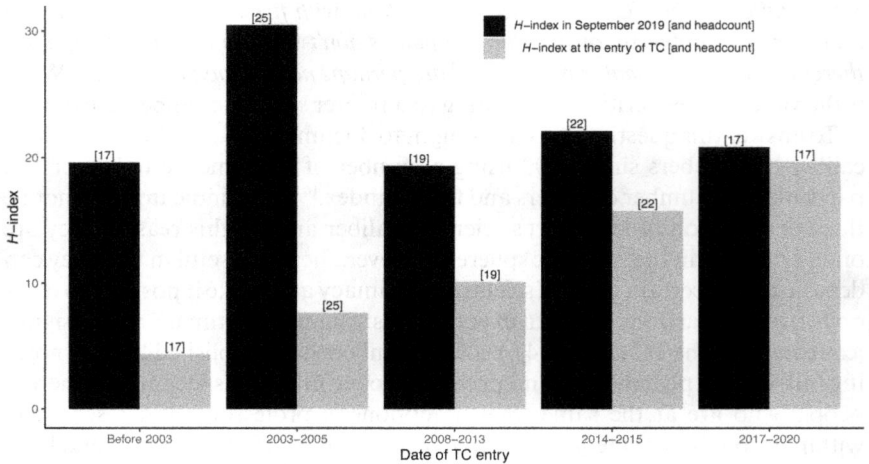

Figure 4.7 Average *h*-index in 2019 and average *h*-index on joining the TC, for members since 2000, according to the period during which they joined the TC.

The linear regression analysis confirms that, in 2019, there was no significant disparity between members entering the TC at different periods, either in terms of their *h*-index (Table 4.3, model 2) or the number of publications (model 11), even when controlling for gender, age, and whether or not they were retired (models 3 and 12). Therefore, at the same stage of their careers, members who had entered during different periods have the same degree of scientific legitimacy insofar as it can be measured using standard bibliometric indicators. Moreover, the more time members spend on the TC, the lower their *h*-index (models 6 and 7). This may be explained by the fact that being on the TC entails a great amount of work, which detracts from their capacity to publish papers. Alternatively, it may mean that members publishing more have greater difficulty reconciling expert work and scientific work, and they thus have to leave the TC sooner. Whatever the reason may be, members with less scientific legitimacy determined on the basis of their publication record are those who sit on the committee the longest.

If experts during different terms of membership are of equivalent worth at a given age, was this the case at the time they were on the TC? The very regular growth over time of the average *h*-index at time of entry suggests this is not the case (Figure 4.7). The regression analysis confirms this by revealing that there is a strong positive correlation between bibliometric indicators on entry into the TC and the most recent date of entry (Table 4.3, models 8 and 10). However, this correlation mostly disappears when controlling for age of entry into the TC (models 9 and 14): it is therefore primarily because they were younger when they entered the TC, and had had less time to publish that members who entered at an earlier date had a lower *h*-index or lower number of publications.[17]

Table 4.3 Multiple linear regressions on the h-index and number of publications by TC members since 2000, in 2019 and at the date they joined the TC

	H-index in 2019							H-index on entry into the TC			Number of publications until 2019		Number of publications on entry into the TC	
	Model 1	Model 2	Model 3	Model 4	Model 5	Model 6	Model 7	Model 8	Model 9	Model 10	Model 11	Model 12	Model 13	Model 14
Joined TC in 2000 or before.	−1.41 (7.30)	−3.85 (7.57)		−5.74 (7.57)	−5.74 (7.02)	6.24 (8.31)		−15.29 (4.43)***	−8.63 (4.73)+		−1.35 (33.47)	4.70 (34.78)	−43.71 (16.95)*	−20.73 (18.36)
Joined TC in 2003 or 2005	8.82 (6.69)	6.59 (7.09)		1.71 (7.02)	1.71 (7.57)	17.31 (8.02)*		−12.01 (4.06)**	−6.10 (4.44)		55.24 (30.68)+	52.96 (32.55)	−33.12 (15.53)*	−11.82 (17.26)
Joined TC in 2008–2013	−2.01 (7.11)	−3.21 (7.43)		−3.30 (7.15)	−3.30 (7.15)	5.32 (7.92)		−9.54 (4.32)*	−4.77 (4.39)		−8.50 (32.58)	−9.70 (34.14)	−29.78 (16.49)+	−12.71 (17.06)
Joined TC in 2014 or 2015	0.44 (6.88)	0.71 (7.16)		0.71 (6.89)	0.71 (6.89)	6.83 (7.34)		−3.92 (4.17)	−0.07 (4.39)		18.74 (31.51)	24.09 (32.91)	−0.97 (15.95)	14.25 (17.05)
Joined TC in 2018	Ref.	Ref.		Ref.	Ref.	Ref.		Ref.	Ref.		Ref.	Ref.	Ref.	Ref.
Woman	−6.36 (5.41)	−6.82 (5.55)		−3.90 (5.22)	−4.37 (5.41)	−6.06 (5.33)	−7.06 (5.39)	−1.00 (3.22)	0.12 (3.26)		−40.84 (25.50)		−8.87 (12.50)	
Age in 2019	0.56 (0.33)+	0.50 (0.35)		0.64 (0.32)*	0.65 (0.35)+	0.65 (0.33)+	0.45 (0.34)					1.23 (1.60)		
Younger than 66 in 2019	8.67 (7.04)	7.79 (7.43)		9.15 (6.75)	8.99 (7.21)	9.03 (6.93)	5.34 (7.27)					26.09 (34.14)		
Age when joined TC for the first time									0.31 (0.15)*	0.40 (0.16)*			0.89 (0.60)	
Younger than 66 when joined TC for the first time									−5.47 (5.14)	−7.29 (4.84)			−22.41 (19.96)	
Time spent into the TC (years)						−0.10 (0.05)+	−0.16 (0.06)*							
Total amount 2013–2019 (k euros, normalized)			0.08 (0.02)***	0.08 (0.02)***						0.02 (0.01)				

*** $p < 0.001$; ** $p < 0.01$; * $p < 0.05$; + $p < 0.1$.

Source and field: See Figure 4.6.

A paradox thus emerges. The assertion that experts who are very closely linked to the industry have greater scientific legitimacy can be verified in our sample of 100 individuals, considered synchronously. The *h*-index and the number of publications in 2019 are indeed positively correlated to the sum of the amounts received from the pharmaceutical industry between 2013 and 2019, including for equal gender, age, and period of recruitment (models 4 and 5). However, the experts selected more recently to participate in the TC have acquired greater scientific legitimacy upon their entry into the TC, while having structurally fewer links with companies than their predecessors. The explanation of this paradox may lie in changes to the recruitment strategy of the HAS. In recruiting older members (who had thus had more time to publish and acquire citations) from 2014, it compensated and even overcompensated for the potential deficit of scientific legitimacy caused by the major effort between 2005 and 2011 to counter-select members with too many industry links. Changes to the recruitment process for TC members have thus invalidated the connection between experts' scientific reach and the quantity of industry links.[18]

Conclusion

Our study on the TC members shows that the policy to prevent COIs launched in the 1990s really did have an impact. It did so within a few years, from the mid-2000s. This was when the declarations of experts working for the health agencies became public, and above all, when the health agency hosting the committee implemented rules for managing COIs. Since then, members of the committee have had structurally fewer industry links, or at least fewer evident, declared links. Despite this, they are no less scientifically reputable than those who came before them. On the contrary, on entering the committee, their scientific reach assessed using several bibliometric indicators appears broader. In recruiting experts who are less linked to the industry, those responsible for their selection have succeeded in putting an end to the correlation, as verified in our sample, between closer industry links and better scientific reputations. The inclusion of increasingly older members might be the reason for this disassociation. The recruiters would thus have killed two birds with one stone by integrating people who are both less connected to the industry, as they are more often retired, and have a better scientific reputation. This transformation of experts' profiles due to tighter control of potential COIs is probably not the only effect. Experts who have fewer industry links may differ from their predecessors for example when it comes to the relationship with medicines and the approach used for evaluating the clinical benefit of drugs, where clinical criteria and biostatistical indicators are confronted with one another.

Notes

1. The 2002 law on "patients' rights and the quality of the health system" and decree 2007-454 dated March 25, 2007 on agreements and links between companies and the members of certain medical professions, and modifying the French Public Health Code.
2. Law 2011–2012 dated December 29, 201,1 on strengthening the safety of medicines and health products.
3. Senate Social Affairs committee hearing, February 3, 2016.
4. Until 2000, a significant number of the members were "proposed" by the health insurance funds, the medical and pharmaceutical councils, and the union of pharmaceutical industries (*order dated July 24, 2000*, on nominations to the Transparency Committee, *Journal officiel*, July 28, 2000). This category of members was abolished in 2003. From 2015, a few members were also selected not for their scientific expertise but as representatives of patients' associations.
5. We would like to thank Adélaïde Bargeau for her help in gathering the socio-biographical data and Thomas Breda for his advice on regression models.
6. <https://www.has-sante.fr/jcms/c_1729421/en/transparency-committee>
7. The Transparence Santé data were collected via the Eurosfordocs.fr website in November 2019 (before data for the second semester of 2019 were available), by searching for members using their first and last names. To eliminate homonyms, the data were cleaned up using the individuals' ID numbers in the national health professionals listing (RPPS), their address, and their specialization.
8. We managed to find the exact age of the majority of the 100 members (not including representatives of patients' associations), from documents available online, such as the French universities' online library catalog SUDOC, which often indicates the date of birth of authors of a thesis or other publication. However, for a little under half of the members, dates of birth had to be estimated. We deduced these from dates of other career events (entrance into higher education, start of internships with the Paris hospitals, thesis viva, or opening of a private practice), on the basis of the usual length of time between birth and one of these events. The proportion of members whose date of birth was unknown was almost the same for all our different groups of new committee members.
9. This date was chosen because it was in the middle of the period being studied (2013–2019).
10. Of the 100 members we selected, 4 were removed from this analysis of interest links: 1 member because of his advanced age (77 in 2013, 4 years older than the next oldest member) and 3 members who died before 2013 or shortly afterward.
11. Amounts attributed directly to health professionals came to approximately €1.4 billion between 2013 and mid-2019. Doctors, who numbered approximately 220,000, received 94 percent of this sum (Cour des comptes, 2016, p. 66).
12. Since we had the data for all the members and therefore knowledge of the "universe" we were studying (rather than just a sample), we could have considered that the differences between the means and the regression coefficients could be interpreted as such, and that it was not necessary to use statistical tests to justify their significance. However, we chose here to use statistical tests, standard deviations, and significance thresholds. This is a more standard approach, especially in economics. It is considered that the process being studied consists of a selection, in this case, the members of a committee among a pool of potential candidates, and that this selection could be better studied if what can be considered our sample under this approach were larger. It is a way of taking into account the randomness in the selection process. This approach is often preferred, for example, in studies on wage discrimination where the authors have access to all the data concerning the companies they are studying.

13. The underlying assumption of our conclusions is that these effects remain comparable over the whole of the period studied.
14. We only have knowledge of the amounts declared by and paid directly to the TC members. Indirect benefits or payments that may have been channeled through a structure that acts as a screen are beyond our reach. These transparency provisions may lead to "pooled" financial transfers by professional associations or foundations (Cosgrove et al., 2016), leading to "institutional conflicts of interest" (Krimsky, 2019). Thus if an expert is employed by the industry or works on an ad hoc basis for a consultancy firm, he or she will not appear in the Transparence Santé database.
15. The retirement age varied slightly over the period under study, but was around 66 for doctors.
16. An author's h-index is represented by the number of papers (h) with a citation number $\geq h$.
17. There are uncontrolled structural effects, such as the possible increase in the number of papers over time (observed in economics for example), which might cause an increase in a member's h-index when it is examined on a more recent date. However, they are probably not significant enough over a 15-year period at most (between the entry dates 2003 and 2018) to invalidate conclusions, as the correlation observed is strong.
18. Using a diachronic analysis approach, there is no longer any link between the h-index and the number of papers published on entry into the TC and the amounts received by members (model 10).

References

Cosgrove, L, Vannoy, S, Mintzes, B and Shaughnessy, AF (2016) 'Under the influence: the interplay among industry, publishing, and drug regulation', *Accountability in Research*, 23(5), pp. 257–279.

Cour des comptes (2016) *La prévention des conflits d'intérêts en matière d'expertise sanitaire*. Communication à la commission des affaires sociales du Sénat.

Hauray, B (2018) 'Dispositifs de transparence et régulation des conflits d'intérêts dans le secteur du médicament', *Revue française d'Aaministration publique*, 165(1), pp. 49–61.

Hérail, E (2015) 'Les conflits d'intérêts en droit pharmaceutique', *Revue générale de droit médical*, 21, pp. 145–153.

Krimsky, S (2019) *Conflicts of interest in science: how corporate-funded academic research can threaten public health*. New York: Hot Books.

Le Pen, C (2018) 'Une (brève) histoire de la Commission de la transparence', *Revue française des affaires sociales*, 3, pp. 111–127.

Nouguez, E and Benoît, C (2017) 'Governing (through) prices: the State and pharmaceutical pricing in France', trans. Jacobs-Colas, A, *Revue Française de Sociologie*, 58(3), pp. 399–424.

Tabuteau, D (2010) 'L'expert et la décision en santé publique', *Les tribunes de la santé*, 27(2), pp. 33–48.

Part II

Physicians and the framing of prescription practices

Conflicts of interest in medical practice

Causes and cures

Marc André Rodwin

What are conflicts of interest?

"Conflict of interest" (COI), an idea that emerged in Anglo-American law of trust and fiduciaries, has Roman law antecedents (Frankel, 2010; Rodwin, 2011). In the 20th century, it became important in the law of finance (securities, banking, corporations), government employment, and the law regulating lawyers and other professionals (Rodwin, 1995, pp. 179–211). Since then this concept has also been used outside of fiduciary law when there are issues of ethics.

The idea underlying COIs is simple: it is implicit in the principle that individuals cannot judge their own case because that would mix two incompatible roles, that of the participant and the judge. Judges are supposed to be unbiased when deciding a case. However, they cannot be neutral when they decide a case that pits themselves – or member(s) of their family – against another party. Similarly, judges who have strong financial ties or a close friendship with one party in a court case are likely to be biased. Other government officials also exercise authority that affects the public and have obligations to make decisions fairly, and to fulfill their public mission impartially despite their personal interests. Yet administrators and public servants sometimes have personal interests that can bias their decisions. Likewise, physicians, pharmacists, and other professionals working in the public and the private sectors have obligations to serve the interests of designated parties or to perform certain public functions. Yet these professionals sometimes have a personal stake in matters that can cause them to favor their own interests over the interests of their patients, clients, or other parties they are supposed to serve.

Definitions

Fiduciaries are individuals entrusted to serve the interest of another party and who are held to the highest legal standards of conduct (Rodwin, 1995, pp. 179–211; Frankel, 2010). The law does not permit fiduciaries to promote

10.4324/9781003161035-5

their own interests, or the interests of third parties. It requires them to be loyal to the party they serve, to act diligently, and to account for their conduct. To advance these goals, the law regulates COIs. It often prohibits fiduciaries from entering into situations that create COIs, requires that they cease the activity that creates a COI, or that they disclose their financial interests so that COIs can be identified and eliminated or managed. Today, public policy also regulates the COIs of parties that are not fiduciaries.

According to standard legal usage, a COI arises whenever activities or relationships compromise the loyalty or independent judgment of an individual who is obligated to serve a party or perform certain roles. There are two broad types: (1) conflicts between an individual's obligations and their financial or other self-interest; and (2) conflicts resulting from an individual's divided loyalties, dual roles, or conflicting duties, sometimes referred to as conflicts of commitments (Peters, 2012, p. 3). For example, a physician who dispenses medication has a financial conflict: the incentive to increase income through prescribing clashes with the obligation to prescribe in the patient's best interest. A physician who enrolls one of his or her patients in a clinical trial has a divided loyalty conflict: the duty to act in the patient's interest diverges from the goal of research, which is to advance scientific knowledge (Angell, 2015, p. 18).

Most dictionaries distinguish between financial and dual loyalty conflicts (Webster's, 2001) but some do not (*American Heritage Dictionary of the English Language*, 1969).[1] These dictionaries reflect the way the term has been used in Anglo-American law, and in the policies of many international organizations (Rodwin, 1995, pp. 179–21; 2019). Consider, for example, the Organization for Economic Co-operation and Development (OECD), which focuses on COIs of public sector actors (Rodwin, 2018a).[2] It says that "'a conflict of interest' involves a conflict between the public duty and private interests of a public official, in which the public official has private-capacity interests, which could improperly influence the performance of their official duties and responsibilities" (Bertók, 2003, pp. 24–25; OECD, 2005, p. 13).

As noted, COIs constitute a problem because they compromise an individuals' *loyalty* to the mission or parties they are supposed to serve, as well as compromising their *independent judgment* (Rodwin, 1995, pp. 179–211. Consequently, COIs increase the risk that individuals will not perform their duties as they should, or even cause them to breach their obligations. The least serious form of breach could be professional neglect: the public employee might perform below the customary level of competence, diligence, or effectiveness. Even worse, public servants may knowingly exploit their position. Extreme disloyalty presents more dramatic danger but is easier to identify. Situations that compromise independence, loyalty, or judgment more subtly occur more frequently but are harder to recognize.

COIs do not constitute a breach of duty. COIs can influence action, but they are not acts, and do not constitute a breach of trust. Although law or ethics may require individuals to not enter into COI situations, this is only a measure to prevent acts considered wrong in themselves. Furthermore, COIs are distinct from conflicting interests. Multiple interests often pull people in different directions. But unless such conflicting interests compromise an individual's or party's *obligations*, no COI exists.

Some distinctions

Potential and apparent conflicts

The OECD uses the term "potential conflict of interest" for situations in which an official would have a COI if there were certain changes in their official work activities or activities outside of work, such that the individual would then have a conflict between these work duties and personal interests (Bertók, 2003, p. 58).

The OECD reserves the term "apparent conflict of interest" for situations where it appears to many observers that a public official's private interests could improperly influence their performance of professional duties, but where in fact there is no conflict because arrangements have been made for the official to stand aside from all decision-making related to the activities in which the official would have a conflict (Bertók, 2003, p. 58).

For example, a public servant with an ownership interest in a private firm has a potential COI because the public servant has a private interest in the success of the firm that might conflict with the official's exercise of her duties. However, if the public servant works in the transportation ministry and is an investor in a pharmaceutical firm or pharmacy, the public servant's work is unlikely to affect the private firm or vice versa. If the public servant is reassigned to work in a bureau that approves the marketing of medicines or that regulates pharmacies, then financial interest will likely create an actual COI. The test is whether the performance of public duties can influence decisions in favor of the business in which the public servant has financial ties.

Similarly, an individual who works in a pharmaceutical affairs bureau and whose sister manages a pharmaceutical firm has an apparent COI because it appears that the official's duties will conflict with his interest in helping his sister's firm. It remains an apparent rather than an actual COI if arrangements have been made so that the official will not participate in any decisions that affect the firm in which his sister is a manager.

COIs of professionals in the private sector

Professionals working in private practice can have COIs when they serve on government commissions or advisory boards or offer expert advice to public officials. Under these circumstances, these professionals perform public functions and are expected to act as if they were public employees. Yet these professionals might have financial interests affected by the outcome of their public decision and might perform their public functions in ways that promote their private interests.

Furthermore, professionals can have COI arising from their usual private practice work. Physicians and pharmacists have professional obligations to act in the best interests of their patients and to comply with professional norms. Nevertheless, these professionals earn their living by performing their professional work and their personal financial interests can create an incentive for them to write prescriptions, offer advice, or otherwise make decisions that promote their personal financial interests over the interests of their patients or customers.

Institutional COIs

An "institutional conflict of interest" exists when an organization performs two or more roles that can conflict (Bertók, 2003, p. 66; Field and Lo, 2009, Chapter 8). This typically occurs when the institution has financial interests that can cut against an institutional mission or activity. Some writers also hold that when an institution's senior official has financial interests that can affect institutional policies, this situation also creates an institutional COI (Association of American Universities, 2001; Field and Lo, 2009). However, the financial interests of senior officials in an organization can also be analyzed as reflecting their individual COIs.

In the United States, many universities and hospitals have joint ventures with for-profit firms to conduct research and commercialize products derived from their research (Barnes and Florencio, 2002; Krimsky, 2004). The university or hospital will share profits or royalties from products derived from the research (Krimsky, 2004). Meanwhile, these universities have a mission of promoting inquiry and public access to knowledge and obligations to oversee the integrity of their researchers and to monitor their financial COIs. In this situation, the university has a financial interest in the research outcome that can conflict with its educational and research mission (Emanuel and Steiner, 1995). For example, if an institution conducts research to evaluate a pharmaceutical product while earning income from the product's sale, those two activities conflict.

Intellectual and non-financial conflicts are not COIs

Some writers draw attention to so-called intellectual or non-financial conflicts and argue they should both be addressed identically. They argue that intellectual interests and points of view are COIs because they can create bias and propose to regulate them (Saver, 2012). Others, in contrast, would reduce or cease oversight of financial conflicts (Rosenbaum, 2015).

Richard Saver has penned one of the most articulate discussions of non-financial conflicts.[3] He defines "non-financial interests" as "any non-financial source of bias that can unduly influence primary research goals" (Saver, 2012, p. 468). However, the law does not currently treat these as COIs. And for good reason (Rodwin, 2018a).

Treating intellectual conflicts as COIs would unmoor the concept from its original meaning, making it merely another phrase to describe bias (Rodwin, 2018a). Although intellectual interests can cause bias, this does not mean that they constitute COIs and should be regulated as such.

Certainly, a predilection for a hypothesis and intellectual commitments can influence a person's work and interpretations. Yet these tendencies, revealed in publications and routine scientific debate, effectively counters intellectual bias. In contrast, a researcher's financial interests are often unknown. And studies show that financial conflicts influence results, especially industry-supported studies. Furthermore, having researchers with diverse intellectual perspectives enriches scientific inquiry. Although the desire for recognition can affect a researcher's conduct in undesirable ways, these interests cannot be eliminated. In contrast, financial conflicts are an unnecessary source of bias.

Expanding the COI concept to include all potential sources of bias would make it a less practical tool. There is no effective way to eliminate most intellectual conflicts. Furthermore, non-financial interests are widespread, so the scope of regulation would greatly increase. It is hard to conceive of professionals ever lacking an interest in their reputation, career advancement, promotion, job security, or receiving honor. Regulating these potential sources of bias using a COI framework will impose heavy burdens on professionals and institutions. On the other hand, financial COIs can generally be avoided or eliminated and are not an inherent or useful part of intellectual activity.

Strategies to cure or manage conflicts of interest

Three main strategies are used to cure or manage COIs (see Table 5.1 and Rodwin, 2011, p. 207) (I use both the phase *cure* and *resolve* a conflict of interest to refer to changes that eliminate the COI rather than mitigate its effects). For the purpose of illustration, we will assume the individual with a COI is a public servant or a health professional working in a public hospital. However, the basic framework applies to other individuals who have COIs and are employed in the private sector.

The first strategy is to *prevent the COI from occurring* or to *eliminate it if it arises*. This can be done by organizing the work of government authorities in ways that preclude key actors from entering into situations in which they would have a COI. Alternatively, when individuals have a COI, the individual or their employer can eliminate the conflict.

Table 5.1 COIs of public servants: Intervention points

PREVENTION -Before public servant act	REGULATION -During the period in which the public servant is acting	SANCTIONS/RESTITUTION -After the public servant has acted
Prohibit public servants from entering into situations with COIs **Disclose** COIs	**Supervise** conduct of public servants and limit their discretion	**Penalize** public servants for violations of trust **Compensate** those harmed if public servants abuse their trust

The second strategy is to *regulate the conduct of key actors who have COIs*. This requires identifying key actors with COIs, then supervising their conduct. Overseeing the conduct of a conflicted actor can sometimes mitigate COIs. Reducing the discretion of key actors can decrease the risk that they will act in ways that are biased or breach their trust. Furthermore, if public authorities monitor the conduct of conflicted actors and suspect they have acted inappropriately, the authorities can overrule their decisions.

The third strategy is to allow individuals to have COIs but to impose sanctions or provide restitution when public servants or publicly employed professionals breach their duties. This approach assumes that the risk of being sanctioned will deter misconduct and that sanctions and restitution provide adequate remedies when public employees breach their trust.

The advantage of policies that preclude COIs from occurring is that they avoid the risks that COIs create. However, rules that preclude COIs usually also restrict activities that are beneficial. For example, a rule that prohibits public employees from engaging in any outside remunerative activity might also preclude government employees from supplementing their income from activities that do not create COIs. A public employee in the pharmaceutical affairs department will not have COIs when she spends her weekends writing magazine articles on films and popular culture.

A more nuanced approach would eliminate COIs only after they arise. This approach restricts activities only when they are necessary to resolve the conflict. For example, an employee who reviews applications to market new medicines has a potential COI if she has a relative who works for Wonderpharma. When Wonderpharma submits an application to market a new medicine and the application is one the employee would normally review, the employee's potential COI becomes an actual COI. The disadvantage of waiting until a conflict actually arises is that such a strategy relies on the ability to identify the conflict and take appropriate action. However, such a COI might not be identified if administrators cannot monitor and analyze the financial interests of employees.

The advantage of employing policies that oversee conflicted actors is that these policies would not preclude potentially beneficial activities that might give rise to COIs. However, overseeing the activities of conflicted actors usually requires the use of significant resources, and it is difficult to properly execute.

Policies that rely on sanctions and restitution avoid the preclusion of wide categories of activities as a preventive measure. They also avoid expending resources to monitor the conduct of conflicted actors. Despite these benefits it is often difficult for administrators to identify breaches of trust, and sanctions often fail to provide an adequate remedy. Moreover, while sanctions can provide a remedy for breach of trust, they cannot provide remedies when the COI results in biased government decisions.

The need to assess the significance of a COI

COIs are widespread. Some are minor and can be ignored without much risk of harm. But there is no simple way to determine to what degree a COI compromises an individual's loyalty or independent judgment. In each case, we must review the facts and context to reach a conclusion. When a declaration of interests reveals a potential or actual COI, then officials are responsible for assessing its significance and deciding what action to take (Rodwin 2018a, b; Rodwin, 2019a).

Some COIs are more serious than others. We can reasonably expect that the risk posed by compromising financial ties increases as the amount of money increases. As a practical matter, public policy often accepts the presence of certain small financial COIs in order to focus on more significant ones. However, research shows that even small gifts often create gratitude and generate reciprocity (Regan, 1971; Dana and Loewenstein, 2003; Friedman and Rahman, 2011). Hence there are also grounds to restrict the existence of small ties.

We should ask several questions. How strong or direct are the conflicts? What is the probability of inappropriate behavior? What kinds of risks are posed? How serious might the consequences be? What effect would measures to eliminate or manage the conflict have on other goals? (See Box 5.1).

Some employees might play such an important role in decision-making that it is prudent to manage even their *potential* COIs in order to avoid potential problems (Bertók, 2003, p. 58). However, not all COIs are of the same importance. In some cases, the responsible official might conclude that the COI is so small that no action needs to be taken aside from its disclosure to promote transparency.

When a significant COI arises, however, public officials need to take action to either resolve or manage the conflict. It is often tempting for responsible officials to assume that rules on COIs should be waived because the government employee or private sector expert is essential and there is

---

Box 5.1 Analyzing COIs: a checklist

I **Is there a COI?**

    1 Who is the actor and what is his/her designated role?
    2 To whom does the actor owe a legal or ethical duty?
    3 What is the nature of that duty or obligation?
    4 Does the actor have a financial tie, a secondary activity, or a secondary role that creates a risk that the actor will not fulfill his/her duty?
    5 When the actor exercises professional discretion, can the actor promote his/her own financial interest or the financial interest of a third party?

II **How significant is the COI?**

    1 Is the financial incentive for the actor so strong that it may cause him/her to behave in ways that promote his/her own self-interest or that of a third party?
    2 How much discretion does the actor have in making professional decisions?
    3 What are the potential risks/harms that can result if the actor is biased in exercising his/her discretion or if the actor violates his/her duties?

III **What policy options exist to eliminate, mitigate, or help manage the COI?**

Consider at least these kinds of options:

1 Changes in the organization and financing of medical care
2 Separation of professional roles or activities
3 Restrictions on having certain financial ties or relationships
4 Oversight of professional activity to reduce discretion or monitor performance
5 Disclosure of financial ties to allow patients and other parties to protect themselves or to facilitate monitoring and management of professionals with a COI
6 Remedies after a breach of duties (such as restitution to individuals harmed and penalties for individuals who violate their duties)

---

no way to resolve or manage the COI. In most cases, this is not true. There should be few, if any, waivers of rules and when they occur, the basis for the decision should be justified in writing and made public.

Identifying COIs

Designated officials, trained to recognize COI (such as an attorney working in the government's office of legal affairs, or an official designated to oversee the ethics of government personnel) need to analyze declarations of interest filed by employees in order to identify potential and actual COIs. They should distinguish between financial interests that are related to the employee's work and those that are not. Some governments, however, prohibit all outside employment or remunerative activity as a precautionary measure (Maskell, 2012).

Identifying COIs requires comparing the individual's work responsibilities to their personal interests and outside activities. The first step is to identify the employee's work duties. Employees can have COIs when they are involved in government decisions such as setting general policies, granting authorization to market pharmaceutical products, approving the conduct of pharmaceutical firms through inspection of manufacturing, or participating in the awarding of contracts and licenses or permits. Employees can also have COIs when they have access to confidential information.

It is important to examine the scope of an employee's duties. Certain high and middle-level employees can affect government policy on a wide range of matters or exercise power or influence over other employees. When these employees have conflicting outside interests, it can affect a broad scope of government activity. In contrast, other employees often have a narrowly defined scope of authority or power and have fewer opportunities for COIs.

After identifying the kinds of decisions that the employee can influence, responsible officials should examine the employee's declarations of interest to ascertain whether he or she has personal financial interests that might give rise to a COI (see Box 5.2). Responsible officials should look at the individual's: (1) personal financial interests and investment and ownership interests, including royalties, patients, and other sources of income; (2) financial interests and activities of family members which should be imputed to the employee; (3) gifts and other benefits received from private interests; (4) supplemental employment outside of public service; (5) private sector appointments and unpaid work performed for private entities; and (6) employment after leaving government service. Reviewers need to ask whether the employee participates in work that could affect those private enterprises and whether the employee's interest in the private enterprise can affect their public employment activities. Declarations of interest can also reveal that employees have received gifts or grants from businesses related to their work or from individuals employed in those businesses (OECD, 2005, p. 44–48). Some governments prohibit public employees from accepting any gifts (Raile, 2004). When public policy does not prohibit all gifts, it typically requires their disclosure so responsible officials can respond appropriately (OECD, 2008).

Most countries prohibit public employees from accepting gifts of any value from individuals or firms engaged in activities related to the employees' work (Raile, 2004; OECD, 2008; Rodwin, 2011, pp. 11–16). However, some countries allow certain kinds of gifts or grants to support publicly employed physicians, researchers, or other employees. For example, France

---

Box 5.2 Sources of COIs of public employees

1   **Personal financial interests and investment and ownership interests**
    The employee's investment and ownership interest or other financial interests that conflict with work duties can be a source of COI. There is a risk that an official who invests in or owns an entity that can be affected by his/her work will use his/her work position to favor his/her investment interest
2   **Financial interests and activities of family members**
    The employee's family members' financial interests and affiliations can be a source of COI. These family members include the employee's spouse, fiancé(e), or the individual with whom he or she cohabits, along with his or her parents and any siblings or children.
3   **Gifts and other benefits received from private interests**
    Public officials who receive gifts, grants, favors, or other benefits from private entities might act to help those private entities
4   **Supplemental employment outside of public service**
    Sometimes the law allows public employees to engage in part-time employment or other remunerative activities in the private sector. Some of these private remunerative activities can interfere in the official's performance of his/her public duties
5   **Private sector appointments and unpaid work performed for private entities**
    Public officials might serve on a board or advise a private entity without compensation on matters that concern their work activity. There is a risk that the officials will use their access to government information to favor one entity over another or that in performing their public duties they will favor the entity with which they have an affiliation
6   **Employment after leaving government service**
    This can create a COI in two ways. First, while working in the public sector, the official might try to secure a job in the private sector by granting special favors to a regulated firm. Second, after leaving public service, the public official might use confidential information obtained while publicly employed to benefit the private firm

---

allows pharmaceutical firms to pay for transportation and lodging for physicians to attend professional meetings and continuing medical education events so long as the physician and pharmaceutical firm disclose the financing and follow certain rules (Rodwin, 2011). Some countries allow public employees to accept business hospitality, such as a meal, if the value falls below a certain threshold.

Some governments prohibit public employees from engaging in any remunerated outside employment (Maskell, 2012). When public employees are permitted to engage in limited outside employment, certain work can create

COIs. For example, working part-time for a pharmaceutical firm will typically create a COI for employees in government ministries that oversee pharmaceutical policy. In contrast, working part-time for a company outside the pharmaceutical sector would not.

Declarations of interest might also reveal certain unremunerated activities that create COIs. For example, a government employee who serves on the board of a firm or not-for-profit organization can develop relationships with those private sector entities that could lead the employee to favor that organization. This typically creates a COI if the ministry in which the employee works regulates the private sector organization with which the government employee is affiliated.

Responsible governmental authorities should also review the post-employment activities of certain government employees to determine if they comply with COI rules that governed their public employment. Governments often restrict employees for a designated number of years from representing any private sector actor in matters before the agency in which they used to work.

Institutional conflicts of interest

The following five steps need to be taken in order to identify an institutional COI: (1) specify the organization's mission and its activities; (2) list the organization's financial interests and its source of funds (including all revenue, grants, royalties, and ownership interests); (3) list the organization's affiliations with other organizations; (4) review the institution's mission, activities, financial interests, and affiliations to see if there are *potential* conflicts among them; and (5) finally, ask whether combining these activities could compromise the performance of any one of them. Also, ask whether the institution's financial interests could bias the performance of its activities or pursuit of its mission.

Resolving individual COIs of public employees

Two main strategies can be employed to resolve a COI: (1) change the compromised employee's relationship to the private interest; or (2) change the compromised employee's work activities.

1 Change the compromised employee's relationship to the private interest
   - *Divest the private ownership interest*: The employee can sell their ownership or investment interest in the private entity. Severing the financial ties eliminates the COI
   - *Terminate the relationship with the private entity*: The employee can resign from the board or cease other relationships with the private entity in order to end the conflict

- *Place the employee's investment interests in a blind trust*: The employee can place his stock or other investment in a blind trust managed by an independent party that has no contact with him. This will prevent the employee from controlling his or her investments while in a position to make decisions that can affect those investments. The trustee has the authority to manage the investment portfolio through sales and purchases. This option is typically used for high-level public officials who own stock in publicly traded firms

2   Change the compromised employee's work activities

- *Resign*: The employee can end her public employment and thereby end the conflict
- *Recusal*: The employee can withdraw from participating in any governmental decisions that can affect his private financial interest
- *Reassign work duties*: The employee's duties can be changed so that she does not work on activities that can affect her private interests. The employee can be reassigned to work in a different division or her work duties can be modified in other ways
- *Restrict access to information*: The government can limit the employee's access to information that might be used to advance his private interests

Typically, when government officials work on general policy and regulatory matters it makes sense to preclude their COIs. This is because it is difficult to separate particular work activities and decisions that can affect the official's private interests from work activities that do not. It is usually not administratively feasible to cope with the conflict by restricting only discrete employment activities. Resolving the conflict requires severing the employee's financial tie to the private enterprise or changing the employee's work responsibilities. In contrast, when public employees do not work on general policy matters but work on making discrete decisions that only concern particular firms, it is often possible to distinguish *potential* from *actual* COIs. This makes it feasible to change the employee's work responsibilities in order to preclude a potential COI from becoming an actual COI.

Sometimes government policies restrict public employees who work in a regulatory capacity from having any financial ties with a regulated industry, so as to preclude even potential COIs. Alternatively, governments could minimize restrictions and permit financial ties that create potential COIs if it is possible to separate the employee's activities that can affect the firms with which they have a financial tie from activities that will not affect the firm.

Resolve institutional conflicts of interest

Institutional COIs can be resolved in the following ways: (1) change the institution's responsibilities to eliminate conflicting roles; or (2) terminate the institution's financial ties that create a COI.

Manage conflicts of interest

When it is not feasible to resolve COIs, they can be managed to reduce the risk of bias or misconduct. The main way to do this is to supervise the conflicted employee to reduce the risk that the employee will abuse the public's trust. The employee's supervisor can check on her performance and modify his decisions if the employee acts inappropriately. It is worth noting that this kind of supervision is costly, burdensome, and difficult to do well. There is a significant risk that the planned oversight will be done ineffectively (Lexchin and O'Donovan, 2010). Furthermore, written plans for supervision can create the appearance that the COI is being effectively managed when in fact it is not. Supervision as a safeguard is used with varying degrees of success outside of public employment.

American universities oversee the COIs of clinical researchers who have financial interests in the research (Rodwin, 2019b). The preferred practice is to bar individuals who have financial interests in a particular medicine or method of therapy from conducting research that evaluates it. However, sometimes the university allows the individual to participate in such research, subject to certain restrictions. The conflicted researcher might be allowed to participate, but not to direct the research. Alternatively, the university might set up a committee to monitor the research and data produced (Field and Lo, 2009). If the COI can affect the enrollment of human research subjects then the university might require the presence of a patient representative to monitor the process of enrolling research subjects and obtaining their consent. The effectiveness of these practices remains unevaluated and there is significant reason to believe that they often are not effective (Rodwin, 2019b).

The limitations of disclosure as a means to address conflicts of interest

Declarations of financial interest provide information necessary to identify whether an individual has a COI. Consequently, the law and organizational rules often require such disclosure. Although disclosure of financial interests does not eliminate COIs, they are necessary in order for managers to take steps to cure the conflict, either by precluding the conflicted actor from participating in activities where they have a conflict or by requiring the conflicted actor to terminate their financial relations that create the COI. Alternatively, managers can take other steps to oversee the conduct of the conflicted employee. In addition, if administrators fail to take action to cure the conflict, individuals who depend on a professional can decide to terminate their relationship as a means to protect themselves.

In short, disclosure of financial interest plays a role in addressing COIs. Regrettably, many people incorrectly believe that disclosure cures

COIs. The limitations of disclosure as a management tool become apparent when we examine its role in patient–physician relationships (Rodwin, 1989).[4]

Some people argue that requiring physicians to disclose their financial interests will cause them to change their behavior. They presume that, when the public is informed, many physicians will not engage in compromising financial arrangements and those that do are unlikely to betray their patients' trust. They believe that disclosure is simple, inexpensive, preserves patients' and physicians' autonomy, and patient choice.

Disclosure is appealing because it prohibits nothing and requires no oversight or changes in the organization of medical practice. It appears to be cost-free. Like a talisman, it resolves problems by incantation. Policies that rely on disclosure assuage physicians' conscience, console the public, relieve policymakers from confronting difficult choices, and shift the burden to patients. But rather than resolve COIs, disclosure typically fails to address them effectively (Moore and Loewenstein, 2004; Cain, Loewenstein, and Moore, 2005; Moore et al., 2005).

It is far easier to write rules that mandate disclosure than to make it occur. Consider physician disclosure of COIs to their patients. Most patient–physician discussions are private, so how are public authorities to monitor physician compliance without adding the burdensome oversight whose absence supposedly makes disclosure preferable to other approaches? Should there be sanctions for all failures to disclose, or only when patients come to harm? What sanctions are appropriate?

One way to promote disclosure is to require physicians to have patients read and sign a form that reveals their COI. Hospital physicians already ask patients to sign forms to document that they have disclosed the risks and benefits of the proposed treatment and obtained their informed consent. However, these forms protect physicians from liability more effectively than they inform patients, who usually read them just before surgery, long after they have decided to undergo it. Patients and physicians typically view the rapid reading and signing of these forms as a formality, not an opportunity for discussion.

The use of COI disclosure forms will be even less helpful and more burdensome than informed consent forms. Surgery is an infrequent, dramatic event that alerts patients to risk; patients may have time to reflect between the time a physician first discusses surgery and when it occurs. In contrast, situations that raise COIs occur much more frequently. Patients are likely to pay less heed than they do for surgical consent.

What, when, and how to disclose?

Physicians could reveal their COIs at several points. Should they do so once, or routinely? Physicians could reduce their burden by having patients read and sign disclosure forms only at the beginning of the relationship. But that would diminish the information's value. Most patients cannot anticipate what services they will need and their relation to a physician's COI. Patients will not find COIs related to potential medical problems as important as when they concern current treatment. By the time physicians make medical decisions colored by COIs, patients may have forgotten the previous disclosures.

Physicians can present information in ways that do not help patients. Should we monitor what physicians say to ensure that they accurately and effectively disclose their financial interests? Studies of disclosure for informed consent reveal that patients often do not understand the information provided. New information seldom leads patients to reconsider proposed treatments. Detailed written forms sometimes obscure understanding (Grundner, 1980; Faden and Beauchamp, 1986; Appelbaum, Lidz, and Meisel, 1987).

If the aim is to give patients objective information and appraisal of their risk, a neutral party should disclose the COI. Empirical studies indicate that individuals often disclose information selectively in ways that promote their interests. Moreover, individuals' own perspectives affect how they report information. Studies show that individuals perceive their own motivations and behavior positively and believe that they are fairer than average (Messick et al., 1985). Physicians with COIs rarely believe that they compromise their patients' care and will disclose their COIs in ways that support this conclusion.

Physicians can reveal their financial arrangements in ways that do not alert patients to the risks. They can portray their COIs as innocuous, or imply that because they supply the services that they recommend, they have expertise and can ensure quality care. Discussing their COI in this way is akin to advertising. Rather than make patients proceed cautiously, it will encourage them to accept the arrangement. Indeed, if disclosure effectively alerted patients to the limits of physician loyalty and their biases, it might undermine trust and damage the relationship.

We know from psychological experiments that the framework in which people make choices affects their decisions and that the same information presented in contrasting contexts produces different decisions. It may be possible to regulate the written information that patients receive; but it will be much harder to regulate the context in which it is presented – the patient–physician relationship. Patients turn to physicians for advice and expect them to act on their behalf. The relationship requires trust, which means that most patients will follow their physician's advice. Moreover, people typically follow the requests of authority figures (Milgram, 1974). Studies also show that individuals prefer to agree with and say yes to people whom they know and like (Cialdini, 1993). Transference increases these tendencies (Katz, 1984).

Many people acknowledge that physicians might be affected by COIs, but few believe that their own doctors would be (Gibbons et al., 1998). Patients are likely to downplay COIs that physicians disclose. Experiments reveal that individuals discount the risk of bias when warned and that they have difficulty ignoring information provided even when they are aware it is not reliable (Wilson and Brekke, 1994, p. 117). When physicians inform patients that their advice may be biased, this message clashes with patients' understanding of the relationship since they trust their physician. This cognitive dissonance is usually resolved by discounting the COI.

Disclosure does not create satisfactory choices. How should a patient react upon learning that her physician has an incentive to prescribe a test because he supplies it? The patient can refuse to take the test, but that would interfere with her treatment and disrupt the relationship. Alternatively, the patient could obtain the test from another provider, but that might make both parties feel uncomfortable. A greater drawback is that obtaining the test from another provider does not resolve the problem. If the incentive leads a physician to recommend a test inappropriately, the patient still receives an unnecessary test if she obtains it elsewhere.

The patient could consult another physician regarding whether she needs the test. This costs time and money, delays treatment, and undermines patient–physician trust. Studies show that individuals are less likely to search for alternative products and services when time is important or they are ill-equipped to assess the differences (Hibbard, Slovic, and Jewett, 1997). When time is crucial, patients are unlikely to exercise this option. Moreover, physicians consulted for a second opinion are reluctant to contradict the initial recommendation unless they have a different medical opinion on the whole problem. The patient could end the relationship with her conflicted physician. That, too, is costly, especially when the patient has a chronic medical condition that requires continuing attention, or has had a long-standing relationship with her physician.

If physicians routinely supply ancillary services that they prescribe, patients will be unlikely to question the practice. People tend to perceive behavior as appropriate if they see others following the same pattern (Festinger, 1950, p. 271). When public policy allows physicians to recommend and supply services, merged roles become prevalent. Then patients who prefer physicians without financial COIs might not be able to find one.

The negative effects of disclosure

Disclosure may lull the public into believing that this response is sufficient, thereby encouraging medical practice with COIs. Physicians may conclude that they are relieved of further responsibility. This would shift the responsibility from physicians to patients. Is it fair to require individual patients to cope with this burden?

Disclosure sometimes protects physicians from liability and might reduce their obligation to act in their patients' interests. Physicians can argue that because they revealed their conflicts, patients should be barred from complaining about their effects. If courts accept this argument, disclosure will replace a fiduciary model of patient–physician relations with caveat emptor. Disclosure has sometimes had this effect. Cigarette manufacturers used disclosure of health risks to limit their liability to smokers (Cipollone v. Liggette Group, Inc., 1986). The US Supreme Court held that the Food, Drug, and Cosmetic Act's regulation of medical devices preempts state tort laws, thereby barring patient liability suits against manufacturers (Riegel v. Medtronic, Inc., 2008). Courts might similarly interpret rules that require the disclosure of COIs to preempt patients' suits against physicians.

Since disclosure does not end practices that create COIs or create effective means to oversee physicians, it is insufficient for protecting patients. Still, it offers some benefit when the activity that creates the COI is valuable, there are no good alternative means to supply it, and the risk from the COI is small.

Conclusion

COIs create risks that weaken good medical practice because they compromise the loyalty and independent judgment of medical professionals and other actors who oversee medical practice. The law has developed tools to help identify COIs that then allow steps to be taken to cure the conflicts, by eliminating them or to mitigate and manage them. These measures, however, usually entail some costs. It makes sense for policymakers to organize medical practice in ways that preclude COIs from arising when this is possible because this is typically less costly and more effective than trying to deal with COIs once they arise.

Notes

1. On this question, see for instance (Rodwin, 2018a; Rodwin 2018b, pp. 186–188).
2. The OECD uses the traditional legal definition. Some writers have attempted to redefine COIs, with confusing results.
3. Saver's list of conflicting non-financial interests includes an individual's interest in "career advancement", "tenure and promotion", "enhanced reputation, professional honors and prestige, access to power", as well as "intellectual or political predispositions", "intellectual passion", "investigative zeal", "a reluctance to antagonize powerful faculty investigators", and "social relationships formed in […] research […], ranging from collegial to competitive to hierarchical" (Saver, 2012, p. 468).
4. This section draws on Rodwin (1989); Rodwin (2011a, pp. 215–219); and Rodwin (1995, pp. 213–219).

References

American Heritage Dictionary of the English Language (1969) American Heritage Publishing: Houghton Mifflin.

Angell, M (2015) 'Medical research on humans: making it ethical', *New York Review of Books*, December 3 [online]. Available at: http://www.nybooks.com/articles/2015/12/03/medical-research-humans-making-it-ethical/ (Accessed: January 27, 2021).

Appelbaum, PS, Lidz, CW and Meisel, A (1987) *Informed consent: legal theory and clinical practice.* New York: Oxford University Press.

Association of American Universities (2001) *Report on individual and institutional financial conflict of interest* [online]. Available at: http://ccnmtl.columbia.edu/projects/rcr/rcr_conflicts/misc/Ref/AAU_CoI.pdf (Accessed: January 27, 2021).

Barnes, M and Florencio, PS (2002) 'Financial conflicts of interest in human subjects research: the problem of institutional conflicts', *The Journal of Law, Medicine & Ethics*, 30(3), pp. 390–402.

Bertók, J (2003) 'Managing conflict of interest in the public service: OECD guidelines and overview', *OECD* [online]. Available at: http://www.oecd.org/gov/ethics/48994419.pdf (Accessed: January 27, 2021).

Cain, DM, Loewenstein, G and Moore, DA (2005) 'The dirt on coming clean: perverse effects of disclosing conflicts of interest', *The Journal of Legal Studies*, 34(1), pp. 1–25.

Cialdini, RB (1993) *Influence: science and practice.* 3rd edn. New York: William Morrow and Company.

Cipollone v. Liggett Group, Inc., 789 F.2d 181 (3d Cir. 1986).

Dana, J and Loewenstein, G (2003) 'A social science perspective on gifts to physicians from industry', *JAMA*, 290(2), pp. 252–255.

Emanuel, EJ and Steiner, D (1995) 'Institutional conflict of interest', *New England Journal of Medicine*, 332(4), pp. 262–268.

Faden, RR and Beauchamp, TL (1986) *A history and theory of informed consent.* New York: Oxford University Press.

Festinger, L (1950) 'Informal social communication', *Psychological review*, 57(5), pp. 271–282.

Field, MJ and Lo, B (eds.) (2009) *Conflict of interest in medical research, education, and practice.* Washington: National Academies Press [online]. Available at: http://www.kumc.edu/Documents/coi/TOC.pdf (Accessed: January 27, 2021).

Frankel, TT (2010) *Fiduciary law.* New York: Oxford University Press.

Friedman, HH and Rahman, A (2011) 'Gifts-upon-entry and appreciatory comments: reciprocity effects in retailing', *International Journal of Marketing Studies*, 3(3), pp. 161–164.

Gibbons, RV, et al. (1998) 'A comparison of physicians' and patients' attitudes toward pharmaceutical industry gifts', *Journal of General Internal Medicine*, 13(3), pp. 151–154.

Grundner, TM (1980) 'On the readability of surgical consent forms', *New England Journal of Medicine*, 302(16), pp. 900–902.

Hibbard, JH, Slovic, P and Jewett, JJ (1997) 'Informing consumer decisions in health care: implications from decision-making research', *The Milbank Quarterly*, 75(3), pp. 395–414.

Katz, J (1984) *The silent world of doctor and patient.* Baltimore: Johns Hopkins University Press.

Krimsky, S (2004) *Science in the private interest: has the lure of profits corrupted bio-medical research?* Lanham: Rowman & Littlefield.

Lexchin, J and O'Donovan, O (2010) 'Prohibiting or "managing" conflict of interest? A review of policies and procedures in three European drug regulation agencies, *Social science & medicine*, 70(5), pp. 643–647.

Maskell, J (2012) Outside employment, 'moonlighting', by federal executive branch employees. Congressional Research Service.

Messick, DM, et al. (1985) 'Why we are fairer than others', *Journal of Experimental Social Psychology*, 21(5), pp. 480–500.

Milgram, S (1974) *Obedience to authority: an experimental view.* New York: Harper and Row.

Moore, DA and Loewenstein, G (2004) 'Self-interest, automaticity, and the psychology of conflict of interest', *Social Justice Research*, 17(2), pp. 189–202.

Moore, DA, et al. (2005) *Conflicts of interest: challenges and solutions in business, law, medicine, and public policy.* Cambridge: Cambridge University Press.

OECD (2005) 'Managing conflicts of interest in the public sector: a toolkit' [online]. Available at: https://www.oecd.org/gov/ethics/49107986.pdf (Accessed: January 29, 2021).

OECD (2008) *Managing conflict of interest: frameworks, tools, and instruments for preventing, detecting and managing conflict of interest.* Proceedings of the 5th regional seminar on making international anti-corruption standards operational [online]. Available at: https://www.oecd.org/site/adboecdanti-corruptioninitiative/40838870.pdf (Accessed: January 29, 2021).

Peters, A (2012) 'Conflict of interest as a cross-cutting problem of governance' in Peters, A and Handschin, L (eds.) *Conflict of interest in global, public and corporate governance.* Cambridge: Cambridge University Press.

Raile, E (2004) *Managing conflicts of interest in the Americas: a comparative review.* Washington: US Office of Government Ethics [online]. Available at: https://www2.oge.gov/web/oge.nsf/0/63AFE8A872F928F285257EA6006557B4/$FILE/36d75c57a708473ca786a10c264797783.pdf (Accessed: January 29, 2021).

Regan, DT (1971) 'Effects of a favor and liking on compliance', *Journal of Experimental Social Psychology*, 7(6), pp. 627–639.

Riegel v. Medtronic, Inc., 552 U.S. 312 (2008).

Rodwin, MA (1989) 'Physicians' conflicts of interest: the limitations of disclosure', *New England Journal of Medicine*, 321(20), pp. 1405–1408.

Rodwin, MA (1995) *Medicine, money, and morals: physicians' conflicts of interest.* New York: Oxford University Press.

Rodwin, MA (2011a). *Conflicts of interest and the future of medicine: the United States, France, and Japan.* New York: Oxford University Press.

Rodwin, MA (2018a) 'Attempts to redefine conflicts of interest', *Accountability in Research*, 25(2), pp. 67–78.

Rodwin, MA (2018b) 'Conflicts of interest in medicine: should we contract, conserve, or expand the traditional definition and scope of Regulation', *J. Health Care L. & Pol'y*, 21, p.158–88.

Rodwin, MA (2019a) 'Conflict of interest in the pharmaceutical sector: a guide for public management', *DePaul Journal of Health Care Law*, 21(1), pp. 1–32.

Rodwin, MA (2019b) 'Conflicts of interest in human subject research: the insufficiency of US and international standards', *American Journal of Law & Medicine*, 45(4), pp. 303–330.

Rosenbaum, L (2015) 'Beyond moral outrage—weighing the trade-offs of COI regulation', *New England Journal of Medicine*, 372(21), pp. 2064–2068.

Saver, RS (2012) 'Is it really all about the money? Reconsidering non-financial interests in medical research', *The Journal of Law, Medicine & Ethics*, 40(3), pp. 467–481.

Webster's Unabridged Dictionary (2001) New York: Random House.

Wilson, TD and Brekke, N (1994) 'Mental contamination and mental correction: unwanted influences on judgments and evaluations', *Psychological Bulletin*, 116(1), pp. 117–142.

Chapter 6

In whose best interest? Framing pharmacists' and physicians' (conflicts of) interest in the French market for generic drugs

Etienne Nouguez

Since the end of the 1980s, generic drugs have been a subject of worldwide attention. Presented by their promoters as a means of treating a large number of diseases at a lower cost and thus as a solution to the problems of financing treatment in both developed and developing countries, they have been criticized by their detractors as counterfeit products whose quality, safety, and efficacy are questionable (Greene, 2014; Nouguez, 2017; Quet, 2018). The introduction of these copies to the French drug market is quite recent. While they represented barely 3% of all drugs sold in pharmacies in 1999, they now account for one third, still far behind the United States' 84%, the United Kingdom's 83%, Germany's 80%, and the 48% average of the 19 main countries of the Organisation for Economic Co-operation and Development (OECD, 2019).[1]

Drug prescribing was one of the first topics addressed by scholars investigating conflicts of interest (COIs) within the medical field (Rodwin, 1995; 2011; Latham, 2001). Indeed, physicians occupy a specific position at the meeting point of many conflicting interests. In most cases, they choose the drugs that the patients will acquire and consume, and these choices are a source of benefits and risks for patients, income for manufacturers and distributors (wholesalers and pharmacists), and expenses for (public and private) insurance schemes and, to some extent, patients. In addition to the interests of these actors, drug prescribing holds a series of interests for the physicians themselves: first, a therapeutic interest, since drugs are the main recourse for treating a large number of the problematic situations they encounter (Freidson, 1988); second, a professional interest, since medications play an essential role in the dependence of patients and third parties on doctors and in the legitimation of professional expertise and efficacy (Starr, 1982); and third, a financial interest, since pharmaceutical companies and (public and private) insurance schemes are seeking to influence these prescriptions by developing financial incentive systems for doctors (Latham, 2001). However, research has rarely explored the potential COIs of other healthcare professionals such as pharmacists. This is probably due

10.4324/9781003161035-6

to the fact that pharmacists are perceived as an executing profession, whose actions are derived from medical prescriptions, and they are thought of as mere links in the drug distribution and sales chain. However, pharmacists have the originality of being both a health profession and a commercial profession and as such are subject to COIs (Aïach, 1994). In the medical context, identifying and qualifying COIs surrounding drug prescriptions are both obvious and problematic. It is obvious if one draws on the standard definition of COI as a situation in which a professional's judgment or action concerning his or her primary interest is likely to be unduly influenced by an interest qualified as secondary (Davis and Stark, 2001; Field and Lo, 2009; introduction of this book). A physician may (or may not) prescribe a drug because he or she considers that it is in the patient's best interest or because he or she has in mind other interests such as those of the pharmaceutical companies, the insurance schemes, or his or her own self-interest. But qualifying and identifying COIs is also problematic as this relies on what and who define primary and secondary interests and the conflicts between them (Davis and Stark, 2001; Rodwin, 2011). For example, the "restriction logic" identified by Rosman (2010) as dominant among Dutch general practitioners (GPs), who try to prescribe as little as possible, can be interpreted as serving first and foremost the interest of the Dutch health insurance schemes, but Rosman shows how it also responds to the desire of Dutch GPs not to expose patients to drugs seen as just as or more dangerous than the disease itself. Conversely, the "reparation logic" associated with the majority of French GPs, who prescribe a lot of drugs, can be seen as the result of the influence of pharmaceutical companies on physicians, but Rosman emphasizes that it also responds to an overestimation by doctors of the comparative risks of the disease in relation to the risks of the drugs and a desire to reinforce their status and to manage the fatigue of consultations (Rosman, 2010). This comparison shows both the multiple reasons for prescribing and the various trade-offs made by doctors between those reasons, which the notion of COI may seem unable to encompass.

Generic drugs offer a particularly heuristic case for questioning COIs, because they are theoretically supposed to align all interests surrounding drug prescription: they are legally defined as "substantially similar"[2] to the original drugs and are therefore supposed to have exactly the same benefit/risk profile for patients as their original counterpart; they are less expensive than the original drugs and therefore save money for patients and (public and private) insurers; and they do not hinder innovation, since they do not reach the market until the patent on the original drug expires, many years after it is marketed, and thus allow insurers to finance innovative drugs that reach the market. The prescription or dispensation of these copies should therefore be self-evident for physicians and pharmacists and it is their refusal that could be interpreted as the result of a COI. However, the development of generic drugs has given rise to a paradoxical framing of COI in the media and in political and professional fields. Although pharmacists have increased their substitution rate (which measures the share of generic drugs in the sales of drugs that can be copied) from 18% in 1999, the first year when the right to substitute was introduced, to more than 80% today, they have been questioned on numerous occasions because of the higher margin they make when selling these copies. On the other hand, although GPs and moreover specialists have not become very invested in prescribing generics or have even opposed them, they have been questioned very little for possible COIs. How can this paradoxical framing of COIs around the (non-)prescription of generics be explained?

To answer this question, I will focus on how the prescription choices of physicians and the substitution choices of pharmacists are "framed" (or not) as COIs in the relationships they establish with pharmaceutical companies, France's (public) national health insurance scheme (hereafter NHI), patients, and other healthcare professionals. I take up the notion of "framing" from the research on social movements (Benford and Snow, 2000; Gusfield, 1996) that defines these framings both as rhetorical motives for argumentation and justification and as the cause and consequence of relations of alliance and opposition between actors. I will first analyze the framing of the prescription and substitution of generic drugs from the perspective of the financial interests of healthcare professionals, pharmaceutical companies, and the NHI (1). I will turn then to the controversies surrounding the qualification of the health benefits and risks related to the prescription and substitution of generic drugs (2). Finally, I will highlight the central role of inter- and intra-professional relationships in the framing of professional interests and the prescription or substitution of generic drugs (3).[3]

Generic drugs and financial (conflicts of) interest

In many books and articles devoted to COIs in medicine, the focus is on the financial ties between physicians and pharmaceutical companies or insurance companies. The development of generics in France offers a heuristic case to discuss this notion. The NHI and the generic companies have developed many financial incentives to push pharmacists to increase their substitution of original drugs for generics, and to a lesser extent, to push physicians to prescribe these generics. But should the growth of generic sales be considered as the result of a financial COI?

Strong financial interest in substituting generics for original drugs

The right to substitute introduced on December 23, 1998, by the Social Security Financing Act (LFSS) for 1999, is today described by all observers as the key to the development of generics in France. By giving pharmacists the power to substitute the original drug prescribed by doctors with a copy, Parliament has not only reconfigured relations between healthcare professionals, but also the alliances between both professions, pharmaceutical companies, and the NHI. Unprecedentedly, a health policy was initiated without or even against physicians.

The public authorities have set up a preferential margin system to encourage pharmacists to increase substitution. The amount of margin guaranteed to pharmacists by the state is the same for the generic drug and the original drug, i.e., a percentage of the original drug Manufacturer's Price Outside Taxation (MPOT). But beyond these legal provisions, the right to substitute has given pharmacists a big market power. As generic drug companies offer a similar range of perfectly substitutable products, their prices are all that they have to seduce pharmacists. Since the beginning of the 2000s, they have engaged in a "discount war", outbidding each other with so-called "business cooperation services" officially paying for the services provided by the pharmacist to the company – such as the distribution of leaflets to patients, the installation of displays and posters advertising generics, or the provision of statistical information on sales – but really intended to "buy" market share in the pharmacy. These discounts were valued in 2006 by the High Council for the Future of the National Health Insurance (HCAAM) at around 25% of the MPOT. In the 2000s, by combining all margins, pharmacists were able to recover a margin on the sale of generics that was thrice that obtained from the sale of the original drugs. In 2004, they achieved a total remuneration of €1.2 billion, representing more than two-thirds of the €1.7 billion in sales generated by generics listed in the Official Repository of Generic Drugs (which regroup the original drugs and their generics) and "only" €415 million, one-fifth of the €1.9 billion sales of original drugs listed in the Official Repository.

This margin system has been the subject of two types of criticism. As early as 2001, the General Directorate for Competition Policy, Consumer Affairs and Fraud Control (DGCCRF) reported practices deemed illegal by generic companies: not only did they pay discounts above the legal cap set at 10.75% of MPOT, but some of them also paid pharmacists the remuneration intended for wholesaler–distributors. The DGCCRF considered that the payment of the wholesaler's margin to the pharmacist in the context of the purchase of generics online constituted an "overfee" that had to be "returned to Social Security by reducing the public price by the difference in the margin". The DGCCRF thus carried out inspections in pharmacies in 2000 and 2001, resulting in criminal charges being brought against pharmacies for exceeding the authorized legal discounts, which could lead to a maximum fine of 10,000 francs (€1,500) for each infraction committed. Considering that it was the main driver of generics growth, the government turned a blind eye to these practices until 2006 when it gradually lowered the price of generic drugs (from 80% of the original drug MPOT in 2000 to 40% since 2012) and original drugs (–15% upon the arrival of the first generic drug and –25% after 2 years in 2006; –20% upon the arrival of the first generic, and –38% after 18 months since 2012), which reduced the pharmacists' margin and transferred a significant part of the savings on generics from pharmacists and pharmaceutical companies to the NHI. While reimbursed expenses for generic drugs increased by only 50% between 2004 and 2011 (from €1.7 to €2.6 billion), the savings achieved by the NHI more than tripled (from €380 million to €1.4 billion).

A second (paradoxical) criticism came from the generic companies themselves. For example, Sandoz, a subsidiary of Novartis, experienced the bitter consequences of this race for discounts. Number two worldwide, in 2005 Sandoz occupied third place in the French market for generic drugs with a 14.7% market share, an increase of nearly three points in one year. Nevertheless, its parent company decided to dismiss the director of Sandoz France in November 2006 after the company's auditors found "errors in the evaluation of drug inventories, retrocessions deemed exaggerated to pharmacists under contract with Sandoz and a few other irregularities" (Mamou, 2006, p. 18). The company also said it would have to record an additional charge of $58 million (€45 million) to offset these discrepancies and make up the deficit of its subsidiary – which had sales of less than €300 million. Following this incident, Novartis decided to bring the accounts of its French generics subsidiary back into balance, by strongly moderating the level of rebates granted to pharmacists. The "market sanction" was irrevocable since, between 2005 and 2010, the company dropped from third to the fifth position in the French market with market shares dropping from 14.7% to 5.5%, leading to this disillusioned comment by Sandoz CEO Jeff George:

> We regret that in France there are discount practices for pharmacists that go well beyond what is allowed by law. This is a specific feature of this market that we refuse to comply with. I would rather lose ground by respecting ethics than gain ground by forgetting it. But it's a fact: companies that observe an ethical and legal code are at a disadvantage in France.
>
> (Tonnelier, 2010, p. 18)

Despite these statements, Sandoz seems to have complied once again with this iron law of the French market, given the rise of its market share from 5.5% in 2010 to 9% in 2012.

These criticisms relate to the strong position of pharmacists on the generics market, which has enabled them to recoup a significant part of this market financial product to the detriment of the NHI and the generics industry. But at the same time, these two players have recognized the key role of pharmacists in the development of the market. And although the margins achieved by pharmacists on generics were very high until 2006, they fell sharply afterward with the drop in generic prices. Pharmacists, for their part, presented this higher margin as fair compensation for the delicate work of promoting the financial interests of NHI to patients while ensuring the safety of substitution. Thus, pharmacists attempted to show that substitution was not a source of conflict but of alignment of interests. Although they received an additional margin while delivering a generic drug, they were saving NHI money. And as long as the generics were similar to the original drugs, there was no conflict between the interests of the patient and the interests of the insured, who are one and the same person. Doctors defended a different perception of this tradeoff.

Low but rising financial interest in prescribing generic drugs

Unlike pharmacists, physicians have only become moderately invested in prescribing generic drugs, when they have not opposed it outright. First, they directly prescribed generics very little. Although the GPs committed themselves to prescribing 100% in common denomination (the generic name given by the World Health Organization to the active ingredients of the drug) in 2002, the rate of common denomination prescriptions only slightly increased to reach 14% of GP prescriptions and 5% of specialists' prescriptions in 2010. Second, the 1998 Act on the Right to Substitute enabled doctors to oppose the substitution of a generic drug by handwriting "non-substitutable" next to each drug concerned and justifying this mention by "particular reasons relating to the patient". In 2011, a survey carried out by the NHI on a sample of 12,000 prescriptions estimated the rate of "non-substitutable" mentions at 4.2% of prescription lines. Moreover, 2.6% of the prescriptions analyzed included this mention on all lines, "thus suggesting a systematic practice of mention by the physician". The use of the "non-substitutable" mention thus seemed relatively marginal among physicians in 2011 according to this survey, even if these figures were contested by pharmacists' unions. Third, physicians retained the freedom to prescribe original patented drugs that are not listed in the Official Repository of Generic Groups. Under the influence of original drug companies, many French GPs and specialists transferred their prescriptions to still-patented drugs that were therapeutically equivalent. For example, the share of prescriptions within the Official Repository declined from 52% in 2007 to 39% in 2011 for statins and from 71% to 61% for proton pump inhibitors (PPIs) in France, although the number of drugs listed in the Official Repository had increased during the period (Caisse nationale d'assurance maladie des travailleurs salariés, 2012, pp. 61–62).

This lack of interest or even frank opposition of private physicians to generics is largely explained by their relationship with the NHI and more generally with health economics. Not prescribing generic drugs meant for many physicians questioning the equivalence between generic and original drugs (see below), promoting research and innovation, and above all refusing the intrusion of the NHI into prescribing habits in the name of financial considerations.

While some doctors were very reluctant to accept the right to substitute, presented as an intrusion into the medical monopoly on prescription, others saw it as a virtuous division of labor, allowing them to rid themselves of these economic considerations promoted by the NHI:

> It was more complicated for us when we had the responsibility [to increase the amount of generics we prescribe], because we had the impression, when we had no economic interest in it, that we were the agents of economic regulation. The pharmacist, it's clear: he makes margins, he earns his living, he's going to propose this drug because the relationship of interest is more obvious. [...] What is our interest? It isn't scientific. It isn't in the interest of the patient.
>
> (GP, Paris, 18th arrondissement, 2007)

From the mid-1990s to the present, the government and the NHI have sought to encourage prescribers to incorporate drug prices into their prescribing choices by linking their revenues to targets for drug expenditures. The order of April 24, 1996, passed by the Juppé government introduced a mechanism for "reimbursements [from] doctors according to the way in which targets (fees and/or prescriptions) are exceeded" (Hassenteufel, 2003, p. 129). However, these measures were strongly opposed by the private doctors' unions, who saw them as an attack on freedom and medical autonomy and who successfully used all media, legal, and political means to obtain the cancellation of these measures (Hassenteufel, 2003). After 2002, the government abandoned the principle of financial sanctions for physicians who did not meet the NHI's objectives, switching to a system of financial bonuses for those who met these objectives. The agreement signed in 2002 by the NHI and the physicians' unions made the prescription of generic drugs under a common name a counterpart to the increase in the price of a GP's consultation from €18.50 to €20. Starting in 2009, a performance-based payment system was also introduced, first with the Individual Practice Improvement Contracts (CAPI) from 2009 to 2011, and the Remuneration on Public Health Objectives (ROSP) since 2011. Each of these individual contracts signed between a private physician and the NHI included a prescription target in the Official Repository for the most expensive therapeutic classes. In addition, the NHI created in 2014 a body of NHI delegates (DAM) who visit doctors to give them their personalized prescription profiles, remind them of the commitments made by the unions with the NHI and the recommendations of good practices defined by the French National Authority for Health (HAS), and offer advice on how to change their prescriptions (Greffion, 2007). In this way, the NHI sought to personalize the relationship with doctors and to counter the influence of pharmaceutical companies' delegates on prescribing. Although these policies have not led physicians to actively prescribe generic drugs, they have largely succeeded in neutralizing their opposition to generics.

Physicians have not received the same attention from generics companies. These generics companies had very little incentive to promote their drugs to doctors, since pharmacists were free to replace the generic brand prescribed by the doctor with another brand of their choice. Leading generics companies occasionally promoted their brand to physicians but devoted the bulk of their resources to commercial rebates to pharmacists. Conversely, companies marketing original drugs have intensified their promotion to physicians, either to maintain their market share in the face of the arrival of generics, or to regain market share of unpatented drugs by encouraging physicians to transfer their prescriptions to their still-patented drugs.

Whether we look at physicians or pharmacists, we seem to see not a COI but a progressive alignment of the financial interests of the various players around the promotion of generics, which would allow the NHI to make savings, while providing additional revenues to generics companies, pharmacists, and physicians. In this operation, the only interests harmed seem to be those of the companies marketing the original drugs, but this harm to their interests can be legitimized by the fact that they benefited from patent protection for many years before being genericized. However, this idyllic picture has been regularly disturbed by challenges over the equivalence between generic and original drugs. If generic drugs are not "good" copies, is there not a risk that health professionals will sacrifice the interest of patients for financial considerations?

Generic drugs and public health (conflicts of) interest

Numerous studies on COIs present them as harming patients' health. When a physician's relationship with an insurer or pharmaceutical company leads him or her to prescribe or not to prescribe an examination, medication, or intervention, this has consequences (positive or negative) for the patient's health (Latham, 2001; Rodwin, 2011). But can the choice of this or that brand of a drug be described as a problematic decision for the health and therefore the interest of patients?

Promoting equivalence or hierarchy between drugs?

Since their introduction at the end of the 1990s, generic drugs have been the subject of numerous suspicions and even denunciations as to their lesser quality, safety, or efficacy on the part of physicians or patients. In three surveys conducted in 2011, 2013, and 2016, the proportion of respondents who felt that generics were not "as safe" as the original drugs rose from 29% in 2011 to 40% in 2013, before dropping to 25% in 2016. Similarly, the percentage of those who felt that they were not "as effective" rose from 23% in 2011 to 31% in 2013, before dropping back to 23% in 2016. In the 2016 survey, the 500 GPs and 1,005 patients surveyed had moderate confidence in generic drugs (giving them average scores of 6.6 and 6.8 out of 10 respectively) while the 500 pharmacists surveyed had high confidence in them (8.7 out of 10 on average).

Many reasons have been put forward by physicians and patients to justify their mistrust of generics. The first reason is related to the relationship between the look of generics, which may differ to a greater or lesser extent from that of the original drugs, and their unobservable "essence", which is guaranteed to be similar by public health authorities. For some patients and doctors, this cheaper look is both a practical problem (generics can be more difficult to "cut" into pieces, to swallow, and so on) and a logical one: Isn't it a sign of lower intrinsic quality? The second reason is related to the lower price of generics and the reputation of the companies that market them (Podolny, 2005): If generics are much cheaper than the original drugs, is it because they are produced less rigorously? A third reason is that some patients experienced a lesser efficacy or new side effects that they or their doctor attribute to generic drugs.

Some original drug companies nurtured these doubts, using scientific marketing (Gaudillière and Thoms, 2015) to denigrate generics to doctors. For example, Sanofi-Aventis was condemned by the French Competition Authority to pay a €40.6 million fine and ordered to publish an insert in *Le Quotidien du médecin* and *Le Quotidien du pharmacien* for "having engaged in a practice of denigrating generic competitors of Plavix® on the French market for clopidogrel sold in ambulatory care" (Autorité de la concurrence, 2013, p. 120).[4] Despite the arrival of 11 generic competitors between September and October 2009, Sanofi-Aventis managed to maintain a significant market share 2 years later, both for its originator (38% market share in volume at the end of 2011) and for its own generic marketed by its subsidiary Winthrop (30% of the generic clopidogrel market and 21% of the total market in volume at the end of 2011). According to the French Competition Authority, this "atypical" trend compared to trends in other similar generic groups is explained by "the very large number of 'non-substitutable' mentions affixed by physicians to Plavix® prescriptions" (12.6% of the prescriptions examined by the NHI study) (Autorité de la concurrence, 2013, p. 90) and by pharmacists' preferential use of Sanofi's own generic rather than the generic brand that they usually sell. This strategy was based on a three-point argument distributed in August–September 2009 to the departments in charge of training the company's delegates. The first argument was based on the two patents[5] held by Plavix® to cast doubt on the perfect substitutability between Plavix® – or its own generic sold by its subsidiary Winthrop – and the generics marketed by other companies. Once the doubt was instilled on the bioequivalence between copies and originals, a second argument put forward the severity of the disease treated with clopidogrel and the risk of death of the patient. Finally, a third argument put forward the responsibility of the physician or pharmacist in the event of an accident or death that could result from the prescription and substitution of a drug not marketed by Sanofi-Aventis.

Indeed, physicians and pharmacists have gradually come to distinguish between "common" and easily substitutable drugs, such as antibiotics, which have little practical and symbolic attachment from patients and few complaints, and "sensitive" drugs that are more difficult to substitute, such as anxiolytics or antiepileptics, because they are subject to strong practical and symbolic attachment and give rise to various complaints from patients about their lesser efficacy or greater dangerousness (Nouguez, 2017). More generally, French physicians opposed the idea of a possible commensuration between the health and financial stakes, the latter only intervening at the margins, when the patient is entirely satisfied with his or her medication, whatever the basis for this satisfaction.

A similar reasoning applies to French doctors' preference for newer, patented me-too drugs that nevertheless have similar indications and risk–benefit balance to older, generic drugs. Above, I mentioned the case of proton pump inhibitors (PPIs), particularly Mopral® (omeprazole) and Inexium® (esomeprazole), both marketed by AstraZeneca. I asked physicians about their preferences for PPI prescriptions and two polar positions emerged in the interviews. On the one hand, some doctors presented Inexium® (a more recent drug) as a marketing stunt that would bring no benefit to patients but would only allow the pharmaceutical company to slow down the progression of generics. On the other hand, some doctors echoed the arguments of Astra-Zeneca's delegates, according to which the use of Inexium® would make it possible to treat patients more quickly and efficiently and would ultimately allow the NHI to save more money (by limiting the duration of the drug's intake or the number of medical consultations) than prescribing older genericized drug.

These two polar types of physicians differ in their relationship to the drugs they prescribe and to the influences of the drug company, through scientific marketing (Gaudillière and Thoms, 2015), and the NHI, through prescription guidelines. It is less a matter of interest than a matter of confidence in the information and recommendation conveyed by these two influencers. But these doctors also have to position themselves in relation to the patients. Should they treat all the patients in the same way or make some exceptions?

Promoting equivalence or hierarchy between patients?

Doctors and pharmacists also adapted the situation to the patients they were dealing with. Thus, two categories of "difficult to substitute" patients have been reported to me by professionals: "fragile" and "troublemaker" patients.

Fragile patients are those whose compliance with medication is considered by healthcare professionals to be at risk. These are patients suffering from cognitive impairment or who used to recognize their medications from superficial markers (brand name, color of the box, or shape of the tablet) and who would be exposed, in case of misunderstanding, to the risk of under or overdosing on their medications. Other "fragile" patients are those who have developed a particularly strong symbolic or practical attachment to their usual medication and who may stop taking it if they find the generic less convenient or effective. This is the case, for example, of patients taking an anxiolytic, antidepressant, antiepileptic, or opioid substitution therapy, medications that have a strong placebo effect and that may cause compliance problems. Aware of these possible difficulties, the pharmacists' unions "are committed [in 2012], within the framework of the national agreement with the NHI, to ensuring the stability of dispensing for people over 75 years of age, for a certain number of drugs used to treat chronic pathologies: type 2 diabetes, hypercholesterolemia, arterial hypertension, chronic heart failure …" (Ministère des solidarités et de la santé, 2016).

Doctors and pharmacists also had to deal with patients they describe as "troublemakers" who are willing to openly provoke a ruckus if one tries to give them generic drugs. Faced with this resistance, a large majority of doctors have tried to avoid conflicts by delegating to pharmacists the "dirty work" (Hughes, 1962) of convincing patients of the benefits of substitution, or by putting the words "non-substitutable" on the prescription at the patient's request. Pharmacists oscillated between confrontational and avoidance strategies depending on the size of the queue, the fatigue of the day, or the verbal aggressiveness of the patient.

This power struggle shifted in favor of generics during the 2000s and 2010s as a result of two joint movements. First, doctors and pharmacists committed themselves individually and through their unions to meet increasingly higher targets for prescribing and dispensing generics in exchange for financial bonuses. Then, the public authorities put in place financial measures aimed at making recalcitrant patients pay the price of their refusal of generics, either through a partial delisting of the price differential between original and generic drugs as of 2003 (only for the least substituted drugs), or the deferred reimbursement of prescriptions in case of refusal of substitution as of 2006 (Nouguez, 2017). However, the fact that many doctors and pharmacists gave in to pressure from patients has revealed another source of COIs around generics: professional competition and hierarchy.

Generic drugs and professional (conflicts of) interest

As various works in the sociology of medicine have shown, the position of physicians in a private practice or in a hospital has consequences on the interests they value. Freidson (1988) suggested that doctors working in individual practices or part-time in hospitals tend to favor the appreciation of patients over that of their colleagues, because it is in their interest to attach themselves to the patient in order to maintain their activity and because they operate far from the eyes of their colleagues. Conversely, hospital physicians tend to favor the appreciation of their colleagues, because their careers within the hospital depend much more on the judgment of peers and department heads than on the judgment of patients (Freidson, 1988, Chapter 6). The same issues are played out around the prescription and substitution of generic drugs, which are deeply influenced by inter- and intra-professional relationships.

Professional competition and interests in generics

Generic drugs have been an enabler and catalyst for inter- and intra-professional competition. The choice of drug was initially the subject of a major jurisdictional struggle (Abbott, 1988) between physicians and pharmacists, leading to the establishment of a relatively complex division of labor between subordination (from pharmacist to physician) and competition for prescription control. Thus, some physicians did not hesitate to use the term "non-substitutable" as a means of restoring their control over prescribing.

> The delegates who make the generics no longer come to see us, they have no interest, since it is the pharmacist who does the substitutions. [...] It's a matter of money between the delegates and the pharmacists, we have nothing more to say. [...] I no longer control the prescription: I'm going to prescribe a drug and it will be substituted and I won't even get a say on it, unless I put "do not substitute".
>
> (GP, Bas-Rhin, 2008)

But this competition has also pitted pharmacists and doctors against each other. Although generic substitution is highly remunerative for them, pharmacists have long practiced generic substitution sparingly for fear that patients would leave them for a more conciliatory pharmacy. Some pharmacists have even used non-replacement as an argument to attract patients who are refractory to generics and to compensate for the loss of profit on margins by increasing sales. To prevent this competition between pharmacists from hindering the development of substitution, the unions and the NHI entered into agreements leading to the monitoring of substitution rates in dispensing pharmacies and possible sanctions against pharmacists who do not ostensibly practice substitution or do not apply the measures decided at the national level, such as the measure conditioning the third-party payer (i.e., the advance payment of drug costs by the pharmacist) on the acceptance of generics. On July 30, 2012, local NHI and pharmacist unions agreed to sentence a pharmacy in Deux-Sèvres to "one month of exclusion from the NHI listing"[6] (between September 15 and October 15, 2012) for not having reached the target of 60% substitution that had been set for the end of 2011 – its substitution rate had risen from 29% at the beginning of 2011 to 50% in December 2011 against an average of 82% in the department and 80% in the other pharmacy in the village (Durand, 2012).

Although they mention it less often and in non-commercial terms, physicians have also been confronted with competition issues around the prescription of generics. Prescribing drugs is indeed a way for doctors, particularly specialists, to build up and maintain patient loyalty, and even to justify fee overruns. By comparing the substitution rates reported by the NHI with socioeconomic and health data on the population and data on the supply of care in the French departments, I showed that the diffusion of generics was all the more pronounced when the density of pharmacists and specialist physicians and the fee overruns were low and when income inequalities within the population were limited (Nouguez, 2017). To put it another way, generics are promoted by pharmacists and consumed by middle- and lower-class patients, whereas original drugs are promoted by specialist physicians and acquired by upper-class patients.

Professional hierarchy and interest in generics

This competition is embedded in a strong hierarchy of healthcare professionals. I have already emphasized how much substitution required the pharmacist to assert his or her brand over that of the physician, and thus to challenge the hierarchy established between the two professions (Hughes, 1951). However, the same dynamic concerned the different professional segments (Bucher and Strauss, 1961), with patients and professionals considering hospital doctors to have a higher status than ambulatory care doctors, and specialists to have a higher status than GPs.[7]

A very large proportion of the prescriptions made by GPs consist of prolonging medications already taken by the patient, by "copying" the previous prescription, whether it was issued by them or by a colleague. Like substitution, which involves the respective authorities of the physician and the pharmacist, this practice of renewing a prescription may involve the respective authorities of the prescribing physician and other physicians who have previously left their "mark" on the prescription (Coleman, Katz, and Menzel, 1966). Some GPs may then choose to erase themselves behind the mark of their colleagues, and thus avoid a conflict, while others will oppose it, even if it means being on the receiving end of the anger of their patients or colleagues.

Original drug companies have relied on this statutory hierarchy to encourage prescription transfers to their medications and thus limit the competition from generics. If we take the case of Inexium®, AstraZeneca offered its new drug at a very low price in all hospitals[8] in order to have it referenced by hospital pharmacies and prescribed by hospital doctors. The laboratory thus hoped to influence the prescriptions of GPs and compensate for the hospital's loss of income by increasing sales in ambulatory care.

> Most people who go to the hospital for an ankle sprain, they get a splint and come out with an anti-inflammatory and Inexium®. Why are these [drugs] given out? Because, in the emergency services, as in all hospitals in France and Navarre, the pharmaceutical industry has done its job well, so much so that in the hospital pharmacies there is Inexium® and so the hospital pharmacist says to the doctors: "If you prescribe a PPI, prescribe Inexium® instead". In addition, there are the companies' delegates who arrive with their miniskirts and, all excited that a glamorous delegate has shown up, the interns are all in favor of Inexium®.
>
> (GP, Drôme, 2008)

My analysis of NHI data shows that this strategy has largely paid off: Inexium® prescriptions increased from 3% in 2002 to 43% in 2010 at hospital discharge, and from 5% to 29% in ambulatory care. GPs were less inclined to use Inexium® than hospital doctors, but the influence of the latter was nonetheless strong, along with that of the company's delegates.

Although these situations and practices cannot strictly speaking be considered as COIs, they are nonetheless representative of the way in which relations between health professionals constitute an essential determinant of the interests and prescriptions of these professionals, and therefore an essential lever of influence of the industry, and to a lesser extent of the NHI, on these interests and practices.

Conclusion

Following this analysis of the issues raised by the prescription and substitution of generics in France, it would appear that there are many conflicting interests and few COIs (Latham, 2001). When choosing the generic drug or the original drug, doctors and pharmacists must in fact arbitrate between the financial and health interests held by numerous actors: pharmaceutical companies (of generic and original drugs), the NHI, patients, and other prescribers. But the presence of these different conflicting interests is not sufficient to characterize the prescription of an original drug or its generic copy as resulting from a COI. Indeed, pharmacists make a higher margin on the sale of generics and thus serve the interests of the NHI and the generic companies. But this does not mean that they have abolished any consideration for the health of their patients, as their caution in substitution for fragile patients or sensitive drugs has shown. Similarly, although physicians have long enjoyed no financial incentive to prescribe generics and have regularly justified their preference for the original drug by a primacy of health over any other consideration, they have sometimes made this prescription a means of attaching themselves to an easier patient (and one more likely to pay overcharges), settling their accounts with the NHI or pharmacists and sometimes promoting pharmaceutical companies engaged in research and development.

The analysis of the case of generics, therefore, invites us to shift the question of COIs to that of the relations of influence in which prescribers find themselves. What separates doctors and pharmacists is not so much the framing of their interests, which we have seen to be (increasingly) similar, as their position and their relations with all the players who try to influence their prescriptions: pharmaceutical companies, the NHI, patients, and other professionals. A specialist doctor charging fee overruns is thus more "likely" than a GP charging the agreed fee to be confronted with patients of a higher class, to have strong links with the original drug companies and weak links with the NHI, and to be in competition with other specialists or GPs for control of that patient. His or her preference for branded prescriptions of original drugs that are patented or labeled "non-substitutable" is a result of his or her position in this network of influences. Conversely, a pharmacist practicing in a rural area is likely to have the same strong links with the NHI and generic companies as a pharmacist practicing in a large metropolis. But he or she is more likely to benefit from captive and less demanding patients, less competition from other pharmacies, and stronger personal links with the few GPs located near his or her pharmacy.

In this sense, the analysis of the interests at stake in the prescription of generic drugs constitutes a call to return to the etymology of interest: to be between multiple actors and values whose articulation is problematic.

Notes

1. It is important to note that some of these differences between countries result from differences in the sources and scope considered. In France, for example, paracetamol or aspirin-based drugs are not listed in the Official Registry of Generic Groups, which "amputates" the share of generics in the market by several points. Based on data provided by IMS Health and using a definition of generics that was "comparable across countries", the Ministry of Health obtained a 47% share of generic drugs in the total market volumes in France compared to 64% in Germany, 66% in the United Kingdom, and 75% in the United States in 2013 (Plan national de promotion des génériques, 2015).

2. A "substantially similar" drug is defined as a drug with the same composition of active ingredients (in quality and quantity), the same dosage form and the same bioavailability in the body as the reference drug. For a presentation of the controversies in the United States around the equivalence between generic and original drugs, see Greene (2014).

3. This chapter draws on a 5-year empirical research project (2004–2009) that involved 8 weeks of observations in pharmacies, 150 interviews with various actors, and analysis of archives and statistical data provided by the NHI. For a more in-depth presentation of this research, see Nouguez (2017).

4. Sanofi-Aventis appealed this decision at the Paris Court of Appeal, which dismissed the appeal on December 18, 2014 and ordered the company to pay the legal costs of the French Competition Authority. The company announced that "it is considering an appeal to the Court of Cassation".

5. The first patent protected the "salt" used in Plavix®, clopidogrel hydrogen sulphate, until February 16, 2013; the other, initially valid until February 17, 2017 and extended by a supplementary protection certificate until February 16, 2022, protected the indication in the treatment of acute coronary syndrome (ACS) by dual therapy combining clopidogrel and aspirin. The French Medicines Agency, consulted by the laboratory in 2009, ruled that neither of these two patents constituted an obstacle to the substitution of generics for Plavix®.

6. Since anything this pharmacy sold would not be reimbursed by the NHI, this was akin to closing the pharmacy for one month.

7. The choice of "specialties" by medical students according to their ranking following the sixth-year national exam gives a good estimate of this symbolic and statutory hierarchy of doctors. General medicine is at the bottom of students' choices along psychiatry and public health, whereas cardiology, radiology, or dermatology are at the top of the list.

8. Unlike drugs sold in pharmacies, the prices of drugs in hospitals are not set by the state but are negotiated in tenders. This gives pharmaceutical companies more leeway to play with these prices.

References

Abbott, A (1988) *The system of professions: an essay on the division of expert labor*. Chicago: University of Chicago Press.

Aïach, P (1994) 'Une profession conflictuelle : la pharmacie d'officine'in Fassin, D and Aïach, P (eds.) *Les métiers de la santé: enjeux de pouvoir et quête de légitimité*. Paris: Anthropos, pp. 309–338.

Autorité de la concurrence (2013) *Décision no 13-D-11 du 14 mai 2013 relative à des pratiques mises en œuvre dans le secteur pharmaceutique* [online]. Available at: http://www.autoritedelaconcurrence.fr/pdf/avis/13d11.pdf.

Benford, RD and Snow, DA (2000) 'Framing processes and social movements: an overview and assessment', *Annual Review of Sociology*, 26(1), pp. 611–639.

Bucher, R and Strauss, A (1961) 'Professions in process', *American Journal of Sociology*, 66(4), pp. 325–334.

Caisse nationale d'assurance maladie des travailleurs salariés (2012) *Propositions de l'Assurance maladie sur les charges et produits pour l'année 2013*. Paris: CNAMTS.

Coleman, JS, Katz, E and Menzel, H (1966) *Medical innovation: a diffusion study*. Indianapolis: Bobbs-Merrill Company.

Davis, M and Stark, A (eds.) (2001) *Conflict of interest in the professions*. Oxford: Oxford University Press.

Durand, F (2012) 'Une pharmacie sanctionnée car elle vendait trop peu de génériques', *Le Nouvel Observateur* (AFP), August 31.

Field, MJ and Lo, B (eds.) (2009) *Conflict of interest in medical research, education, and practice*. Washington: National Academies Press.

Freidson, E (1988) *Profession of medicine: a study of the sociology of applied knowledge*. Chicago: University of Chicago Press.

Gaudillière, JP and Thoms, U (eds.) (2015) *The development of scientific marketing in the twentieth century: research for sales in the pharmaceutical industry*. London: Routledge.

Greene, JA (2014) *Generic: the unbranding of modern medicine*. Baltimore: John Hopkins University Press.

Greffion, J (2007) 'Convergence (ou mimétisme) entre des modèles professionnels publics et privés: le cas des délégués de l'assurance maladie (DAM)', *Revue sociologie santé*, 27, pp. 153–172.

Gusfield, JR (1996) *Contested meanings: the construction of alcohol problems*. Madison: University of Wisconsin Press.

Hassenteufel, P (2003) 'Le premier septennat du plan Juppé. Un non-changement décisif', *Le carnet de santé de la France 2003*, Dunod, pp. 121–147.

Hughes, EC (1951) 'Mistakes at work', *The Canadian Journal of Economics and Political Science/Revue canadienne d'economique et de science politique*, 17(3), pp. 320–327.

Hughes, EC (1962) 'Good people and dirty work', *Social Problems*, 10(1), pp. 3–11.

Latham, SR (2001) 'Conflict of interest in medical practice' in Davis, M and Stark, A (eds.) *Conflict of interest in the professions*. Oxford: Oxford University Press, pp. 279–301.

Mamou, Y (2006) 'Novartis enquête sur des irrégularités comptables de sa filiale Sandoz France', *Le Monde*, November 21, p. 18.

Ministère des solidarités et de la santé (2016) 'Cas particuliers' [online]. Available at: https://solidarites-sante.gouv.fr/soins-et-maladies/medicaments/professionnels-de-sante/medicaments-generiques-a-l-usage-des-professionnels/article/cas-particuliers#:~:text=Chez%20les%20personnes%20%C3%A2g%C3%A9es%20et, qu'il%20remplace%2C%20etc.

Nouguez, É (2017) *Des médicaments à tout prix: sociologie des génériques en France*. Paris: Presses de Sciences Po.

OECD (2019) *Panorama de la santé 2019* [online]. Available at: http://www.oecd.org/fr/sante/systemes-sante/panorama-de-la-sante-19991320.htm.

Podolny, JM (2005) *Status signals: a sociological study of market competition*. Princeton: Princeton University Press.

Quet, M (2018) *Impostures pharmaceutiques. Médicaments illicites et luttes pour l'accès à la santé*. Paris: La Découverte.

Rodwin, MA (1995) *Medicine, money, and morals: physicians' conflicts of interest*. Oxford: Oxford University Press.

Rodwin, MA (2011) *Conflicts of interest and the future of medicine: the United States, France, and Japan*. Oxford: Oxford University Press.

Rosman, S (2010) 'Les pratiques de prescription des médecins généralistes. Une étude sociologique comparative entre la France et les Pays-Bas' in Bloy, G and Schweyer, FX (eds.) *Singuliers généralistes: sociologie de la médecine générale*. Rennes: Presse de l'EHESP, pp. 117–131.

Starr, P (1982) *The social transformation of American medicine: the rise of a sovereign profession and the making of a vast industry*. New York: Basic books.

Tonnelier, A (2010) 'Les génériqueurs qui observent la loi sont désavantagés en France'. Interview with Jeff George, CEO of Sandoz', *La Tribune*, March 12, p. 18.

Chapter 7

The politics of industrial transparency

Constructing a database on the pharmaceutical funding of the health sector

Henri Boullier and Jérôme Greffion

For several years now, the health sector has seen a substantial rise in so-called transparency mechanisms. In keeping with the principles of open government, an initial series of measures took the form of "institutional transparency" with the opening up of public data (Coglianese, 2009; Moore, 2018). This government-led "data-driven transparency" (Birchall, 2015) purportedly offers a way of improving the traceability, auditability, and performance of public healthcare against a backdrop of declining public resources and managerialized healthcare policies (Bevan and Hood, 2006; Blomgren, 2007). However, the health sector is also the locus of another form of transparency with very different aims, particularly the re-establishing of trust in medicines among citizens and consumers. This trust has waned considerably in the wake of health scandals such as those involving Vioxx® or Mediator®, which revealed the extent to which health agencies, pharmaceutical companies, and physicians are structurally bound up together in conflicts of interest (COIs).[1]

This second form of transparency is based on the mandatory disclosure of information otherwise unknown to State agencies about the links between the private sector and health professionals. Experts' disclosure of their interests to the health agencies on whose committees they sit[2] is thus supposed to guarantee independence – although some consider the latter to be minimal (Lexchin and O'Donovan, 2010). More recently, this second type of transparency has taken an original form through websites disclosing the financial ties between industry and actors in the health sector: physicians, medical students, pharmacists, patient associations, healthcare professional associations, healthcare organizations, the media, etc. (Grundy et al., 2018). In June 2014, the French government launched the website Transparence Santé (Transparency in Healthcare) making all this information accessible. As the home page states, "this transparency initiative, run by the Ministry of Health, aims to preserve the necessary relationship of trust between citizens, public service users, and the various actors in the healthcare system".[3]

10.4324/9781003161035-7

Between 2012 and September 2020, the database, which can be accessed via the website, registered over 18.5 million disclosures corresponding to a total of 6.5 billion euros. A similar website was also launched in 2014 in the United States, making health one of the main areas of development of a new form of transparency that we call "industrial transparency", in which the disclosed data is produced by the targeted industries – in our case the pharmaceutical companies.

This chapter analyzes the process through which the promise of transparency embodied by the Transparence Santé website was fulfilled. In unpacking this process, we show the respective roles of the State, companies, and civil society actors in contemporary policies on the disclosure of industry data. In so doing, we follow the lead of studies that have focused on the political and organizational dimensions of the development of information infrastructures (Bowker and Star, 1999; Denis and Pontille, 2012) and we take up questions raised by "critical transparency studies" (Alloa and Thomä, 2018), a research field that has explored the implications of transparency in terms of government disengagement and the outsourcing of disclosed data processing (Birchall, 2015). As we shall see, data disclosure does not necessarily result in greater transparency, not to mention accountability, insofar as the data in question cannot automatically be used or analyzed. The journalists who tried to draw on the Transparence Santé website soon encountered a range of difficulties: there are mistakes in some of the data published, several hundred million euros are not properly allocated, and it is impossible to obtain an overview of the sums in question (Hecketsweiler and Ferrer, 2017). We show that the Transparence Santé tool reproduces the model of "institutional transparency", promoting a voluntary form of regulation, but this time targeted at, and operated by, economic actors – thus embodying "industrial transparency".

The study on which this chapter is based was carried out between late 2018 and late 2019. Our aim was to retrace the process through which the database was constructed, paying close attention to the technical choices that determined its development, to the actors involved, and to the difficulties encountered. During this investigation, we met and interviewed nine people, sometimes several times, who were directly involved in developing the database. These respondents, with whom we conducted interviews lasting between one and four hours, were legal experts, computer scientists, and project managers at the Ministry of Health, the French association of pharmaceutical companies Les Entreprises du médicament (LEEM), and the French government's open data agency Etalab. We also attended numerous weekly meetings held by the association EurosForDocs over the course of more than a year and had more informal discussions with several of its members. In addition, we draw here on a substantial body of technical literature that includes decrees but also technical manuals produced by the ministry and by LEEM, who drafted a series of documents analyzing the database for its members. Finally, we examined all press articles published on the subject of the Transparence Santé database.

Managing influence by disclosing interests: The origins of the Transparence Santé database

Over the past ten years, a wide range of tools have been put in place to document situations of COI that are likely to affect politicians, public experts, and civil servants. Since 2011, the European Union has had a "transparency register" on which all interest groups (lobbying firms, companies, NGOs, think tanks, etc.) that "directly or indirectly influenc[e] the formulation or implementation of policy and the decision-making processes of the EU institutions" are inventoried. The European register currently includes around 6,300 companies, 3,100 NGOs, and over 830 consultancies specializing in European legislative processes (European Commission, 2020). In France, similar arrangements have been put in place by means of a public register of lobbyists (répertoire des représentants d'intérêt). It is run by the Higher Authority for Transparency in Public Life (Haute Autorité pour la transparence de la vie publique), an organization that is also tasked with publishing the declarations of the assets owned by public officials. Transparency mechanisms have thus become an increasingly common response to regulating the lobbying of politicians, administrations, and regulatory agencies.

However, the field of healthcare shows that the problem to which these transparency measures are supposed to provide an answer – in this instance, the influence of the pharmaceutical industry – is far more long-standing (on this, see Kefauver Committee, 1951; Comanor, 1966) and extends beyond the political and administrative spheres. From as early as the 1970s, physicians came together to criticize the ties that the pharmaceutical industry sought to create with researchers and healthcare professionals. This chorus of dissent resulted in the creation of organizations capable of producing information about medicines without funding from the pharmaceutical industry (e.g., the journal *Prescrire,* first published in 1981, and the Cochrane Library, since 1993). It also gave rise to activist associations specialized in fighting COI (e.g., No Free Lunch in the United States, founded in 2000) and in championing independent medical training (Formindep in France, founded in 2004). In this context, public authorities and healthcare actors progressively set up a multitude of systems (the mandatory disclosure of interests before being able to publish in certain journals, the obligation to fill out a "public declaration of interests" before being able to sit on certain public expert committees, etc.) that promised to make the links between industry and health professionals more transparent in order to limit situations of COI.

In the 2010s, transparency mechanisms changed in nature, and databases were developed offering exhaustive lists of "private" financial ties between pharmaceutical companies and health professionals (Hauray et al., introduction; Grundy et al., 2018). In France, the creation of the Transparence Santé website was closely linked with the Mediator® scandal.[4] This appetite suppressant, marketed since 1976 as an adjuvant antidiabetic, was withdrawn from the market in 2011 for having caused the deaths of several hundred people. The investigation into the causes of the tragedy revealed systemic conflicts in the health sector. Xavier Bertrand, Minister of Health at the time, proposed a radical reform of the regulatory framework for the safety of medicines, introducing a series of new requirements aimed at fighting COIs (Légifrance, 2011). The most emblematic measure, which resulted in the Transparence Santé website, mandated that pharmaceutical companies make all their financial ties with health professionals public (Hauray, 2018).

When the "Bertrand Law" was adopted in 2011, the rules governing how financial ties were to be made public remained vague. Article 2 of the law, devoted to new transparency measures, stipulated that pharmaceutical companies were "obliged to make public the existence of *agreements*" (in other words, contracts) signed with a series of actors (professionals, associations, students), but also, above a certain threshold, the *benefits* – whether "in kind" or in cash (meals, travel expenses, etc.) – that they gave to these actors.[5] Many other aspects, however, remained to be defined by decree, such as the threshold above which *benefits* had to be made public, the precise nature of the information to be provided regarding *agreements*, and even the timeframe and modes of publication.

Implementing transparency: An unfinished process

When the "Bertrand Law" was adopted at the end of 2011, the conditions under which private industry data were to be made public had not yet been determined. Months later, the idea emerged of setting up a website that would make accessible the huge database constituted by pharmaceutical companies, following the model of the American Physician Payments Sunshine Act of 2010.[6] Two factors disrupted the development of this tool, however. First, LEEM raised the issue of trade secrets and confidentiality with a view to influencing how detailed the data made available by the website would be. Then, technical, budgetary, and organizational constraints further complicated the development of the Transparence Santé website, which was finally launched in the summer of 2014.

Negotiating the content of the database with pharmaceutical companies

The year after the "Bertrand Law" was passed was a key moment. The Ministry of Health began preparing the decrees determining exactly how this new healthcare transparency policy would be applied. Looking at the mobilization of the pharmaceutical industry around article 2 of the law during this period and at the compromises it managed to strike with the ministry over the course of regular exchanges reveals the substantial leeway that the industry benefited from when it came to determining the conditions under which the policy would be applied.

One question that remained unresolved in the law adopted in late 2011 was that of the threshold (i.e., the amount of money) above which *benefits* granted by pharmaceutical firms would need to be declared. This threshold had very practical implications both for the authorities and for the pharmaceutical companies: a low threshold implied registering a very large number of transactions (e.g., meals out, breakfasts in hospitals, etc.), if not all of them, and would also inflate the quantity of information that had to be entered into the future database. Representatives of the pharmaceutical industry told us that they had argued in favor of setting this threshold at €30, which presented the dual advantage of being the same amount as the value of gifts usually considered of "negligible value" (according to France's competition and fraud control authority) and of avoiding the publication of excessive numbers of small transactions.[7] The ministry, however, decided instead to set the amount "as low as possible" with a view to exhaustiveness, excluding only the smallest of transactions such as coffees.

According to a legal expert involved in drafting the decree, in the aftermath of the Mediator® crisis her team "could not take into account"[8] the issue of the workload that a low threshold would represent for companies. Such a concern seemed entirely trivial in light of the scale of the scandal. The administration, therefore, decided to opt for a threshold of €10, seen as a way of ensuring almost total transparency regarding the *benefits* granted by companies to other actors in the health sector, even though this would result in far more work for the companies.

Despite this setback for the industry, regular contact with staff at the Ministry of Health was maintained by legal experts from LEEM. From 2012 onwards, they produced a series of circulars in which they outlined their suggestions for interpreting the provisions relative to the transparency of interests. Between 2012 and 2017, the Department of Regulatory Affairs prepared seven long notes of between 10 and 67 pages in which LEEM's legal experts provided their analyses of the law, as well as a detailed account of their negotiations with government representatives. Their intention was to influence how certain measures would be interpreted when the legal texts governing their application were drafted, with a view to limiting the normative constraints weighing upon companies in the sector.

A good example of the way in which the pharmaceutical industry used the notion of trade secrets to influence the implementation of the 2011 law's transparency measures can be seen in the process leading to a typology of the content of *agreements* signed with health professionals. In late 2016, the Directorate General for Health (Direction générale de la Santé, DGS) prepared an *arrêté* (order) intended to offer a more detailed definition of the "precise subject matter" of research contracts linking pharmaceutical companies to health professionals. The aim was thus to drive companies to disclose not only the monetary value of the *agreements* in question and their beneficiaries but also what exactly they were funding. LEEM's legal experts contacted the DGS to ensure that the content of these research contracts would remain confidential:

> For us, publishing the subject matter of the contracts wasn't conceivable, in terms of local attractiveness, international competition, etc. But things were cleared up quickly, because the logic wasn't one of publishing the contracts in and of themselves, but rather one of defining categories.[9]

LEEM understood that what the DGS required was a series of categories, in other words, a list of "types" of expenses, linked to *agreements*. The organization, therefore, prepared a typology of *agreements* that it sent to the DGS with a view to feeding into the *arrêté* at its draft stage. LEEM proposed 18 categories (ranging from "purchase of scientific documentation" to "conference registration fees", "hospitality", and "training" [LEEM, 2017]), all of which were retained in the *arrêté* published in March 2017. This new example illustrates how public authorities partly relied on the pharmaceutical companies to design this new disclosure tool and how the latter were also put in charge of recording the financial ties connecting them to other actors in the sector. While the whole process was "collaborative", it also illustrates how companies managed to reap the benefits of this situation: it gave them the capacity to influence how transparency principles were applied in practice, for example by defining the typology of *agreements* that best suited their needs with a view to making the recording process easier and to safeguarding what they believed fell into the category of trade secrets.

Developing a transparency tool with limited resources

Alongside the drafting of legal texts stipulating how the law would be enforced, the plan to set up a one-stop website soon emerged. Immediately after the law was passed, the industry still knew nothing about the technical modalities according to which *benefits* and *agreements* would be made public. The office of the new Minister of Health, Marisol Touraine, exhumed an idea that had first been discussed by parliamentarians in 2011, i.e., the idea of setting up a centralized database combined with an openly accessible website. In May 2013, a decree made this idea official and outlined "the nature of the information that must be made public by companies [...] via a one-stop public website", specifying that "this information is made available to the public free of charge and in an accessible format, and is updated every semester" (Légifrance, 2013). In the months that followed, the ministry staff also had to determine the website architecture, find a service provider to manage the project, and oversee its roll-out.

Creating the public website was a real challenge for the actors involved for at least three reasons. The first difficulty lay in the urgency with which it was designed. While the idea of a one-stop website emerged as early as 2012, the CNIL (France's data protection agency) was consulted on the issue of using personal data and then took more than a year to draft its opinion. Despite this extended timeframe, Touraine's office still deemed the publication of *benefits* to be a political priority that should be implemented as soon as possible. The May 2013 decree thus stipulated that data about signed *agreements* and granted *benefits* should be published from June 1, 2013, onwards, should include all transactions from 2012, and should appear on the websites of the pharmaceutical laboratories while the one-stop website had yet to be launched. For the ministry, this transitional period was not intended to last long and it was, therefore, important to put in place a system that allowed industry actors to register their disclosures as soon as possible. The IT project was ultimately completed over only a few months, between autumn 2013 and spring 2014, during which time the service provider had to be chosen, discussions had to take place with both industry actors and professional bodies to collect their requests and remarks, and a test version of the site had to be launched.

A second difficulty concerned the limited financial resources allocated to the website. When the Transparence Santé website development began, it was just one IT project among others and the funds available to the Ministry of Health were limited. The people in charge of the project had to negotiate, sometimes on a case-by-case basis, funding for certain functions or modules to improve the interface, the quality of the data, or certain errors. The head of the IT project told us in an interview, for example, that she had not managed to obtain funding to develop a module that would have made it possible to systematically check the identity of the associations listed as beneficiaries by companies. According to her, this was typically the sort of function that would have avoided the duplications that today make the database difficult to navigate and use. The website was allocated a budget of €500,000, which seems relatively limited when compared to the €1.5 million allocated to the site hosting public disclosures of interests by experts working for health agencies. The latter project, while similar, in fact seems far less complex, at least insofar as it concerns a much smaller volume of data which are far more homogeneous. However, its development (and thus its budget) no doubt benefited from the fact that its end users – civil servants and public experts – were directly involved in the implementation process, whereas the end users were absent from discussions about the Transparence Santé tool.

The limited human resources allocated to the one-stop website further complicated its development and publicization. At the end of 2013, during the most intense phase of the website design, only two people from the ministry were assigned to project management. They were only working on this part-time and had limited IT skills (one was a legal expert by training and the other an administrative assistant with one year's training in IT). The external service provider in charge of website development proper was also working with a small team, comprising only a project manager and a developer. In addition to the project being carried by a small number of people, its management was further complicated by the turnover of personnel, partly because the IT service provider was taken over by a bigger group and partly because, at the ministry, the project manager left for another position. When the website was launched the following spring, these human and organizational resources faced additional cuts. Indeed, after the launch in early 2014, only one legal expert from the ministry devoted a small amount of her time to providing support to companies as they entered information into the database that would then appear on the website. According to her own description, in the absence of additional resources, this task essentially consisted of providing a "hotline" managing companies' initial registration on the website.[10]

Taking an approach invoking the principles of open government – broadly inspired by the philosophy of open-source software – public authorities disclosed not their own data but that of a sector, with a view to providing transparency and, ultimately, to restoring citizens' trust by enabling them to monitor the practices of that sector. At least this is what can be deduced implicitly from the ministry's approach in creating a minimalist tool for data access. Although the relationships between health professionals and the pharmaceutical industry were not directly transformed, public authorities did make them visible thanks to the Transparence Santé website in the hope that doing so would offer a safeguard against the harmful consequences of drug manufacturers' strategies of influence.

Making the promise of transparency more effective: The work of activist groups

When the Transparence Santé website was launched in 2014, the data provided by companies could be consulted but transparency was far from effective. Despite the satisfaction reported by administrative staff involved in the development phase, the website still suffered from a certain number of flaws linked to the functions it offered and the quality of the information to which it gave access. Transparency nevertheless became more tangible following pressure and voluntary work on the part of activist engineers and computer scientists, defending, in particular, open-source software and the principles of open government. Thanks to their mobilization, the industry data was made downloadable and more user-friendly via an alternative website.

External pressure and release of all the data in the form of a database

Although from the outset, the ministry's tool did include an option allowing the public to download all the data, this option remained deactivated. Until 2016, any use of the data for statistical processing remained impossible. However, despite its concerns linked in particular to the CNIL's requirements, the ministry eventually changed its position thanks to the interventions of, first, an association specialized in promoting the opening up of public data and, second, Etalab, the administration responsible for coordinating governmental strategy with regard to open data.

As soon as the website was launched, members of the association Regards Citoyens started to campaign for the possibility to use the information in the database. Regards Citoyens was founded in 2009 and is made up of IT specialists and IT engineers whose objective is to reinforce "civic engagement by promoting open access public data and the re-use of that data"[11] through the furthering of "open content licensing and open-source formats".[12] In 2014, several members or sympathizers of this association took on the task of breaking through the Transparence Santé website's IT protections in order to collect all the data via crawlers, so as to make them available to the public as a complete set. They took this opportunity to clean the data substantially, for example bringing together all the ties of one given professional under one single identifier (despite spelling mistakes in last names, for example). When this data was first posted online, presenting a name-based summary, the Ministry of Health soon found out. The project manager was concerned because it revealed security issues with the website:

> If the CNIL found out, we were done for. [...] We'd failed in our duty to ensure security, protection. Luckily, we managed to find the email address of the person behind it and we sent him a beautiful letter reminding him what he was exposing himself to if he did not remove the database the very minute he received that message.[13]

Shortly afterward, Regards Citoyens made a summary of the amounts spent by pharmaceutical firms available to the public, highlighting the total value of *benefits* paid out and the companies spending the largest amounts.[14] This overview was then reported by the press. Most importantly, although all the data had been made available, they had been "reluctantly" anonymized by the association, so they were not, strictly speaking, open data. This was framed as a militant act designed to push the ministry itself to release the information as open data.

According to the ministry staff, while this initial step taken by the association was somewhat embarrassing, it also revealed the wealth of data collected and the value of the statistical analyses that they made possible:

> We saw what he'd done with the data he'd got hold of and it was fascinating. And we said to ourselves that it would, indeed, be good if people could use it. Only at that point we were supposed to be preventing the database from getting out into the open.[15]

This episode gave greater weight to the initiative of an Etalab IT specialist when he approached the ministry several months later, asking them to make all the data available to download as a set. While the ministry's position remained similar to that of the CNIL, stating that personal data could not be shared, both administrations began thinking about how the database content might be shared as a whole. The Council of State (Conseil d'État), consulted on this matter, did not disapprove of the initiative but concluded that there was no legal framework to govern the dissemination, and above all the use, of this information. Two legal experts at the ministry then began working on designing a specific license for the Transparence Santé data, restricting the ways in which it could be used. They stipulated that the database could be used freely for personal ends, but any online use would require respecting the same data protection regulations as the original database. This approach was ratified by the 2016 Health Law and since then the Transparence Santé database has been fully downloadable via Etalab's website.

It was therefore under pressure from actors outside the ministry that the data were made accessible and analyzable. Other outside actors, working in the same circles, then took a further step toward delivering on the promise of transparency.

Creation of a more effective tool to present and process the data

For many years, Regards Citoyens itself processed statistics for investigative journalists or for Formindep. However, its volunteers wanted to design an ergonomic tool that would allow researchers, journalists, or ordinary citizens to visualize and use the data themselves. The lack of resources may explain why the ministry did not pursue this particular avenue to provide a tool that would clean data, allow easier searches, or enable data to be visualized. Its tool was not designed for these purposes and its position was instead to leave this task to others.

> We don't have the resources, internally, to develop these kinds of very fancy tools. And in fact that's why the transparency was put in place: to allow those who do have the resources to help us. [...] It's a way of calling for help. And if, afterwards, they want to sell us the application at a reasonable price, we'll be happy to take it.[16]

A tool for promoting the use of the data emerged at the initiative of a data scientist – an engineer from one of France's prestigious *grandes écoles* – who discovered the existence of the Transparence Santé website, along with its potential and its flaws, via the press in early 2018. He decided to develop a website called EurosForDocs, inspired by the American website Dollars for Docs. In order to secure help from other volunteers, he embedded his project within the "Data for Good" collective, whose developers and data scientists use data science to "provide associations with cutting edge technological tools to increase their societal impact".[17] These IT specialists, often from *grandes écoles*, use their skills to further a project with a final goal that they find more palatable than that of their own well-paid jobs. On average, their involvement with EurosForDocs lasts a few months. The collective's main priority was to simplify access to existing data, in particular by allowing partly cleansed data to be presented more clearly and by enabling ad-hoc statistical analyses to be carried out.[18] For its founder, this tool was mainly designed for journalists and researchers wanting to examine the data from a variety of different perspectives. In September 2020, 4,000 accounts had been opened to access this tool with approximately 10 daily connections. Both these figures represent a sharp rise compared to the previous year.[19]

This is how engineers and IT specialists involved in collectives championing open data, transparency in public life, or open-source software drew on their IT skills – which were of a far higher level than those available internally at the Ministry of Health – and managed to deliver on a promise of transparency that had thus far only been partially fulfilled. Their work made the data available in the form of a (cleaner) database and also made them much easier to use. It is probably no coincidence that there was a subsequent rise in references to the transparency database in the press.

The tool's main use: Financial ties and COIs made increasingly visible by the press

For the most part, the general public is not aware of the Transparence Santé website. The number of users who connect to it, as a consequence, is very low (300 per day). Certain State bodies – health agencies, first and foremost – have developed a greater interest in these data and consequently in a tool such as EurosForDocs, which can help them to monitor the interests disclosed by their experts. However, the main quantifiable use of the data is by the press. Regularly, and increasingly, the press uses those data to examine the ties between health professionals and the pharmaceutical industry. Most often, it draws attention to *benefits* received by individual physicians who are cited by name. It is rare to see more in-depth investigations, and there is currently very little academic research on these data.

Our analysis of press use of the data is based on a corpus created by searching in the Europresse database[20] for articles published in France and including the terms "Transparence Santé" or "EurosForDocs" (in their different forms). Once duplicate entries and off-topic articles had been excluded, this corpus comprised 303 articles published between 2013 and 2020 (see Figure 7.1). Generally speaking, press interest in the Transparence Santé data has increased steadily over time; with a sharp rise in 2020 (over 125 articles were published during the first 7 months of the year). A quarter of the articles (81) were published by the daily national press (including on their websites) – first and foremost *Le Monde* (23 articles) – and by the news agency Agence France-Presse. A small number (30) appeared in weekly or monthly national magazines (in particular, *La Tribune* and *L'Express*). The vast majority of the articles were from the daily regional press.

If we turn now to how these articles refer to the transparency database and its data, using text-mining tools they can be broadly grouped into six classes[21] according to their lexical similarities. The content of these classes can be summarized based on their ten characteristic documents and on their most frequent terms. The first group (57 articles, published from 2014 to 2017) refer to criticism of the Transparence Santé database, whether in terms of its ergonomics, the lack of actual amounts of money mentioned for the *agreements*, or the impossibility of downloading the data. Its articles voice the concerns of various organizations (Regards Citoyens, Formindep, the national physicians' association) and relay the critical report produced by France's revenue court (Cour des Comptes) in 2017 concerning "the prevention of conflicts of interest in matters of health expertise" and examining the implementation of the Bertrand Law.

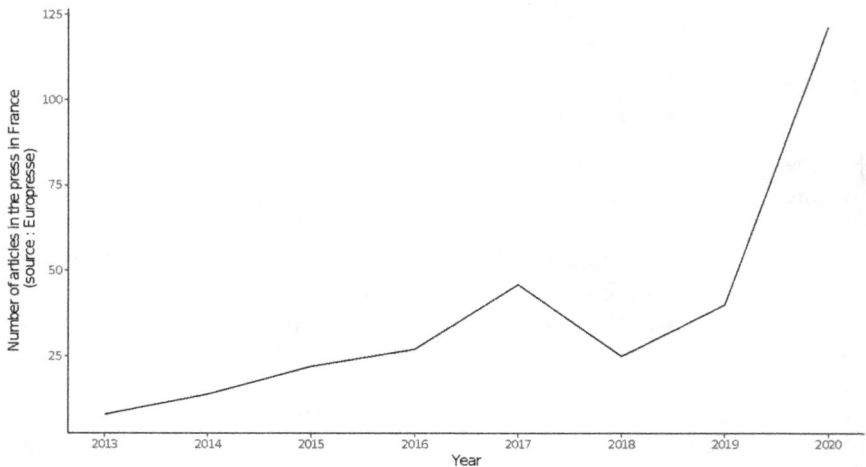

Figure 7.1 Number of articles focusing on the Transparence Santé website and published in the French press, by year of publication.

This first group, just like the second fairly heterogeneous group (108 articles), also contains articles published in 2018–2019, reporting on the campaigns by groups using the Transparence Santé data to point to the COIs of people whose positions they exposed. Two examples illustrate this: first, a complaint by an anti-corruption association about experts at the National Authority for Health (Haute Autorité de Santé) denouncing by the same token the fact that the institution had not consulted the database; second, opposition from physicians to the Human Papilloma Virus (HPV) vaccine based, in part, on the exposure of the links between the vaccine's proponents (physicians, learned societies, the media) and its manufacturers. Sometimes the journalists themselves used the data, revealing, for example, the sums spent by a homeopathy manufacturer to train and influence physicians at a time when State reimbursement for its products was potentially about to be withdrawn, or underlining the links between a company selling an alternative breast cancer treatment and the physicians publicly promoting this kind of treatment.

The content of this type of article is similar to that of a third small group (17 articles, mainly published from 2015 to 2017 in the national press) focusing on the pharmaceutical company Servier or its drug, Mediator®. The Transparence Santé data were analyzed to point to persisting financial ties between this company and the world of cardiology (physicians or learned societies), the medical specialism within which the prescription of Mediator® fell. Once again, Formindep's points of view were foregrounded. This association was also behind a revelation that was widely covered in the national press: a physician belonging to future president Emmanuel Macron's campaign team had many interests tying him to Servier. This case, described as a problem of COI, led to the person resigning from the campaign. In general, Mediator® was widely mentioned in this corpus on the transparency data (in one article in three) and the same is true of Servier (one article in six).

The last three classes are extremely homogeneous. The fourth group (81 articles published in January 2020, in 15 regional daily newspapers) corresponds to a large local investigation, conducted by a collective of data journalists. The articles describe financial ties in 2018 between pharmaceutical companies and university hospitals (and their physicians), as well as the measures implemented to find out about and oversee these ties. Several articles point to problems with how clean the Transparence Santé data were and the lack of subsequent monitoring of their accuracy. The journalists used the EurosForDocs website, recognizing its usefulness in making the data accessible, although they only cited it in the page dedicated to their methodology. Immediately after this investigation, an opinion piece in *Le Monde* written by a group of physicians, including Irène Frachon, suggested a series of measures to fight COIs in the medical sphere, including the requirement for donations to associations to be "redistributed to each of their members and registered in the national database by name" so that they would appear in the Transparence Santé database and for checks to be conducted on the comprehensiveness of disclosures.

The fifth series of articles (25 published in June and July 2020) focuses on the controversy around the use of hydroxychloroquine in treating COVID-19. They refer to the accusations of COI made by Didier Raoult, a physician championing the treatment, against its opponents in the medical world, particularly during a hearing at the Assemblée nationale (French parliament). He used the Transparence Santé database and the EurosForDocs website to underline its opponents' ties to Gilead, a company manufacturing a competing product. Certain journalists pursued this analysis using the same means to examine the links between Gilead and researchers working on infectious and tropical diseases.

Finally, one last small group of articles (15) from November 2019 reported the conclusions of a research paper published in the *British Medical Journal* (BMJ) by a group of physicians, some of whom had close links with Formindep (Goupil et al., 2019). The authors showed that the French general practitioners who receive the most gifts tend to have the most costly and least efficient prescribing patterns. This is one of the rare academic publications to have used the Transparence Santé database on a large scale, along the same model as prior studies conducted in Anglo-American countries, the most recent of which no longer draw on private sector databases but rather on the public sector databases that arose from the Sunshine Act (e.g., Perlis and Perlis, 2016).[22]

What this analysis of the press shows is that since the development of the EurosForDocs website, the Transparence Santé website data have been mentioned regularly and increasingly often by the media reporting its use either by physicians voicing criticisms, by associations such as Formindep, but also by journalists themselves. These different actors have used this data to shed light on various situations of COI, whether of a structural or a more one-off nature, giving rise to "scandals" in certain medical subsectors and therapeutic fields or concerning certain public figures and associations.

Conclusion

This chapter is in line with social science research that has studied the institutionalization of disclosure policies and practices in a multitude of domains and professions (Fung, Graham, and Weil, 2007; Schudson, 2015). This scholarship has discussed the kinds of transparency produced by the institutionalization of openness (Heald, 2006), while also providing critical analyses documenting both the limits of the "fuzzy" promise of transparency and its ability to make things visible without holding anyone or anything accountable (Birchall, 2011; Ananny and Crawford, 2018). This chapter wanted to contribute to this field of research by looking more closely at the invisible work performed "behind the scenes" to develop transparency tools, in the spirit of research on the politics of information infrastructures (Bowker and Star, 1999). To do so, we decided to follow in detail the development of a transparency tool targeted at, and largely operated by, the pharmaceutical industry.

We focused on a new system for disclosing data that has recently appeared in the healthcare sector, in the shape of websites providing inventories of the pharmaceutical funding of healthcare professionals. The example of France's Transparence Santé website, designed by the Ministry of Health and made accessible to the French public in 2014, shows that the people behind its construction had to make compromises with the demands of the pharmaceutical industry, obviously reluctant to divulge data that it considered sensitive, while also developing a website with limited resources. Activist groups that were unsatisfied with the end result then mobilized to deliver more effectively on the promise of transparency, endeavoring to make the data more accessible by improving the quality of the database and developing an alternative website that was more functional than its original iteration. Journalists have since made increasingly regular use of these data in their analyses of financial interests in the health sector, suggesting that the process has at least in part delivered on the promise to provide greater transparency regarding the ties between the pharmaceutical industry and health professionals.

The case of the Transparence Santé project thus allowed us to document a new form of data disclosure that we have called "industrial transparency". This form of transparency is based on private-sector data and aims to make strategies of influence visible, thereby restoring the trust of the public, following a logic that is quite similar to that of the mechanisms set up to reveal the lobbying of politicians by private parties. One of the merits of our example, however, is that it involves massive data, with tens of thousands of people involved and millions of transactions. The case raises, in sharper relief, the question of the role played by public authorities in achieving this form of transparency. In the process we analyzed, the State appears to be relatively disengaged, and, sometimes, to remain in the background. In the end, its ambitious disclosure project suffered from a number of flaws, with little to no monitoring of registered data, no tools to facilitate its use, and data remaining the property of the companies. The authorities did, however, succeed in creating a single website, whereas the companies would have preferred to publish the details of their transactions on their respective websites. After some struggle, this design made it possible for third parties to make actual use of the dataset. This example, therefore, enabled us to explore the hypothesis that the mechanisms of industrial transparency in fact allow the neoliberal state to regulate the private sector at a marginal level, limiting its own investment while outsourcing the responsibility for processing and monitoring the disclosed data.

Notes

1. See introduction and Chapter 1 of this volume.
2. See Chapter 4 in this volume.
3. <https://www.transparence.sante.gouv.fr/>
4. See Chapter 9 in this volume.
5. Here we thought that *benefits* and *agreements* (voluntarily in *italics*) were the best way to translate the original terms: "avantages" and "conventions".
6. This law was adopted in 2010 at the same time as the Affordable Care Act (also known as Obamacare) and aimed to improve the transparency of financial ties between pharmaceutical firms and healthcare providers. It gave rise to the launch of Open Payments, an ambitious database providing an inventory of these ties: <https://openpaymentsdata.cms.gov>.
7. Interview with a former legal officer at LEEM, May 2019.
8. Interview with a legal expert from the Ministry of Health, March 2019.
9. Interview with LEEM's legal officer, March 2019.
10. Interview with a legal expert at the DGS, October 2018.
11. The association's statutes.
12. The association has, in particular, developed tools making it possible to follow the activity of French members of parliament, changes in law during their parliamentary career, and lobbying at the French parliament, via summaries of the people given audiences by parliamentarians.
13. Interview with a legal expert at the Ministry of Health, March 2019.
14. <https://www.regardscitoyens.org/sunshine/>
15. Interview with a legal expert at the Ministry of Health, March 2019.
16. Interview with a legal expert at the DGS, October 2018.
17. <https://www.meetup.com/fr-FR/Data-for-Good-FR/>
18. <https://www.eurosfordocs.fr/presentation>
19. Figures provided by EurosForDocs.
20. This database is not exhaustive and does not contain all French press publications. The investigation conducted in 2018 by the online magazine *Basta !* and the Multinationals Observatory, entitled "Pharma papers", is therefore not part of our corpus.
21. We used the R.TeMiS (R Text Mining Solution) package (https://cran.r-project.org/web/packages/R.temis/index.html) on our corpus to create a vocabulary table, from which function words were removed. We then used hierarchical clustering to identify six classes based on the principal components drawn from a correspondence analysis run on this table.
22. Along with two other publications: one unpublished, seeking to calculate the impact of benefits and payments on prescriptions (Farvaque, Garcon, and Samson, 2020); and the second published as a "pre-proof" (Roussel and Raoult, 2020), showing a correlation between the stance taken by physicians in the hydroxychloroquine debate and the extent of their private interests in Gilead.

References

Alloa, E and Thomä, D (2018) *Transparency, society and subjectivity: critical perspectives*. London: Palgrave MacMillan.

Ananny, M and Crawford, K (2018) 'Seeing without knowing: limitations of the transparency ideal and its application to algorithmic accountability', *New Media & Society*, 20(3), pp. 973–989.

Bevan, G and Hood, C (2006) 'What's measured is what matters: targets and gaming in the English public health care system', *Public Administration*, 84(3), pp. 517–538 [online]. Available at: https://doi.org/10.1111/j.1467-9299.2006.00600.x (Accessed: January 25, 2021).

Birchall, C (2011) 'Introduction to "secrecy and transparency": the politics of opacity and openness', *Theory, Culture & Society*, 28(7–8), pp. 7–25.

Birchall, C (2015) 'Data.Gov-in-a-box': delimiting transparency', *European Journal of Social Theory*, 18(2), pp. 185–202 [online]. Available at: https://doi.org/10.1177/1368431014555259 (Accessed: January 25, 2021).

Blomgren, M (2007) 'The drive for transparency: organizational field transformations in Swedish healthcare', *Public Administration*, 85(1), pp. 67–82 [online]. Available at: https://doi.org/10.1111/j.1467-9299.2007.00634.x (Accessed: January 25, 2021).

Bowker, GC and Star, SL (1999) *Sorting things out: classification and its consequences*. Cambridge: MIT Press.

Coglianese, C (2009) 'The transparency president? The Obama administration and open government', *Governance: An International Journal of Policy, Administration, and Institutions*, 22(4), pp. 529–544 [online]. Available at: https://doi.org/10.1111/j.1468-0491.2009.01451.x (Accessed: January 25, 2021).

Comanor, WS (1966) 'The drug industry and medical research: the economics of the Kefauver Committee investigations', *The Journal of Business*, 39(1), pp. 12–18.

Denis, J and Pontille, D (2012) 'Workers of writing, materials of information', introduction to the special issue 'The invisible workers of the information society', *Revue d'anthropologie des connaissances*, 6(1), pp. 1–20.

European Commission (2020) Transparency register and the EU [online]. Available at: https://ec.europa.eu/transparencyregister/ (Accessed: January 25, 2021).

Farvaque, E, Garçon, H and Samson, AL (2020) '"Je ne tromperai jamais leur confiance": Analyse de l'influence des laboratoires sur la relation médecin-patient en France', Discussion paper LEM (Lille Economie Management) 2020-07 [online]. Available at: https://lem.univ-lille.fr/fileadmin/user_upload/laboratoires/lem/Doc_travail_2020/DP2020-07.pdf (Accessed: January 25, 2021).

Fung, A, Graham, M and Weil, D (2007) *Full disclosure: the perils and promise of transparency*. Cambridge: Cambridge University Press.

Goupil, B, Balusson, F, Naudet, F, Esvan, M, Bastian, B, Chapron, A and Frouard, P (2019) 'Association between gifts from pharmaceutical companies to French general practitioners and their drug prescribing patterns in 2016: retrospective study using the French Transparency in Healthcare and National Health Data System databases', *BMJ*, 367(l6015) [online]. Available at: https://doi.org/10.1136/bmj.l6015 (Accessed: January 25, 2021).

Grundy, Q, Habibi, R, Shnier, A, Mayes, C and Lipworth, W (2018) 'Decoding disclosure: comparing conflict of interest policy among the United States, France, and Australia', *Health Policy*, 122(5), pp. 509–518 [online]. Available at: https://doi.org/10.1016/j.healthpol.2018.03.015 (Accessed: January 25, 2021).

Hauray, B (2018) 'Dispositifs de transparence et régulation des conflits d'intérêts dans le secteur du médicament', *Revue française d'administration publique*, 165(1), pp. 49–61.

Heald, DA (2006) 'Varieties of transparency', *Proceedings of the British Academy*, 135, pp. 25–43.

Hecketsweiler, C and Ferrer, M (2017) 'Les ratés de la base de données publique transparence Santé', *Le Monde,* October 12, 2017.

Kefauver Committee (1951) 'Organized crime in interstate commerce', final report of the U.S. Senate's Special Committee to Investigate Organized Crime in Interstate Commerce, August 31.

LEEM (2017) 'Transparence des liens. Publication de l'arrêté relatif aux conditions de fonctionnement du site public unique', Circular n°17-0131, April 7, 2017.

Légifrance (2011) 'Loi n° 2011–2012 du 29 décembre 2011 relative au renforcement de la sécurité sanitaire du médicament et des produits de santé [law strengthening the health safety of medicines and health products]' Official Journal of the French Republic, n°0302 of December 30, 2011 [online]. Available at: https://www.legifrance.gouv.fr/jorf/id/JORFTEXT000025053440/ (Accessed: November 23, 2020).

Légifrance (2013) 'Décret n° 2013–414 du 21 mai 2013 relatif à la transparence des avantages accordés par les entreprises produisant ou commercialisant des produits à finalité sanitaire et cosmétique destinés à l'homme [Decree n°2013-414 of May 21, 2013 relating to the transparency of benefits awarded by companies that produce or market health and cosmetic products for human use]' [online]. Available at: https://www.legifrance.gouv.fr/jorf/id/JORFTEXT000027434029 (Accessed: January 25, 2021).

Lexchin, J and O'Donovan, O (2010) 'Prohibiting or "managing" conflict of interest? A review of policies and procedures in three European drug regulation agencies', Social Science & Medicine, 70(5), pp. 643–647.

Moore, S (2018) 'Towards a sociology of institutional transparency: openness, deception and the problem of public trust', Sociology, 52(2), pp. 416–430 [online]. Available at: https://doi.org/10.1177/0038038516686530 (Accessed: January 25, 2021).

Perlis, RH and Perlis, CS (2016) 'Physician payments from industry are associated with greater medicare part D prescribing costs', PLoS ONE, 11(5), e0155474 [online]. Available at: https://doi.org/10.1371/journal.pone.0155474 (Accessed: January 25, 2021).

Roussel, Y and Raoult, D (2020) 'Influence of conflicts of interest on public positions in the COVID-19 era, the case of Gilead Sciences', New Microbes and New Infections, 38, 100710 [online]. Available at: https://doi.org/10.1016/j.nmni.2020.100710 (Accessed: January 25, 2021).

Schudson, M (2015) The rise of the right to know. Politics and the culture of transparency, 1945–1975. Cambridge: Harvard University Press.

Chapter 8

Scientific marketing and conflict of interest

Lessons from the hormone replacement therapies (HRT) crisis

Jean-Paul Gaudillière

A tale of two crises

In April 1973, the US Food and Drug Administration (FDA) decided to ban the use of the drug DES (diethylstilbestrol), an analog of estrogens, in animal food. DES, a powerful growth enhancer used on a large scale as an additive in the industrial food consumed on US farms since the early 1950s, was thus threatened with a premature death. The origins of this decision were to be found two years earlier in the publication of epidemiological studies showing that when prescribed to pregnant women, the same drug had induced vaginal cancers in their daughters. This discovery triggered a major public controversy about the uses of the drug and its promotion by the chemical industry, which ended, in 1978, with a confirmed ban on its agricultural use (Marcus, 1994; Gaudillière, 2014).

Thirty years later, in January 2003, the same FDA published new guidelines and labels regarding other estrogen preparations, those used for hormone replacement therapy (HRT) during the menopause. The FDA recommended that these no longer be used for preventive purposes, and be prescribed only to women suffering from acute symptoms responsible for serious impairment of their quality of life. In addition, the FDA advised doctors to prescribe these hormones in the smallest possible doses and never for more than five years. These guidelines followed the early termination of the Women's Health Initiative (WHI), a very large cohort study of HRT. The trial was terminated in 2002 before its scheduled end date because the women receiving hormones presented higher risks of cancer and cardiovascular disorders than the women not taking HRT (Writing Group for the Women's Health Initiative Investigators, 2002). The WHI trial and the new FDA guidelines threatened a consensus about the benefits of HRT for the prevention of osteoporosis and cardiovascular disorders that had lasted more than 20 years, leading to the indictment of the pharmaceutical industry.

10.4324/9781003161035-8

These cases are just two of the multiple hormone crises that have occurred in the United States since the 1960s, and in which many common features are apparent. The chemicals considered were similar (estrogens and progestogens) and were produced by the same firms. Uses in both instances were preventive, involving fuzzy boundaries between physiology and pathology. The danger was actually a question of the risk measured as an increased probability of cancer. More importantly, public controversies erupted with the same palette of targets: the regulatory agencies, the medical professions, and the chemical and pharmaceutical industries. Finally, in both instances, a whole series of court actions followed the public scandals.

And yet, when it comes to the visibility of the category of COI in the public discussion of what happened and what was to be done, these controversies do not follow the same pattern. In the 1970s, although chemical and pharmaceutical corporations were criticized extensively, the term was barely used. Conversely, in the 2000s, the producers of HRT preparations as well as their medical partners were regularly accused – in the media and in tort law trials – of biased expertise stemming from deeply entrenched COIs.

This chapter does not discuss the dynamics of public expertise during the 1970s, that is, the ways in which experts' as well as women's voices – which could be heard in debates taking place in Congress, in the media, or in the courts – were highly critical of the industry and/or the medical profession without paying much attention to the notion of COI.[1] It is suffice to say that the social movements of the time were more interested in criticizing medicalization and male-dominated medicine than in the capture of expertise. As Boris Hauray discusses in this volume, COI did not become a central category for analyzing the influence of the industry on medical practice until the following decades. In 1984, the most prestigious medical journal, the *New England Journal of Medicine*, decided to ask its authors to disclose any commercial interests that could potentially affect the opinions or results reported in their articles. This innovation was progressively taken up by all major biomedical journals. From the late 1990s onward, the generalization of disclosure statements in scientific articles and the analysis of documents obtained through litigations fostered the development in medical journals of a quasi-subfield of research on COI. The majority of these articles aimed at demonstrating that collaboration and financial ties with industries impact scientific practices and result in biased evaluation.

To better understand this move toward preeminence, and to discuss the present roles of COI as a category, as well as the price paid for its dominance, this chapter focuses on the debates about the role of pharmaceutical companies in the shaping of our knowledge of HRT and its dangers. It explores the question of influence from a viewpoint emphasizing the collective construction of knowledge, expertise, and public problems. The aim is therefore not to explore all the ways in which the actors of the HRT controversy – above all women's health organizations – problematized the risks of HRT and negotiated prevention, but to offer a two-sided exploration of the judicial archives produced around the compensation trials of the mid-2000s, looking at what they reveal about a) the paths of action taken by drug companies, and b) the uses of the category of COI.

HRT, a controversial therapy

Medical treatment for the menopause has never been a matter of consensus. Until the 1960s, in the United States, gynecologists and endocrinologists were rather reluctant to agree to the idea of systematic interventions. As the historian Elizabeth Watkins recounts (Watkins, 2007), the prescription of HRT started to increase in the early 1970s. Two explanations have been proposed: the mounting investments in marketing and the resulting influence drug representatives gained on general practitioners (GPs); and the growing demand from women who had read about HRT in the women's press or in the feminist press, advocating hormones as ways of liberating women from the constraints of biology (Cooper, 1975).

This emerging legitimacy of HRT was nonetheless seriously challenged when, in 1975, researchers revealed a correlation between the use of estrogens and an increased incidence of endometrial cancer. The National Women's Health Network (NWHN) then allied with the FDA to mandate the producers of HRT preparations to distribute flyers informing the women about these risks. A way out of this first crisis was found only in the 1980s, when experts started to advocate a combined use of estrogens and progesterone in order to benefit from the latter's protective effect against endometrial cancer. Finally, the main explanation for the increasing use of HRT in menopausal women in the late 20th century was the changing meaning of the therapy, from a source of wellbeing to a tool for the prevention of health risks. In the 1980s and 1990s, HRT emerged as a powerful means to avoid age-related pathologies: osteoporosis, cardiovascular disorders, and putatively Alzheimer's disease (Leysen, 1996; Kaufert and Lock, 1997).

However, feminists and the women's health movement contested this generalization. During the 1980s, the NWHN persistently lobbied Congress and the health administration to increase their support for research on women's health, including the evaluation of hormone uses and their long-term effects. In 1991, under the Clinton administration, the National Institutes of Health (NIH) finally launched the WHI, then the largest clinical study in history, which included one branch focusing on HRT (WHI, 1998). The WHI was supposed to end in 2005 but, as mentioned above, in 2002 its main branch, which included women who had not undergone a hysterectomy and had received Prempro®, a drug manufactured by Wyeth, was stopped. Given the number of cancer cases and cardiovascular events reported, the organizers of the trial had come to the conclusion that it was not ethical to pursue the administration of such dangerous substances.

The WHI thus confirmed that HRT could increase the incidence of cancer in treated women – a problem discussed since the 1960s. However, the main surprise of the trial was that HRT was also increasing the incidence of cardiac and vascular adverse events. This opposed all claims grounding the second main motive for the preventive use of HRT – a risk reduction strategy launched in the 1980s on the basis of smaller and non-controlled studies. In addition, in the context of the WHI, HRT also seemed to increase the risk of dementia. Quality of life was moreover barely improved since the only benefit for which statistical significance was demonstrated regarded sleeplessness. The one single piece of good news for the proponents of pharmaceutical treatment of the menopause was the confirmation of HRT's value in reducing the risks of osteoporosis.

The end of the WHI initiated a new hormone crisis in which the main concern was no longer the medicalization of the menopause or women's quality of life, but the merit of drugs in managing health risks and the consequences of aging. Moreover, in contrast to the 1970s crisis, the HRT controversy had immediate and large-scale effects on the market. In the late 1990s, in the United States, Wyeth products accounted for 70 percent of all HRT prescriptions. The 60 million packets that Wyeth sold of its two leading brands – Premarin® (conjugated estrogens) and Prempro® (conjugated estrogens + progestogens) – earned the firm more than $800 million annually. The fall in sales was dramatic: by 2008, Wyeth, which was still in command of the market, was selling only 10 million packets.[2]

Court actions soon followed. In 2009, 8,400 cases were filed against one or the other of Wyeth's products, allegedly for causing breast cancer, strokes, and heart disease. Even if the majority of first instance rulings were in favor of the plaintiffs (with the consequence that Wyeth put aside more than $1 billion in anticipation of settlements), all appeal procedures have still not been exhausted. Judicial archives are therefore in most instances not accessible. In 2008, however, the *New York Times* and *PLOS Medicine*, a biomedical research publication, filed a right of access legal request, which resulted in the release of documents that are now a part of a specific "Prempro litigations" collection within the University of California San Francisco Industry Documents database.[3] These include numerous archives about Wyeth's practices of scientific marketing, and its relationship with a communication firm called DesignWrite (Sismondo, 2018).[4]

The rise of scientific marketing in post-war pharmacy

DesignWrite was much more than a communication partner. Given the breadth of its functions, it is more appropriate to label it a "scientific marketing organization" (SMO) by analogy with the contract research organizations that have proliferated for 20 years in the pharmaceutical sector, becoming obligatory subcontractors of all major drug companies in charge of the organization of their clinical trials (Mirowski and Van Horn, 2005; Sismondo, 2008; 2018). One of the critical consequences of the changing organization of the sector has been the mounting importance of outsourcing practices, especially when research and development are concerned (Gaudillière, 2015). Outsourcing critical steps in the screening of drugs is now considered financially good practice since it makes it possible to: (a) externalize the risks of organizational failure associated with efficacy trials; and (b) reduce costs via competitive bidding.

DesignWrite is a SMO because it organized a vast palette of activities and interventions at the boundary between research and marketing for the benefit of Wyeth. Scientific marketing emerged as a key feature of the drug sector in the 1960s. Operations aimed at influencing physicians' prescription practices escalated during the following decades, becoming a distinct and fundamental feature of health markets and pharmaceutical capitalism (Gaudillière, 2021). Within this context, scientific marketing encompasses two different dynamics (Gaudillière and Thoms, 2015). The first, typical of an economic sector bound to the mediation of professionals, is a systematic mobilization of research results on drugs, their toxicity, and their therapeutic effects, to convince prescribing physicians of a given product's usefulness. The second, which is more general, is the inclusion of market research as a normal component of marketing activities. For drug companies, this has meant not only expanding the surveillance of sales and competitors, the evaluation of publicity campaigns, and the modeling of consumption prospects but also investing in social studies of medical professionals and of their relationship with their patients/clients. Scientific marketing is therefore much more than a mere scaling-up of inter-war drug publicity.

The emergence of scientific marketing practices within the rapidly expanding drug companies of the 1960s and 1970s is just one component of a more all-encompassing adoption of a new model of drug invention, production, and commercialization. The post-war generalization of *screening* as a linear organization of drug development – from the synthesis of candidates' chemicals to the design of publicity material – relied on major structural novelties such as legal acceptance of patenting and its systematic use to ensure a monopolistic control of active substances or the reorganization of clinical research along the model of controlled clinical trials. The rise of scientific marketing was thus based on a palette of new tools taken up by the industry: the organization of expert meetings, the publication of journals mimicking the academic press, and the large-scale recruitment and training of drug representatives who visited the targeted physicians at their consulting rooms.

A case in point from the 1970s is the Swiss industry that has been documented through company archives and that in many ways echoes the pharmaceuticalization of the menopause (Gerber and Gaudillière, 2016). In the late 1960s, the firm Geigy started to subscribe to the monthly bulletin on pharmaceutical sales provided by Intercontinental Marketing Services (IMS). Although costly, this information supplemented in-house numbers to make three levels of accounting possible: (a) comparing the sales of Geigy's products with their main competitors; (b) assessing the size of the "global" psychotropic drugs domain as one single class that included tranquilizers, neuroleptics, and antidepressants; and (c) exploring physicians' motives for prescription, especially the connections they made between products, symptoms, and indications. This decision was integral to a more general transformation of Geigy's in-house research activities, aimed at strengthening the basis for strategic planning by reorganizing the management of products around divisions based on therapeutic classes as overarching units of research, development, and marketing.

In 1966, accordingly, the division for neuro- and psycho-pharmaceuticals, established within the marketing department, prepared an overarching assessment of the market situation in psycho-pharmaceuticals, a key sector for Geigy. The data collected confirmed the strength of the firm in antidepressants, but also revealed its weakness in tranquilizers and – more importantly in the eyes of the authors – in the realm of drugs targeting disorders common in general practice. Such discussions led to an internal reassessment of priorities and, in particular, of the relationship between tranquilizers and antidepressants. By the late 1960s, Geigy's management endorsed the idea that to surpass the success of its first antidepressant (Tofranil®) and ensure future growth of income and profits, the objective was to lessen the divide between the tranquilizer and antidepressant niches; such blurring would best be achieved by inventing an antidepressant that targeted the mild mental complaints encountered in general practice.

As scientific marketing expanded within the newly merged company Ciba-Geigy, more intense coordination between marketing and research began. Two levels were concerned: daily promotion and advertising campaigns involving the selection of clinical data, its shaping and translation into promotional material; and long-term planning, selection of market segments, and specific requests for new trials and/or product development. Specialized committees and tools were established to ensure integrated decision-making. For instance, at weekly meetings in Basel, the heads of both the clinical and marketing departments would discuss products already on the market, as well as those in the clinical trial pipeline. The resulting memos circulated throughout all upper levels of management. They summarized major decisions about the surveillance of sales, the production of publicity material, the organization of campaigns, and the outcome of prioritized trials. Medical marketing information was however given so much priority that an entire "product management information" section was set up. This second-line of coordination focused on the follow-up of trials and the preparation of material for medical representatives. The section was placed under the authority of a physician and a pharmacist. It was responsible for writing regular – almost weekly – information sheets for the managers of the sales force, who would, in turn, use them in meetings with their representatives.

The impact of this combination of technologies can be best appreciated using the example of Ludiomil®, a new antidepressant that Ciba-Geigy introduced onto the market in the early 1970s. In July 1975, while a new Ludiomil® campaign was being prepared, the information material designed by Ciba-Geigy for its representatives targeted a peculiar form of depression called "larved depression". The category "larved" or "masked" depression was not entirely new. It had surfaced in the psychiatric literature in relation to atypical cases, such as depressed states in which the typical triad of depression was difficult to identify owing to the emphasis on somatic symptoms that typified such patients' complaints.

The new profiling of Ludiomil® as an antidepressant with anxiolytic properties specially designed for the treatment of mild or masked depression in general practice was advanced through a major symposium Ciba-Geigy organized in 1973 in St. Moritz, a mountain resort, gathering most European psychiatrists interested in depression and a chosen core of GPs. The entire purpose of the St. Moritz symposium was to discuss masked depression. In spite of their heterogeneous views on etiology, nosology, and treatment, all the participants endorsed the term and agreed that the problem had great importance in routine practice. What is important here beyond the "classic" work with key opinion leaders (KOLs), is that this type of market construction did not translate "clinical facts" into "statements of promotional value", but tried to reveal a new target population, a new need for antidepressants rooted in the existence of a previously invisible (or non-existing) category of depressive patients. The main data for such framing of prescription were therefore not only the clinical trials, but also the market research surveys conducted by the firm, and its inquiries into physicians' diagnostic and prescription practices, which were extensively discussed in St. Moritz and in the ad hoc group for the promotion of masked depression therapy set up after the meeting.

The embedding of scientific marketing within the organization of industrial research, therefore, had three major consequences: (1) the production of a significant body of (industrial) knowledge regarding not only market shares and sales but also the multiple factors influencing prescription patterns; (2) the invention of new means of having the so-called marketing department and clinical research department collaborate with a virtuous circle in which the former's promotion campaigns drew on the results of the clinical investigations coordinated by the latter, while the latter took into account the expectations of the former in the design of their trials; and (3) a new hierarchy among physicians, with the emergence of KOLs, namely the biomedical elite, who were closely associated with the conducting of trials and legitimate enough to influence their colleagues and the experts working for the regulatory agencies (Gaudillière and Thoms, 2013; 2015).

DesignWrite and Wyeth, an SMO at work

In 1996, when Jeff Solomon, the manager in charge of the HRT line at Wyeth approached DesignWrite, the aim was not simply to hire consultants to act as brokers for the publication of scientific articles discussing the advantages of HRT. The first request was for instance the organization of a speakers' bureau, that is to say, a panel of 10 permanent consultants and 300 members identified as medical opinion leaders, preferably involved in the Premarin® trials. These individuals would speak at local events attended by front-line prescribers. Their role would be to discuss the problems associated with the menopause, the benefits of HRT, and the optimization of dosage to fit the needs of individual patients.[5] In the words of DesignWrite, they would "influence physicians to increase HRT, maintain relations with influential prescribers, and test the most compelling information". The functions of the SMO were to select the speakers, organize their meetings and communication events, and prepare documents for GPs including a specific information kit.

On the basis of this experience, DesignWrite became Wyeth's main contractor for the scientific marketing of the Premarin® line of products. By the end of 1999, the negotiation of the 2000–2001 communication plan thus included a broad palette of activities: (a) the writing and placement of 20 articles on various aspects of HRT; (b) the production of new information material for Wyeth's drug representatives, including the circulation of a newsletter on new developments in research; (c) the organization of panels and thematic sessions during major medical conferences; and d) the surveillance of sales, market shares, and novel initiatives from competing firms, with a special eye on the ways in which Wyeth products were described in the medical and pharmaceutical press, in health databases, and online. [6] The proposed contract thus amounted to $2.5 million.

This externalization of activities previously falling in the province of the marketing department included critical aspects of Wyeth's marketing research. In February 1997, following another request by Solomon, DesignWrite drew up a plan to collect new data on the HRT market since – as stated in its proposal – "HRT continues to be a drug [sic] in search of disease".[7] What was at stake was less the optimization of physicians' prescriptions than the crafting of "new marketing alliances", beginning with a radical "expansion of direct publicity to women". To this end, DesignWrite would investigate "women's health care" in general: the list of competing products to monitor included all sorts of alternatives to HRT and the use of synthetic steroid hormones, starting with phytoestrogens and plant medicines. The issues considered ranged from the motives for non-compliance with HRT and doctors' advice or women's views of the menopause, to the reasons for variations in local physicians' prescription patterns.

The alliances hoped for did not only target women, they also included other non-medical actors like health maintenance organizations and pharmacists. In 1998, DesignWrite secured another "surveillance" contract regarding the pharmacists.[8] The point of departure was a new law with a provision on patients' information (the 1996 Health Insurance Portability and Accountability Act) that granted pharmacists a role as advisors, along with the authority to replace brand medicines with generics (unless the prescribing physician had formally banned such substitution). Wyeth then asked DesignWrite to monitor the sources of information used in drugstores: the national pharmacopeia, the various compendia produced by medical and pharmaceutical professional bodies, and the newly created commercial databases on drugs (First Databank and Medi-Span). Again, the aim was not simply regular reviewing but a mandate "to take all means necessary to correct errors and misrepresentations".

One specific event the SMO proposed in 1997 was a "national consensus meeting", with multiple aims: (a) increase the awareness of HRT's positive impact on cardiovascular and cancer risks beyond its well-known effect on the risk of osteoporosis; (b) endorse the growth of HRT prescription as beneficial to health; (c) take the lead in establishing relationships with other sources of prescription guidelines, first of all managed care; and (d) reinforce the scientific status of Wyeth products in order to meet the biggest challenge Wyeth envisioned at the time: the approval of HRT generics by the FDA.

The vision emerging from all these initiatives and reports (all issued before the 2002 crisis) was that of a promising market. DesignWrite thus reminded its client that "only" 12 to 32 percent of potential users were actual consumers, and that a Gallup poll had shown they were poorly informed about the menopause and its issues when they reached that age. The good prospects of the market were not limited to known benefits like reduced risks of osteoporosis or improved quality of life. They relied on the coming results of Wyeth's clinical research focusing on aging with promises of improved cognitive capabilities, or of better care of Alzheimer's disease.

DesignWrite was thus a great help in handling the competition. Wyeth did indeed have two sources of concern: the arrival of HRT generics, and the marketing of a new class of drugs: selective estrogen receptor modulators (SERMs). Outsourced scientific marketing proved a key asset in handling both threats. In both instances, DesignWrite's contribution was to deconstruct their market and "reduce their niche" by playing on the uncertainties and risks these new products presented in comparison with the vast corpus of knowledge acquired on the whole Premarin® line.

For instance, in 1999, the competing firm Duramed was on the verge of putting Cenestin®, a generic of Premarin®, on the market. DesignWrite's campaign to minimize the prescription of Cenestin® was focused on several issues. First, it drew experts' attention to Wyeth's own products' value, with memos emphasizing the very small number of trials on Cenestin® (even though this is an absolutely normal state of affairs for a generic drug).

Second, it highlighted the fact that the FDA marketing authorization did not include the prevention of osteoporosis. In short, as the contract between Wyeth and DesignWrite clearly stated, the motto was: "don't trust anything less than Premarin®".[9] The agreed communication plan thus rested on a weekly surveillance of both products' sales.

One last aspect of the strategy was economic, with initiatives to reduce the financial incentives associated with the use of generics. Wyeth was ready to communicate its willingness to reduce its margin in order to negotiate with pharmacists an increase in their margins on the brand drug without increasing the price paid by patients and/or health insurances. In this way, pharmacists would no longer benefit from the substitution.

DesignWrite's handling of the SERM problem is even more revealing of the mangle of science and promotion in scientific marketing. Wyeth mobilized the SMO in order to "niche" the first SERM – raloxifene. In May 1997 its approval by the FDA for the prevention of osteoporosis was imminent. DesignWrite then offered to coordinate the publication of a corpus of articles covering the whole palette of Premarin®'s uses: osteoporosis, cardiovascular risks, Alzheimer's, colorectal cancer, and presenting Wyeth's flagship drug as the first SERM in history.[10] To niche raloxifene however meant in the first place casting doubts on its efficacy. DesignWrite thus insisted on the uncertainties originating in the raloxifene trials since they did not look at the patients' quality of life but focused on biological surrogate markers. In addition, the SMO took on board the fact that raloxifene was a parent drug of tamoxifen, another analog of hormones, then used for preventing breast cancer recurrence in spite of a ten-year controversy about its cardiovascular adverse effects.

Conclusion: COI, a problematic native category

In spite of this large palette of activities, the public uses of the archives from DesignWrite released in 2009 have paradoxically focused on only one dimension of the SMO's activities, namely ghostwriting and the documentation of individual COIs.[11] For instance, on August 4, 2009, in its main article on the affair, the *New York Times* just described some articles DesignWrite had prepared and channeled into academic publications, indicting the authors who had not been in charge of any aspects of the investigations, as well as the mistaken but reputable journals. The situation was viewed as unethical for two reasons: (a) the misconception originating in the fact that the formal authors were not authors at all; and (b) the evaluation bias and the putative false claims originating in the financial ties between these fictional authors, DesignWrite's employees who did the real job, and Wyeth. Similarly focusing on COI, *PLOS Medicine* used the Prempro® litigation papers in a broader study of the ways in which scientists were or were not disclosing their ties with companies in their publications focusing on a group of experts whose interests were known since they were involved in court cases against off-label prescriptions (Kesselheim et al., 2012). The conclusion was a disturbing but not so surprising recognition that non-disclosure was widespread.

If "scientific marketing" was already in place in the 1970s, at least as an in-house organization, if not as a network of competing "research organizations", why did the category of COI surface as central only during the latest HRT crisis and not during the previous "hormone scares"?

The answer to this question has probably less to do with the existence or non-existence of "COI" as a situation (meaning a system of dense financial and non-financial links between firms and the experts evaluating their products) than with changes in the status of the category. What the history of scientific marketing shows is that its generalization did indeed originate in a regime of knowledge production revolving around the big corporations and their commanding positions in organizing the majority of drug-centered clinical trials. While this form of industrial science did not create a complete monopoly, it definitely did result in strong asymmetries in the ability to frame issues and inquiries, to circulate and make visible specific results, and, finally, to accumulate the means of influencing regulators and prescribers. The process marginalized sources of expertise that had been important when the predominant way of regulating drugs was through medical professionals; for instance, the ability of GPs – who made up the bulk of prescribing physicians – to put forward claims about toxicity or efficacy, based on their daily experience. Finally, the expansion of scientific marketing made the proliferation of "COIs" almost inevitable since virtually the entire monopoly on the production of drug-related knowledge rested inherently on the blending between new industry-led drug research and marketing operations.

When it comes to the controversies about hormonal therapies, the increasing visibility of the category is however linked to two other processes. The first is peculiar to social movements and social critique in this area. In the 1970s, organizations in the women's health nebulae took a keen interest in the medicalization of women's bodies and the domination of men in the medical professions. Twenty years later, after the experience of HIV/AIDS mobilization, the same movements had become more science-oriented, developing their own expertise base and becoming deeply involved in debates about the best ways of reducing (individual and collective) health risks. The obvious consequence was renewed interest in expertise and in the problems of industrial bias. The second transformation process consisted of changes in the use of the category itself, with the mounting importance of COI in the legal and regulatory domains that Boris Hauray describes in this volume.

However, as discussed in the final chapter of this volume, the systemic nature of the problems originating in the industrial/corporate production of knowledge and expertise are barely reflected in the current meanings associated with the category. As a descriptive tool, COI is indeed mainly cartographic: pointing to the existence of links but saying nothing about their specific nature and the modalities of interaction involved. In order to take into account the ways in which industrial knowledge resonates with the processes of market construction and the diverse political economies at play in the logic of influence, one, therefore, needs additional tools.

The historiography and social studies of pharmacy have recently offered a variant of Gramsci's concept of hegemony to this effect (Rajan, 2017; Sismondo, 2018). Introduced to reflect upon the historical dynamics of capitalism and upon the complex, systemic, and dialectical relationship between the economic and the political, hegemony has accordingly been used in two different ways: firstly, as a way to recognize the domination of capitalistic firms and their interests in the framing of our pharmaceutical knowledge; secondly, as an encompassing category to explore the economic, political, and legal dynamics of health appropriation as well as its contestation. This suggests that hegemony may indeed shed some light on "pervasive powers" in the worlds of science, pharmaceuticals, and medicine as it reminds us that "capitalism" is not simply about profit and greed but that the logic of accumulation critically depends upon social and political "regimes of regulation" (Boyer, 2015).

Notes

1. A more in-depth comparison of the two crises can be found in Gaudillière (2020).
2. *New York Times*, "Medical papers by ghostwriters pushed therapy", August 4, 2009.
3. "Prempro litigations", https://www.industrydocuments.ucsf.edu/drug.
4. Sismondo (2018) similarly uses the HRT litigations papers to discuss the practices of ghostwriting and the ways in which contract research organization writers and planners handle key opinion leaders and authors signing the articles they produce.
5. DesignWrite Proposal to Wyeth, "Speakers' bureau meeting", August 6, 1996. Prempro Litigations, UCSF Library Drug Industry Documents.
6. DesignWrite to Wyeth, Proposal "Premarin® communication plan 2000–2001", September 1999. Prempro Litigations, UCSF Library Drug Industry Documents.
7. DesignWrite to Wyeth, Proposal "Competitive intelligence on HRT market", February 13, 1997. Prempro Litigations, UCSF Library Drug Industry Documents.
8. DesignWrite to Wyeth, Proposal "Pharmaceutical compendia surveillance program", April 9, 1998. Prempro Litigations, UCSF Library Drug Industry Documents.
9. Wyeth, PowerPoint presentation "Premarin® preemptive plan", February 11, 1999. Prempro Litigations, UCSF Library Drug Industry Documents.
10. DesignWrite to Wyeth, Proposal "Premarin® publication program", May 15, 1997. Prempro Litigations, UCSF Library Drug Industry Documents.
11. In this case, the medical press included in the PubMed database and the leading US national dailies (*New York Times, Washington Post, USA Today*).

References

Boyer, R (2015) *Économie politique des capitalismes. Théorie de la régulation et des crises*. Paris: La Découverte.

Cooper, W (1975) *Don't change: a biological revolution for women*. New York: Stein & Day.

Gaudillière, J-P (2014) 'DES, cancer, and endocrine disruptors: ways of regulating, chemical risks, and public expertise in the United States' in Boudia, S and Jas, N (eds.) *Powerless science? Science and politics in a toxic world*. New York: Berghahn Books, pp. 65–94.

Gaudillière, J-P (2015) 'Une manière industrielle de savoir' in Bonneuil, C and Pestre, D (eds.) *Histoire des sciences et des savoirs 3: le siècle des technosciences (dépuis 1914)*. Paris: Seuil, pp. 85–105.

Gaudillière, J-P (2020) 'Conflits d'intérêts, science industrielle et expertise dans les controverses américaines sur les usages des hormones sexuelles', *Sciences sociales et santé*, 38(3), pp. 21–47.

Gaudillière, J-P (2021) 'Pharmaceutical innovation and its crisis: drug markets, screening the dialectics of value', *Biosocieties*. Available at: https://doi.org/10.1057/s41292-021-00235-7 (Accessed: June 18, 2021).

Gaudillière, J-P and Thoms, U (2013) 'Pharmaceutical firms and the construction of drug markets: from branding to scientific marketing', introduction to the special issue of, *History and Technology*, 29(2), pp. 105–115.

Gaudillière, J-P and Thoms, U (eds.) (2015) *The development of scientific marketing in the twentieth century: research for sales in the pharmaceutical industry*. Studies for the Society for the Social History of Medicine. London: Pickering & Chatto.

Gerber, L and Gaudillière, J-P (2016) 'Marketing masked depression. Physicians, pharmaceutical firms, and the redefinition of mood disorders in the 1960s and 1970s', *Bulletin of the History of Medicine*, 90(3), pp. 455–490.

Kaufert, P and Lock, M (1997) 'Medicalization of women's third age', *Journal of Psychosomatic Obstetrics and Gynecology*, 18(2), pp. 81–86.

Kesselheim, AS, Wang, B, Studdert, DM and Avron, J (2012) 'Conflict of interest reporting by authors involved in promotion of off-label drug use: an analysis of journal disclosures', *PLOS Medicine*, 9(8), p. e1001280.

Leysen, B (1996) 'The medicalization of menopause: from "feminine forever" to "healthy forever"' in Lykke, N and Braidotti, R (eds.) *Between monsters, goddesses and cyborgs: feminist confrontations with science, medicine and cyberspace*. London: Zed Books, pp. 173–192.

Marcus, AI (1994) *Cancer from beef: DES, federal food regulation, and consumer confidence*. Baltimore: Johns Hopkins University Press.

Mirowski, P and Van Horn, R (2005) 'The contract research organization and the commercialization of scientific research', *Social Studies of Science*, 35(4), pp. 503–548.

Rajan, KS (2017) *Pharmocracy: value, politics, and knowledge in global biomedicine*. Durham: Duke University Press.

Sismondo, S (2008) 'How pharmaceutical industry funding affects trial outcomes: causal structures and responses', *Social Science & Medicine*, 66(9), pp. 1909–1914.

Sismondo, S (2018) *Ghost-managed medicine. Big Pharma's invisible hand*. Manchester: Mattering Press.

Watkins, ES (2007) *The estrogen elixir. A history of hormone replacement therapy in America*. Baltimore: Johns Hopkins University Press.

Women's Health Initiative (WHI) (1998) 'Design of the Women's Health Initiative clinical trial and observational study', *Controlled Clinical Trials*, 19(1), pp. 61–109.

Writing Group for the Women's Health Initiative Investigators (2002) 'Risk and benefits of estrogen plus progestin in healthy postmenopausal women. Principal results from the Women's Health Initiative randomized controlled trial', *Journal of the American Medical Association*, 288(3), pp. 321–333.

Part III

Mobilizations and controversies

"This Corporation Has 'Anesthetized' the Actors in the Drug Chain". Influence peddling and the normality of conflicts of interest in the Mediator® scandal

Solène Lellinger and Christian Bonah

In 2009, the French medicines regulatory agency at the time (the AFSSAPS) withdrew benfluorex (Mediator®) from the market because of its cardiopulmonary side effects. The drug – commercialized by the French pharmaceutical firm Laboratoires Servier – was used to treat diabetes and high cholesterol. It was also prescribed off-label as a weight-loss drug. The Mediator® scandal in France resulted in an overhaul of the country's regulatory system and an internal reorganization of its medicines agency and drug safety policies. As part of this process, the concept of conflict of interest (COI) entered private and public discourse to an extent hitherto unknown in France. Why and how did this concept increasingly come to be used to denounce the injustice of patient harm, to describe and analyze the transgression of norms relating to drug authorization and prescription, and to provide a key concept on which administrative reforms were based? Why and when did COI become, throughout the Mediator® scandal, the key lens through which drug scandals in the French medical sector are viewed and debated? And what are the consequences of placing COI in such a central position in these analyses and debates?

The Mediator® scandal offers an ideal case study through which to empirically explore the development of the concept of COI in France, for a number of reasons. These include the media attention it attracted, the intensity and duration of the scandal, from 2009 to 2021, and its regulatory and legal consequences. Furthermore, it allows us to address – over and above the political, legal, and media points of view – the question of why the concept of COI became so central. Did it supplant other possible ways of framing the debate? And how did COI impact – or not – the medical profession, considered as one of the actors in the drug chain?

At the same time, our analysis is less focused on the press headlines, whistle-blowers, and highly visible actors of the scandal as it is interested in ordinary medical practices and the systemic problems of COI that the Mediator®

10.4324/9781003161035-9

scandal has revealed. Following French writer Georges Perec, we are interested in the *"infra-ordinary"* aspects, a concept he describes as follows:

> In our haste to measure the historical, the significant, the revealing, let us not leave aside the essential: the truly intolerable, the truly unacceptable: the scandal is not the firedamp, it is the work in the mines. Social inequality is not worrying in times of strike, it is intolerable 24 hours a day, 365 days a year.
>
> (Perec, 1989, p. 10)

This chapter focuses on a time window running from the withdrawal of Mediator® from the market (2009) to the opening of the criminal trial of those involved in the scandal. Taking as our starting point the central statement made by the 4 administrative and parliamentary inquiry committees (the Inspectorate General of Social Affairs (IGAS), the Senate, and the National Assembly) conducted in 2011, which examined corporate influence, links and COIs, and illegal influence peddling during the introduction of the drug on the market and the 33 years during which it continued to be sold, we investigate how the trajectory of the concept of COI became central to the framing and analysis of the scandal. In particular, we are interested in better understanding how the concept of COI was perceived by ordinary actors in the drug chain, specifically prescribing physicians, and not only the medicine agency pinpointed by the administrative and parliamentary inquiry committees. And what did the medical metaphor of these actors being "anesthetized" imply in terms of constituting, analyzing, and defusing the scandal from the committees' point of view? Our central claim is that the Mediator® scandal shows how COI individualizes acts, responsibility, and lack of awareness about there being interests at play rather than looking at it as a systemic problem. In other words, we ask what COI – as an analytical concept in its situatedness – sheds light on and what it obscures.

How the concept of COI rose to prominence with the Mediator® scandal

To better understand how the concept of COI became a key issue in France in the context of the Mediator® scandal, we shall focus our attention on the period during which the parliamentary and administrative inquiries were carried out following the immediate management of the crisis in 2010 and before the opening of the criminal trial in 2019. It is during this period that the concept of COI (Abraham and Lawton Smith, 2003; Rodwin, 2011) evolved to become the central analytical framework of thinking.

The chronology of benfluorex can be divided into three phases (see Figure 9.1): the commercial lifespan of the drug from its approval to its withdrawal (1974–2009); the administrative and parliamentary inquiries

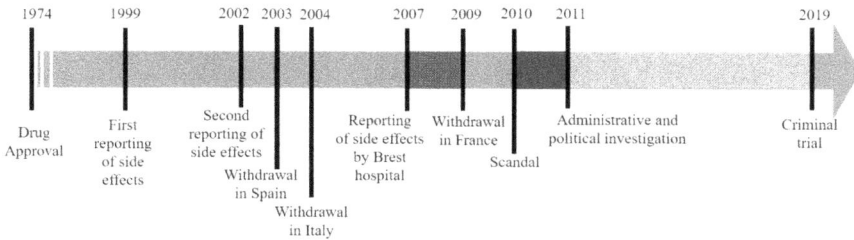

| 1974 | 1999 | 2002 | 2003 | 2004 | 2007 | 2009 | 2010 | 2011 | 2019 |

Drug Approval — First reporting of side effects — Second reporting of side effects / Withdrawal in Spain / Withdrawal in Italy — Reporting of side effects by Brest hospital — Withdrawal in France — Scandal — Administrative and political investigation — Criminal trial

Figure 9.1 Chronology of benfluorex, 1974–2021.

that triggered regulatory changes (2011–2019); and finally the criminal trial focusing on the indictments of specific individuals (2019–2021).

The "S992" molecule was synthesized in 1968 by researchers working at Laboratoires Servier. In 1971, the World Health Organization assigned it the international nonproprietary name "benfluorex". Benfluorex was market approved by the Service Central de la Pharmacie (Bensadon, Marie, and Morelle, 2011b, pp. 628–33) – France's medicines agency of the time – in 1974, under the commercial name "Mediator®" for the treatment of metabolic disorders associated with carbohydrates and fats. The actual market introduction was pursued two years later, supported by a major promotional campaign. This drug started selling gradually in France (see Figure 9.2) and in more than 50 countries abroad including Italy, Spain, and a number of Latin American, Southern Asian, and African countries.

Side effects were first reported in France, in 1999 in Marseille and in 2002 in Toulouse. The reported cases concerned specific valvular heart

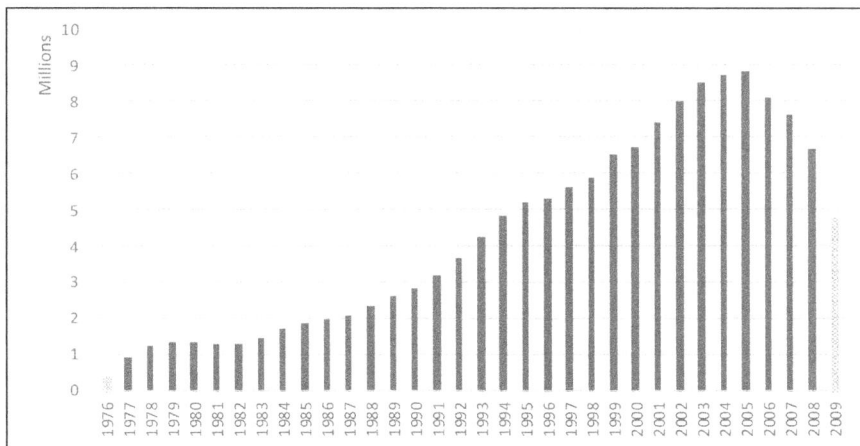

Figure 9.2 Number of packets of Mediator® sold in France by Laboratoires Servier (September 1976 to November 2009).

diseases (VHDs) in patients treated with benfluorex; however, these were not followed up. Further reported VHD cases in Spain and Italy led Servier to halt the drug's commercialization in those countries in 2003 and 2004 respectively, in anticipation of further pharmacovigilance investigations. The drug remained on the market in France and in many other countries in Latin America, Africa, and Asia in particular (see Figure 9.3).

A turning point was reached in France in 2007, when a team from Brest Hospital led by pulmonologist Irène Frachon reported several cases of pulmonary arterial hypertension (PAH) and drug-induced valvular heart disease (DIVHD). Between 2007 and 2009, retrospective adverse reaction data were repeatedly submitted to the AFSSAPS. After considerable resistance from the agency, this eventually led to the drug's withdrawal in November 2009.[1] At this stage, the withdrawal resembled that of any other drug: it was taken off the market, and physicians and pharmacists were simply informed that it was no longer available. Benfluorex users were not informed individually of possible serious adverse effects, in particular DIVHD, of the drug they had been taking. They were therefore ill-equipped to make any link between possible harm and their use of the drug.

A year later, in 2010, the publication of Irène Frachon's book *Mediator 150 mg. Combien de morts?* [Mediator 150 mg: how many deaths?] addressed not only the drug's (non-)safety but raised the hitherto unasked question of the number of benfluorex users who had suffered harm or died as

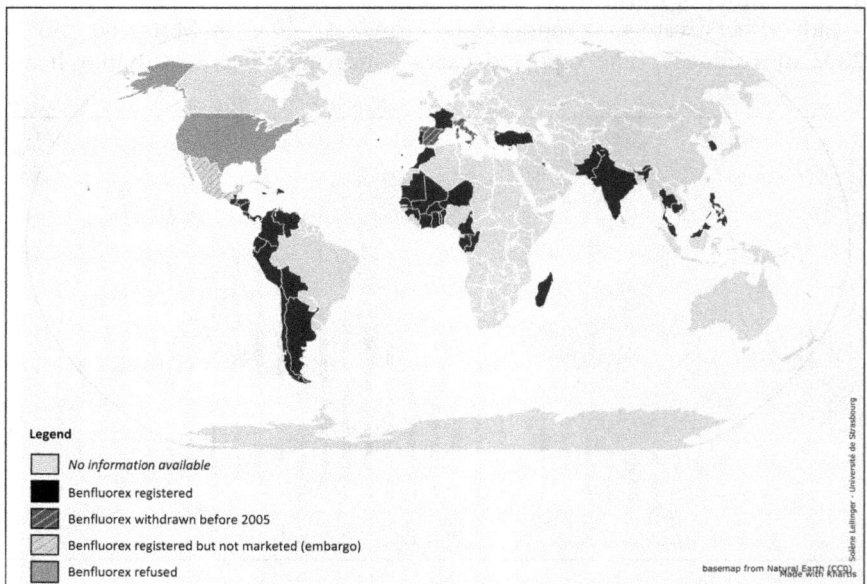

Legend

☐ No information available
■ Benfluorex registered
▨ Benfluorex withdrawn before 2005
▨ Benfluorex registered but not marketed (embargo)
▨ Benfluorex refused

basemap from Natural Earth (CC0)
Made with Khartis

Solène Lellinger - Université de Strasbourg

Figure 9.3 Countries in which benfluorex was being sold in 2009.

a result of using the drug in the light of its delayed withdrawal from the market. The book recounts Frachon's investigation, which led to the withdrawal of benfluorex, and describes the French medicines agency's resistance to the withdrawal. The aim of the book was to "enable people to understand how certain public health decisions are made in France" (Frachon, 2010, back cover). Frachon wrote and decided to publish her book because the drug's withdrawal had been so discreet and had therefore not received much attention in the press. Her motivation was that she "realized that the withdrawal had been carried out without providing any information for potential victims of this drug" (Faure, 2011, pp. 4–5). The book's publication and Servier's attempt to censor it by bringing a defamation lawsuit eventually generated increased media coverage of the drug's withdrawal and the scandal developed. Frachon became the face and the name associated with the withdrawal, thus personifying her struggle to achieve it. At the same time, answers to the question, "How many deaths have there really been?" began to surface, with an initial estimate being given by Flore Michelet in her pharmacy thesis in June 2010, in which she concluded that:

> According to the studies carried out, it would seem that in recent years there have been between 150 and 250 hospitalizations each year in France, directly linked to toxicity of Mediator® and resulting in about 30 deaths. If we multiply this by 30, representing the number of years the drug was on the market, the number of deaths could be between 500 and 1,000.
>
> (Michelet, 2010, p. 106)

From Gérard Bapt's article in the online version of *Le Monde* (Bapt, 2010) and calls by members of parliament for further inquiries, to a survey carried out by the French health insurance fund that backed up Michelet's initial mortality estimates, full disclosure of elements amounting to what would become the Mediator® scandal were finally published in an article entitled "Mediator® could be responsible for between 500 and 1,000 deaths in France" in *Le Figaro* on October 14, 2010 (Jouan, 2010). The withdrawal of Mediator® moved up the media agenda and became a public scandal.

The second phase of what had now become the Mediator® scandal centered on the administrative and parliamentary inquiries that were carried out and that triggered changes in response to evident shortcomings in the regulatory system. The inquiries and subsequent analyses converged to frame the Mediator® case in key terms of interests, COIs, and influence peddling.

On November 29, 2010, the IGAS, a French government agency that supervises public health administrations, was asked by a parliamentary committee and the Minister for Labor, Employment, and Health to investigate the Mediator® case.

The IGAS was established in 1967 as "the French Government's audit, evaluation and inspection office for health, social security, social cohesion, employment and labor policies, and organizations".[2] The IGAS investigation was carried out very rapidly – it took barely six weeks – and was extensive. The committee of inquiry analyzed the regulatory lifespan of benfluorex and identified major dysfunctions in France's medicines regulatory system. The IGAS report concluded in January 2011 in four points:

> Laboratoires Servier has from the onset of the drug's development endeavored to position Mediator® in a manner that is out of step with its pharmacological reality (1);
> The French Medicines Agency responsible for the drug has been inexplicably tolerant of a drug with no real therapeutic efficacy (2);
> The pharmacovigilance system has been incapable of analyzing serious risks that have become apparent in terms of Mediator®'s cardiotoxicity (3);
> Finally, the ministers responsible for social security and health have been slow in managing the withdrawal of medicines that have an insufficient medical benefit, leading in the case of Mediator® to results that are the opposite of those sought (4).
> The committee of inquiry underlines the following three provisos:
>
> - the report concerns a single drug, and even if the committee of inquiry offers a number of basic explanations for the serious failures observed, it warns against any hasty generalization of its analyses;
> - the report recalls the difficult job performed by all those involved in health safety;
> - while the report is, in some of its passages, inevitably technical, the committee of inquiry has constantly borne in mind during its work the tragic human cost. The sick and deceased are the only ones who will be the judges of the debates on which the committee proposes to shed light.
>
> (Bensadon, Marie, and Morelle, 2011a, p. I)

The IGAS report specifically pinpointed first of all the firm's marketing strategy, which presented what was, in reality, an amphetamine as a treatment for metabolic disorders. The three following incriminations, aimed at identifying the dysfunction of a government institution, related above all to the fact that Mediator® remained on the market for more than 30 years. Three sections are devoted to "the agency's incomprehensible tolerance with regard to Mediator®", "serious deficiencies in the pharmacovigilance system", and lastly the "vicissitudes in the reassessment of Mediator®". Three concluding remarks emphasize how Servier acted to keep the drug on the market through a set of influence-peddling actions described as the "anesthetic" of the system. The term "anesthetized" appears in the report's final conclusions:

> To use an expression that came up several times in the testimonies gathered by the committee of inquiry, this corporation "anesthetized" the actors in the drug chain and even, according to two former MAA [marketing authorization applications] committee chairs, "completely pulled the wool over their eyes".
>
> (Bensadon et al., 2011a, p. 121)

The report, published on January 15, 2011, triggered a major reform of France's medicines regulatory system and led to a number of significant legal and administrative changes (Butler, 2011, p. 169). These included the so-called "Bertrand Law" to strengthen the safety of medicines and health products, adopted in December 2011, the demise of the existing medicines regulatory agency (the AFSSAPS), and the creation of a special compensation fund (amending financing law number 2011-900 of July 29, 2011). Last but not least, the report led to a series of legal proceedings and in particular 2 criminal trials that were eventually combined and opened in September 2019, involving more than 4,000 complainants.

Through investigative inquiries, discussion forums, and legislative action, policymakers and medical sector stakeholders, under the impetus of the health minister Xavier Bertrand, pushed an already-existing principle to greater prominence in the debate: that of a public declaration of interests. This principle, together with the introduction of compulsory provisions on transparency (disclosure) imposed on the industry, was held up as a crucial value and a key solution.[3] On the day the IGAS report was delivered, Xavier Bertrand stated: "You are aware of the American system, the Sunshine Act. This same approach will be adopted in France" (Hauray, 2018, p. 54). This political response to what was a major crisis of the health and medicines system was based on a diagnosis that was both medical and political: the disease that needed to be treated was called "conflicts of interest". We have adopted the two definitions of COI proposed by Boris Hauray: the breaches of norms uncovered by the inquiries and investigations relate to a situation where "a person responsible for making a judgment or taking a decision in the interest of others risks being unduly influenced by a secondary interest" (Hauray, 2015, p. 71). And, more generally, the influence of specific interests, in particular economic interests, on health-related knowledge, practices, and policies, and of the implications of their problematic.[4]

The first IGAS investigation was followed by a second one (Bensadon, Marie, and Morelle, 2011c) and, in the same year, by two inquiries carried out for the National Assembly (Door, 2011) and the Senate (Hermange, 2011). The publication of the IGAS report led to an intensification of the media coverage. This in turn sparked a strong response from parliament in the form of the two inquiries, which brought the scandal into the political arena (Figure 9.1). The concept of COI is cited three times in the Senate report:

> A conflict of interest is a situation of interference between a public service mission and the private interest of a person contributing to the exercise of that mission, when that interest, by its nature and intensity, may reasonably be regarded as likely to influence or appear to influence the independent, impartial, and objective exercise of his or her functions.
>
> (Hermange, 2011, p. 89)

> The experts are unaware of the legal scope of the concept of conflict of interest and do not imagine that their relationship with one of the parties could be considered incompatible with the case they are dealing with. The notion of objective impartiality is clearly unknown to most experts, who think of the link of interests only through the notion of subjective impartiality, which is much more restricted.
>
> (ibid., p. 68)

> The lack of a legal culture among scientific experts leads them not to measure all the consequences of a failure to declare interests. For most of the experts who participate in the procedure through their scientific analysis, but who do not take a direct part in the final decision, the notion of conflict of interest still appears to be a bureaucratic formalism.
>
> (ibid., p. 69)

The Senate's inquiry was instigated in response to what was coming to be seen as a "crisis of public confidence in the drug" (ibid., p. 7). The committee of inquiry was chaired by François Autain, and its report was written by Marie-Thérèse Hermange. The National Assembly's social affairs committee set up its own inquiry at almost the same time; the author of its report was Jean-Pierre Door. It was in the discussions and reports of these two inquiries that the concept of "conflicts of interest" made its first real appearance, from which it went on to become omnipresent. Initially, a number of different terms and expressions were used to describe the phenomenon, including "influence", "competition between the public interest and private interests", "link" or "conflict of interests". However, the development of the concept in the course of the inquiries contrasts strongly with its sporadic and marginal use during the first two phases of the scandal. In this political phase, its function changed, and it became the preferred principle for framing the debates. The parliamentary inquiry reports, like the IGAS report, aim to explore and explain the concept, but more importantly, they attribute to it a third function: that of managing the observed dysfunctions.

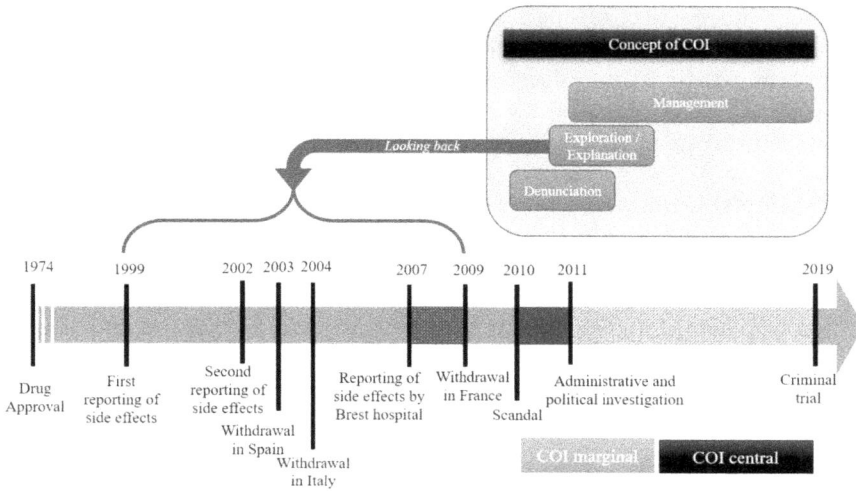

Figure 9.4 Evolution of the concept of COI.

Guarding against COIs implies, in this context, a better management of the systemic and structural influences that tarnish public confidence in the health system.

In the view of the Senate committee, the "anesthesia" is caused by ignorance of the "legal scope of COI". From the initial alert to the parliamentary inquiry reports, COI as a concept moves from a marginal to a central position in the debates. Its status also changes: COI is initially a form of denunciation it becomes a means to explore and explain the scandal, in the second phase, and it finally mutates into a form of crisis management (see Figure 9.4).

The ordinariness, and "normality" of COIs: Perceptions of (little) concerned actors

The reports of the four administrative and parliamentary inquiry committees carried out in 2011 focused primarily – in line with the roles of these administrative and political bodies – on the public health administration and its experts and the relationships between industry and France's medicines agency. However, the actors in the drug chain who the reports suggested had been "anesthetized" comprised many other professionals beyond the industry and the agency. Hundreds of ordinary physicians had been informed about benfluorex, canvassed to evaluate and prescribe the drug, and could have decided – as some, including Georges Chiche in Marseille and Irène Frachon in Brest, did – to follow up and report possible adverse effects.

The concept of COI had begun its administrative, political, and judicial career, as described above. But how did the medical professionals most directly concerned perceive interest links and conflicts? Prescribing physicians had a role as mediators between industry and patient interests, and could in principle be held accountable for individual drug prescription and consumption. The pharmaceutical industry's interest links with the medical profession are wide-ranging. They include sales representatives and their medical visits, sponsorship of medical societies, and advertising in medical journals, as well as gifts and incentives offered to individual physicians including funding for travel and participation in conferences around the world. How were these links, and sometimes conflicts, of interest perceived by these ordinary actors who were part not only of a drug chain but also of the systemic organization of the entire sector of pharmaceuticals and medical devices and services?

On October 4, 2011, the French National Medical Council (CNOM) organized a debate in Paris on "How to restore confidence?" of drug users troubled by the public unfolding of the Mediator® scandal. In the light of the observation that the Mediator® scandal was still causing a stir, CNOM leaders were concerned about the potential damage to physician–patient relationships that COI debates could cause at a very general and systemic level. The CNOM's conclusion was that there was a crisis of confidence, and the political and administrative response in the form of legislative and regulatory reform were both "top-down" responses intended not only to remedy the transgression of societal norms (influence peddling) but also to contain the shockwaves of the Mediator® scandal (the "firedamp" analogy referred to in the quote from Georges Perec). They certainly concern the professional and democratic representatives of physicians and the French population, but they tell us little about the day-to-day perception of practitioners in the field. What did physicians and future physicians think about COI in the context of the Mediator® scandal, especially when CNOM representatives were proclaiming the overall credo of "this concerns all of us" (Legmann, 2011, p. 3)?

To investigate physicians' everyday perceptions of COI in the context of the Mediator® scandal, we conducted a three-part empirical field survey. This aimed to clarify "from the bottom up" what physicians and future physicians thought of the Mediator® scandal, and whether COI played a similarly central role for them. In this section, we describe and compare the results of three surveys: a qualitative survey of second- and third-year medical students; elements of a sociological survey on the practices and perceptions of French cardiologists, as discussed in Solène Lellinger's PhD thesis (Lellinger, 2018); and finally the results of a survey conducted in March 2011 by the communications group BOZ on behalf of the pharmaceutical industry.

In October 2011, out of the 30 second- and third-year medical students interviewed, none were able to say when and where the scandal occurred, to specify the type of drug involved, or to summarize elements of the issue debated in the media over the previous year. At most, the word "Mediator" vaguely evoked a "case" that some of them had heard of. Although limited and qualitatively non-representative, this survey showed that students in their second and third year of medical studies – in other words, future health professionals in the making – knew almost nothing about a case that according to the CNOM "concerned all physicians". In observing the medical students' indifference and their feeling of "not being concerned by the case" we do not seek to criticize them. They had only recently completed an intense and highly competitive year of study that involves thousands of students following distance learning courses, the content of which they have to learn by rote rather than understanding in order to answer sets of multiple-choice questions, the ranked results of which determine whether or not they will get into medical school. These are difficult conditions in which to transmit to students starting out in their profession an attitude that encourages and places value on critical and independent thinking. Our observation of indifference and lack of concern raises the question of when and how to transmit to future practitioners the capacity to feel concerned and to think critically.

Nor is the observation intended to be a fundamental criticism of present-day medical training per se. It aims, rather, to underline the gap that existed between the media's treatment of the case, the statements made by professional and political representatives, and the real-life experience of young, highly motivated future physicians. In contrast to the inquiry report's analysis of "anesthetized" drug chain actors, the medical students seem instead to demonstrate a basic lack of knowledge and information about the political and societal questions that surfaced in the Mediator® scandal. And messages indicating to them that they indeed were (or should be) concerned by drug scandals in their relationship to patients are cruelly missing from medical training programs. Although some medical student associations are actively trying to change practices and to distance the pharmaceutical industry from medical training (AMSA, 2015; Collectif la Troupe du Rire, 2015; Scheffer et al., 2017), they remain, in the light of our interviews, a small minority.

A second survey was conducted in the framework of Solène Lellinger's PhD thesis, entitled "Therapeutic innovation and drug accidents. Sociogenesis of the benfluorex scandal and conditions for the recognition of an emerging pathology: drug-induced valvular heart disease" (Lellinger, 2018). A quantitative and qualitative survey of 173 French cardiologists, administered in the form of an electronic questionnaire and conducted in two steps in 2012 and in 2015, explored four aspects: (1) practitioners' initial and further training; (2) their consulting practice, work, and physician–patient relationships; (3) their diagnostic practice (pathologies perceived as the most frequent and their knowledge of VHDs); and finally (4) their knowledge about DIVHD and their experiences with benfluorex in particular.

The physicians surveyed in 2012 (Group A) were considerably older than those who took part in the 2015 survey (Group B), and they worked mainly in private practice whereas the physicians in the 2015 survey worked predominantly in hospitals.

Asked about their overall perception of the pharmaceutical industry (see Figure 9.5) a majority of the cardiologists surveyed in 2012 (51.39 percent) considered industry information needed to be verified, whereas in 2015, the majority (42.57 percent) said they had conditional trust. Less than 10 percent of cardiologists questioned trusted the pharmaceutical industry whereas roughly one-third were critical of it (31.94 percent for Group A and 24.75 percent for Group B). The survey showed that two-thirds of cardiologists had a critical view of the industry or thought its information needed to be verified. This would appear to contradict the view expressed in the inquiry reports that Servier had "anesthetized" physicians. However, when the cardiologists were asked which sources of information they would use to verify the information produced by the pharmaceutical industry, they showed little awareness of the tools available, giving only a few examples. Between 2012 and 2015, respectively two and five years after the Mediator® scandal, "conditional trust" recovered its position. It has to be said,

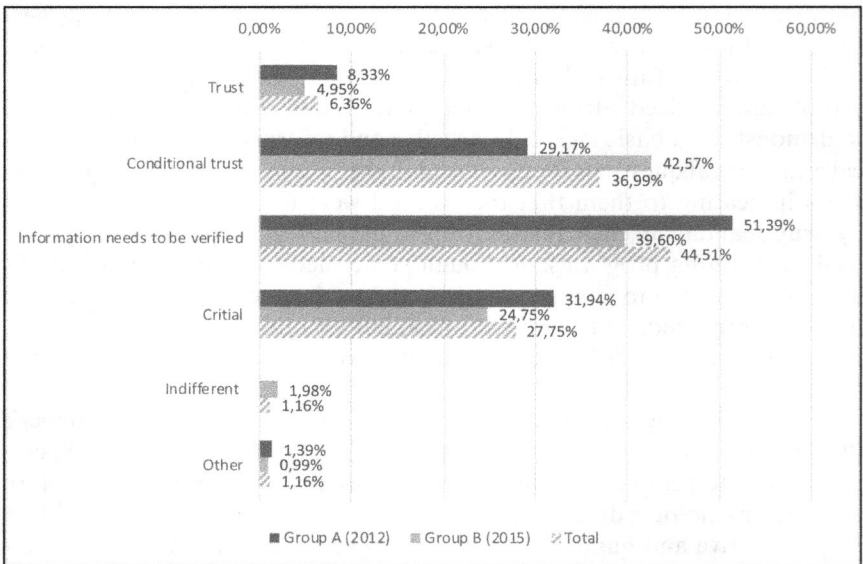

Figure 9.5 Cardiologists' overall perception of the pharmaceutical industry.

however, that although in 2015 nearly half of cardiologists surveyed stated that they trusted or conditionally trusted the pharmaceutical industry, this is at best an approximate result given the different survey population. (Even though the 2015 survey population was younger and more public-hospital oriented, its trust in the pharmaceutical industry was higher than the 2012 survey's population.) The survey indicates that although the cardiologists saw themselves as having a critical or "need to verify" attitude, yet they displayed little knowledge of the sources they could use to exercise this critical attitude, and thus appear to fall short, in practice, of their stated goal. Physicians' overrated self-confidence in their fundamental skills and resources tends to be contradicted by their lack of familiarity with resources available to critically check the information production by pharmaceutical firms. Their overconfidence makes them vulnerable to the corporate efforts to "anesthetize" the actors of the drug chain and dulls their judgment. In other words, physicians sometimes are not only voluntarily misled by pharmaceutical firms, but rather their professional attitude contributes to misleading them.

In the qualitative section of the survey,[5] almost half the cardiologists who answered the question, "How do you perceive the Mediator® case?" considered it to be an important health issue. At the same time, however, the same proportion of them also thought it was a case that had been exaggerated by the media. One practitioner's comments sum up the considerations of a number of cardiologists: "This case is just a smokescreen intended to divert the media from something that was becoming too much of a hot topic (the Dominique Strauss-Kahn scandal) by directing people toward a medical scandal about which they could unanimously agree". Other comments included: "Panem et circenses, there's nothing new about this", and a suggestion that the Mediator® scandal was "much ado about nothing; the small number of valvulopathies probably doesn't justify it". Verbatims such as "We're overdoing it! Hypothetical and wacky variable announcement figures. Let's also stop making cars! 3,500 deaths per year!" or "I've never prescribed the drug. I did not detect any valvulopathy. Patient anxiety. Suspicion of the pharmaceutical industry. Complexity and failure of the AFSSAPS. Abusive mediatization. Do more ultrasound scans and increase my income" indicate the cardiologists' uneasiness and their professional defensiveness. Furthermore, they illustrate not only a lack of the necessary skills and knowledge among those cardiologists who indicated conditional trust and a need to verify information, but – in the case of a fraction of these – that they seem to be merely paying lip service to the notion of verification: "A case that has been very poorly handled by the media and has caused a lot of damage to the image of drugs, whereas the precautions taken by the labs are rather excessive at the moment".

The depth of the cardiologists' trust in and dependency on the pharmaceutical industries is clear from this cardiologist's comment in the 2015 survey:

> This scandal has had lasting negative effects on relations between the pharmaceutical industry and physicians. While it has certainly improved a number of unjustifiable situations, it has above all had a negative impact on partnerships between manufacturers, physicians, and clinical research activities about which there is nothing shocking. All those who had "business" relations with the industry but tried to remain independent in their opinions and prescribing practice have been penalized by the Bertrand Law and its inevitable consequences (the law on transparency). Currently, major COIs persist between some opinion leaders and the industry, in a pseudo-transparency that does not deceive anyone ("interest links" forms abound and they are well filled-in, but it is always the same people who are invited to speak at the labs' symposia). Meanwhile, a sheet has to be signed for every coffee offered by a lab (verified last week at a meeting of therapeutic trial investigators), there is no more funding for publishing scientific posters, and invitations to conferences for young researchers have dried up. We just have the impression that everyone, virtuous or not, will pay dearly for the Mediator® scandal, but that the less virtuous will quickly find a solution.[6]

A coffee, a poster, an invitation to attend a conference – COI situations like these seem normal in a physician's world. From initial medical training to therapeutic trials, collaboration is widespread and unremarkable. As the above quotation highlights, in the aftermath of the Mediator® earthquake, a kind of scale of COIs has arisen, in which a distinction is made between the ordinary, everyday COIs in medical practice and even their normality, and the individual situations pointed at. As the survey results analyzed above indicate, physicians genuinely consider they can verify information and COIs, although their responses as to how they actually do so hint at serious doubts about whether this happens in practice.

Our third field of inquiry into physicians' perception of the pharmaceutical industry follows the lead of an email sent on March 24, 2011, to the entire community of physicians registered with the French Medical Council, inviting them to respond to a survey on the impact of the Mediator® scandal on practitioners' relations with the pharmaceutical industry, their patients, or the health insurance system. The survey was conducted by an organization going by the name of Yssup Research Institute, on behalf of the communications group BOZ. The survey was being conducted as a result of "the news and media coverage of events surrounding the Mediator® affair [that] leads us to wonder about the potential impact of such an affair on healthcare players in their daily practice" (BOZ Group, 2012). It was intended as a tool to "assist a think tank composed of healthcare players and industry leaders". Commissioned by the pharmaceutical industry, the survey aimed to clarify whether and how the Mediator® scandal had altered the relationship between practitioners and the pharmaceutical industry. Of the 676 responses obtained, 55 percent were from general practitioners, while only 1.33 percent were from cardiologists. Forty percent of the respondents said their perception of the pharmaceutical industry had remained good despite the scandal, while 37 percent considered that their view of the pharmaceutical industry had changed (23 percent said that their relationship had always been bad). The survey seems to indicate nevertheless that the case had had little impact on the visits they received from sales representatives and medical representatives, with only 14 percent of respondents indicating that they would like to receive fewer medical visits than before. The responses indicate that physicians had not become more suspicious of what is presented to them during these visits and would continue to participate in studies organized by pharmaceutical companies and to attend their conferences. In terms of their relations with patients, almost half of the practitioners (46 percent) who responded had perceived a change in the attitude of patients, who they said were more worried about the side effects of medical prescriptions. Congruent with the cardiologist survey we conducted, the Yssup survey shows a relatively unchanged everyday reality of pharma–physician partnerships and that physicians considered that their patients were much more worried than they were.

What emerges from these three field surveys is a discrepancy between communication discourse and reality on the ground. The responses of physicians and future physicians seem to indicate what one of the comments sums up fairly well: "The case is exaggerated. I have the feeling that the number of victims is considerably overstated. Media coverage often contains all sorts of nonsense or poorly explained arguments. There is no longer even a presumption of innocence".[7] For different reasons, physicians and future physicians did and do not really feel concerned by the Mediator® case, or question it. They feel remote from it, and as a result, show little interest in the experiences of victims and the potential harm COI could create. There is a disconnect between the importance invested in the concept of COI in administrative, political, and legal circles and the importance attached to it at the level of ordinary practitioners. To paraphrase our quote from Georges Perec, COI was worrying in times of scandal, but "its intolerability [in medical practice], 24 hours a day, 365 days a year" was dismissed by practitioners. COI was associated with individual responsibility, in particular of medical experts and opinion leaders, but not seen as being a systemic problem in the context of physicians' training and their day-to-day work. This conclusion does not, obviously, apply to the entire medical profession, and the methodology used does not guarantee the representativeness of the answers given. This reservation does not, however, disqualify the observation that a major discrepancy exists between the statements made by physicians' representatives – that "this concerns all of us" – and the results of three separate surveys, each of which indicates in its own way that, for many actors in the healthcare sector, the Mediator® scandal was a matter of concern "for others", far removed from them, and above all a matter of concern for another world – that of industry players, politicians, and experts, but not that of ordinary medical practitioners. Although almost one physician in two saw the impact of the scandal in their consulting rooms, reflected in changes in patient behavior, this seems to have had little influence on their own behavior, whether in relation to medical visits, conferences, or studies conducted by the pharmaceutical industry.

Interests, COI, influence peddling, and the law

In parallel with the administrative and parliamentary inquiries described in part one and the field studies investigating ordinary physicians' perceptions in part two, the Mediator® scandal entered the legal arena in the same year – 2011. What was seen by the administrative and parliamentary investigations as a systemic regulatory problem targeting France's medicines agency, and by ordinary physicians as a distant problem concerning individual medical experts, politicians, and opinion leaders, took on a new dimension, that of individual responsibility, in the legal proceedings and criminal trial. Part three of our analysis asks whether the judicial process of individualization of responsibility explains the sidelining of the fact that COI is a systemic problem in relations between the pharmaceutical industry and medical practitioners. In court individualization of responsibility allows other drug chain actors outside the judicial institution to revert the argument of the concept of COI enabling them to distance themselves from the problem, claiming that it concerns solely "other people [those trialed], but not me".

The judicial inquiry opened on February 18, 2011, after several complaints had been filed by benfluorex users since November 2010. Laboratoires Servier was accused of "improperly obtained authorization, deception as to substantial qualities (for the period from 1976 to 1995), deception on substantial qualities causing danger to human health (1995–2009), and fraud". In September 2011, Jacques Servier, the founder and CEO of Laboratoires Servier, was indicted, but his death in April 2014 halted legal proceedings against him. The legal investigation opened on the charge of manslaughter for which Jacques Servier was not prosecuted. In total, around 30 persons or institutions were indicted, including managers at Laboratoires Servier and at the medicines agency. Ten legal entities composing the nebula of Servier firms were represented by their managers.[8] The second group of defendants concerns the French regulatory body (the AFSSAPS) and specifically 13 individuals employed or solicited by the agency, in particular past experts from the agency and its past director. One defendant comes from the political circle, the French parliament. The general indictment of "deception aggravated by the endangerment of mankind as well as charges of interference and illegal taking of interests, complicity, and concealment of these offenses" highlights suggested illicit interactions between two small groups of individuals in industry and the agency.[9] Their suspected influence peddling has led to the two categories of indictment of "manslaughter by manifest breach of a duty of safety or care" and "aggravated intentional injury". The overall perception becomes here one of a very limited number of persons being involved in a nebular conspiracy.

In its indictments, the trial opened on September 23, 2019, clearly indicates that COI is a risk, not a legal charge or fact (see Box 9.1). It is not a judicial concept until acts or events have made the risk of COI real. In terms of law, the categories mobilized are corruption, illegal taking of interest, influence peddling, non-respect of impartiality, and finally what we could understand by "revolving doors" or regulatory capture (Carpenter and Moss, 2014).

In the legal arena, interests and COIs are individualized since they lead to reprehensible acts or events. Courtroom responses in the French legal system thereby transform the systemic problem of COIs between pharmaceutical companies and medical professionals into cases of specific individual misconduct. One result of this is the creation of the situation described in our survey in part two, in which professionals do not see themselves as being concerned by the problem. Another result is that the systemic problem in the relationship between the pharmaceutical industry and the medical profession is reduced to the (somewhat) scapegoat response of pursuing

---

Box 9.1 List of charges filed against the accused in the act of indictment for the Mediator® trial opened on September 23, 2019

- Undue obtaining of authorization
- Fraud
- Misleading information about the substantial qualities and risks inherent in the use of the Mediator with the risk of endangering man
- Manslaughter
- Involuntary injury with total incapacity for work
- Corruption
- Illegal taking of interests and conspiracy to commit the offense of illegal taking of interests
- Concealment of the offense of illegal taking of interests
- Influence peddling
- Unlawful participation of an official in a previously controlled institution

individual "black sheep". This critique of the legal system has been voiced regularly in the past in court suits concerning medical scandals (Kriegel, 2003). From a political point of view, regulatory measures would appear to manage the interactions of a nebulous collection of drug chain actors, while on the judicial side, a few individual cases are brought to court. The French medical journal *Prescrire*, which is independent of the pharmaceutical industry, recently and rightly raised an aspect that had been overlooked in the political and legal investigations: benfluorex prescribers who were nevertheless central actors "anesthetized" in a strategy for managing COIs that used transparency measures (declaration of interest and public consultation) as a defusing technique alongside a few trials where individuals are prosecuted to show an example to others (Prescrire, 2020). On the basis of our survey results, we argue that it would appear that transparency measures and legal prosecution are two public containment responses rather than attempts to actually resolve the COI situations that exist at the heart of the system under which medicines are produced, authorized for the market, and distributed in France.

Conclusion

When analyzed from the perspective of medical students and practitioners, as in this contribution, the Mediator® scandal raises the question of structurally normalized COIs in pharma–physician relationships that are represented as a dichotomy between the parliamentary inquiries on the one hand, where they are defined as industry players "anesthetizing" drug chain actors, and the legal proceedings on the other hand, where individual persons are prosecuted for corruption and influence peddling. When investigated, medical practitioners' perceptions of the admissibility of influence and COIs as part of ordinary professional life have broadly gone unchallenged in the political, judicial, and media accounts of the Mediator® scandal.

And yet they are pertinent to the question of how the industry can anesthetize or corrupt actors in the drug chain. This anesthetizing, understood as "rendering one incapable of resisting or being alert", is made possible and reinforced by the perception of the medical practitioners surveyed, who often see COIs as a problem that affects other people but not their own practice.

Moreover, this distancing and denial are reinforced by the justice system's treatment of legal transgressions, under which individuals – even if they were convicted for evident reasons – at the same time are scapegoated despite the conflict being systemic in reality. In exceptionally severe legal cases, COIs are identified as influence peddling, corruption, or illegal taking of interests. However, putting this with Perec, "infra-ordinary" physicians do not recognize themselves and their everyday practices as being concerned by the transgressions judged.

Notes

1. The withdrawal is described in detail in Solène Lellinger's PhD thesis (Lellinger, 2018, Chapter 4).
2. For more details, see the IGAS website: http://www.igas.gouv.fr/spip.php?article490
3. See Chapter 7 by Boullier and Greffion in this volume.
4. See Chapter 1 by Hauray in this volume.
5. For more details, see Lellinger (2018, Chapter 5).
6. For more details, see Lellinger (2018, Chapter 5). Source: Cardiologist survey 2012–2015, responses coded 193 (2015).
7. For more details, see Lellinger (2018, Chapter 5). Source: Cardiologist survey 2012–2015, responses coded 76 (2012).
8. SAS SERVIER (represented by Olivier Laureau), SAS ORIL INDUSTRIE (represented by Christian Sauveur), SAS LES LABORATOIRES SERVIER (represented by Olivier Laureau), SAS LABORATOIRES SERVIER INDUS-TRIE (represented by Christian Sauveur), SAS BIOFARMA (represented by Olivier Laureau), SARL BIOPHARMA, now SERVIER France (represented by Daniel Molle), SARL ADIR (represented by Emmanuel Canet), SARL IRIS (represented by Emmanuel Canet), SAS SERVIER MONDE (represented by Olivier Laureau), and SERVIER FORSCHUNG UND PHARMA-ENTWICKLUNG GmbH (represented by Christian Bazantay).
9. At the date of submission of this chapter, the trial hearings are closed but the judgment is still pending.

References

Abraham, J and Lawton Smith, H (eds.) (2003) *Regulation of the pharmaceutical industry*. New York: Palgrave Macmillan.

AMSA (2015) *Just-medicine curriculum. Evidence and recommendations for a model pharm-free curriculum*. Chantilly, VA: American Medical Student Association.

Bapt, G (2010) 'Mediator: combien de morts?', *Le Monde*, August 24 [online]. Available at: http://www.lemonde.fr/idees/article/2010/08/24/mediator-combien-de-morts_1402014_3232.html (Accessed: January 27, 2021).

Bensadon, A-C, Marie, E and Morelle, A (2011a) *Enquête sur le Médiator®: rapport définitif*. Paris: IGAS.

Bensadon, A-C, Marie, E and Morelle, A (2011b) *Enquête sur le Médiator®: tome annexe*. Paris: IGAS.

Bensadon, A-C, Marie, E and Morelle, A (2011c) '*Rapport sur la pharmacovigilance et gouvernance de la chaîne du médicament*', Rapport public. Paris: IGAS.

Butler, D (2011) 'France toughens conflict rules', *Nature*, 478(169) [online]. Available at: doi:10.1038/478169a (Accessed: January 27, 2021).

BOZ Group (2012) Impact de l'affaire Médiator en pratique quotidienne. Résultats auprès de 676 praticiens.

Carpenter, DP and Moss, DA (eds.) (2014) *Preventing regulatory capture: special interest influence and how to limit it*. Cambridge: Cambridge University Press.

Collectif la Troupe du Rire (2015) Pourquoi garder son indépendance face aux laboratoires pharmaceutiques? La Troupe du Rire.

Door, J-P (2011) Rapport d'information déposé en application de l'article 145 du règlement par la commission des affaires sociales en conclusion des travaux de la mission sur le Médiator et la pharmacovigilance. Paris: Assemblée nationale.

Faure, S (2011) 'La longue lutte d'Irène Frachon', *Actualités pharmaceutiques*, 50(504), pp. 4–5.

Frachon, I (2010) *Mediator 150 mg. Combien de morts?* Brest: Éditions dialogues.

Hauray, B (2015) 'Conflit d'intérêts' in Henry, E, Gilbert, C, Jouzel, J-N, and Marichalar, P (eds.) *Dictionnaire critique de l'expertise. Santé, travail, environnement*. Paris: Presses de Sciences Po, pp. 71–79.

Hauray, B (2018) 'Dispositifs de transparence et régulation des conflits d'intérêts dans le secteur du médicament', *Revue française d'administration publique*, 165(1), pp. 49–61.

Hermange, M-T (2011) 'Rapport d'information fait au nom de la mission commune d'information sur: "Mediator: évaluation et contrôle des médicaments". Tome 1: rapport', Public report. Sénat, June 28.

Jouan, A (2010) 'Le Mediator serait responsable de 500 à 1000 décès en France', *Le Figaro santé*, October 14 [online]. Available at: https://sante.lefigaro.fr/actualite/2010/10/13/10474-mediator-serait-responsable-500-1000-deces-france (Accessed: January 27, 2021).

Kriegel, B (2003) 'La responsabilité politique et pénale dans l'affaire du sang contaminé en France' in Bonah, C, Lepicard, É and Roelcke, V (eds.) *La médecine expérimentale au tribunal: implications éthiques de quelques procès médicaux du XXe siècle européen*. Paris: EDAC, pp. 359–374.

Legmann, M (2011) 'Pour ne plus jamais revivre le drame du Médiator ...', *Médecins*, 20, p. 3.

Lellinger, S (2018) Innovation thérapeutique et accident médicamenteux. Socio-genèse du scandale du benfluorex (Mediator®) et conditions de reconnaissance d'une pathologie émergente: les valvulopathies médicamenteuses. PhD thesis, University of Strasbourg.

Michelet, F (2010) Utilisation de nouveaux outils en pharmacovigilance: à propos du retrait du Médiator® (benfluorex). PhD thesis, University of Rennes.

Perec, G. (1989) *L'infra-ordinaire*. Paris: Seuil.

Prescrire (2020) 'La quasi-totalité des prescripteurs de Mediator® épargnés par les conséquences juridiques', *La Revue Prescrire*, 40(438), pp. 304–305.

Rodwin, MA (2011) *Conflicts of interest and the future of medicine: the United States, France, and Japan*. Oxford: Oxford University Press.

Scheffer, P, Guy-Coichard, C, Outh-Gauer, D, Calet-Froissart, Z, Boursier, M, Mintzes, B and Borde, J-S (2017) 'Conflict of interest policies at French medical schools: starting from the bottom', *PloS One*, 12(1), e0168258 [online]. Available at: doi:10.1371/journal.pone.0168258 (Accessed: January 27, 2021).

Chapter 10

For science, by science

The emergence and circulation of conflict of interest as a protest repertoire to fight against pesticides

Giovanni Prete, Jean-Noël Jouzel and François Dedieu

Nowadays, the condemnations of the harmful effects of pesticides on human health and the environment are a highly visible political cause in France. Many actors drive this cause, including environmental activists, victims' associations, investigative journalists, law firms, and concerned scientists. Over the past decade, throughout a series of controversies involving numerous substances (neonicotinoids, chlordecone, glyphosate, or succinate dehydrogenase inhibitors), they have criticized the lack of objectivity and the industry ties of the institutions in charge of pesticide assessment at both the national level (ANSES, French Agency for Food, Environmental, and Occupational Health and Safety) and the European level (EFSA, European Food Safety Authority). To denounce these phenomena, they often use the term "conflict of interest" (COI), which has become a central element of their protest repertoire.

This way of framing opposition to pesticides is relatively new in terms of the political history of these substances. French farmers used pesticides on a massive scale starting in the second half of the 20th century. From the 1960s, "pesticides were" part of the effort to modernize agriculture and, as such, received strong support from public authorities. Very soon after their widespread diffusion, these substances were denounced by unions and NGOs who criticized their effects on health and the environment, and the industrialization of agriculture in general. However, activists rarely brought up the pro-industry bias present in the pesticide risk assessment process and in pesticide regulation. The absence of this theme in their mobilization efforts is surprising when we recall that at that time it played a much bigger role in other countries. In the United States, especially, where agriculture already relied even more heavily on synthetic inputs, activists often expressed their doubt that regulatory authorities could act objectively without bending to pressure from powerful corporate interests.

10.4324/9781003161035-10

This transatlantic time difference invites us to examine more closely how the framework used to denounce pesticides evolved over time and circulated in different social contexts. This chapter explores the social conditions that led to the issue of industry influence on pesticide regulation becoming part of anti-pesticide activists' arsenal in France. We highlight three social processes that contributed to the emergence and diffusion of this issue: the institutionalization of risk assessment, the development of investigative environmental journalism, and the professionalization of environmental health advocacy organizations. All three have contributed to the successful framing of the fight against pesticides in terms of COIs. Within this framing, anti-pesticide movements in the United States and in France criticize the way scientific data are produced and used as part of marketing authorization procedures for these products. By doing so, they are helping to change the way pesticides are regulated, but they are also indirectly reinforcing the idea that the best way to control pesticides is to always rely on more science. This chapter is based on a survey conducted in France and the United States, using interviews with various people involved in the controversies surrounding pesticides (activists, researchers, lawyers, risk assessment professionals, victims' groups), as well as archival documents, most of which have been published.

Denouncing COIs in the fight against pesticides: The emergence of the pesticide industry's influence as a prominent issue

As several scholars have shown, the concept of COI emerged decades ago and has been used to describe different issues over time (Parascandola, 2007; Hauray, Chapter 1). Among anti-pesticide activists, this term is often used in a rather broad way to refer to the influence of firms on the regulation of pesticides and their capacity, in particular, to shape the production of scientific knowledge and expertise. This use emerged in the 1970s in the United States, where multiple consumer and environmental activist movements started to condemn pesticide-producing firms' ability to sell dangerous products, and their capacity for influencing risk assessments. These issues would spread internationally only gradually, becoming central in France 30 years later.

The US: The crucible of the denunciation of the pesticide industry's influence on regulation

Pesticides began to be used intensively in the United States at the beginning of the 20th century, encouraged by a coalition of actors working to promote more productive agricultural practices: the US Department of Agriculture (USDA), as well as a host of farmers' unions and researchers in the fields of agronomics and entomology (Whorton, 1974). The USDA was put in charge of approving these products by the Federal Insecticide Act of 1910, which banned the sale of pesticides whose plant protection properties differed from what was advertised on their label. In 1947, the Federal Insecticide, Fungicide, and Rodenticide Act (FIFRA) replaced this law and made it compulsory for industrial firms looking to put a new pesticide on the market to secure a preliminary license from the USDA. These licenses were based on an assessment of the products' health risks for exposed populations and for wild plants and animals.

As the work of various historians and political scientists (Dunlap, 1981; Daniel, 2007) has shown, the birth of the anti-pesticide movement in the United States paralleled the adoption of these early legislations. At first, this movement was made up mostly of agriculture experts and garnered little attention. It began to receive more publicity in the 1960s, at a moment sometimes described as the "toxicity crisis" (Vogel, 2012; Boudia and Jas, 2014). At the time, more and more controversies were coming to light about the health effects of the increasing presence of dangerous substances and technologies in the environment, with pesticides among these. In this respect, the publication of Rachel Carson's book, *Silent Spring* (1962), marked a turning point. It brought worrying information to light about the harmful environmental and health effects of the large-scale use of pesticides in food production and in the environment in general. Carson focuses on one pesticide in particular, dichlorodiphenyltrichloroethane (DDT). Although she mainly discusses its harmful effects rather than the strategies used by the companies that produced it to influence regulation, in a few passages she refers to this wider issue. Indeed, she criticizes the chemical industry's influence on university agriculture laboratories and on the USDA. To describe this influence, she does not use the term "conflict of interest" but talks about the "biases" in favor of industry displayed by many scientists assessing the harmfulness of these products.

Such themes went on to become central to the political debates that followed the book's release. A bestseller, *Silent Spring* received significant television coverage (Kroll, 2001), leading President Kennedy to assert his position on the matter. He claimed to stand with Carson, and in 1963 he created a special panel of the President's Science Advisory Committee to study the issue of pesticides. Congress also held a series of hearings, with the purpose of debating the conditions of the sale of pesticides and their risk assesment. The USDA received regular criticism, especially for its clear unwillingness to share the information in its possession about the harmful effects of pesticides with other administrative bodies (Bosso, 1987). At the end of the decade, a report from the Government Accountability Office sharply criticized the way the USDA had implemented the FIFRA, as well as its inability to effectively limit the environmental and health impacts of pesticides. In 1970, a new administration was created to assess pesticide risks and to authorize their sale in the place of the USDA: the Environmental Protection Agency (EPA). This was followed in 1972 by an overhaul of the FIFRA legislation, on the initiative of President Nixon. These institutional responses aimed to make pesticide risk assessment more objective, a clear response to the publication of *Silent Spring* and its political aftermath.

Questioning the influence that agricultural economic interests had on the institutions charged with regulating plant protection industry became a central issue for the actors involved in the fight against pesticides. Some of these actors were agricultural scientists who had long been engaged in denouncing the negative effects of these substances in particular. Among these was Robert Van den Bosch, a professional entomologist who had testified during the first major hearings against DDT in the late 1960s and early 1970s. In *The Pesticide Conspiracy*, a book published in 1978, he uses the term "pesticide mafia" to refer to the chemical industry's influence on the USDA and on entomological societies. Other players in the rapidly developing environmental movement also took an interest in this issue from the late 1960s. This included the Environmental Defense Fund (EDF), an association founded in 1967 to push for a ban on DDT (Dunlap, 1981). The EDF gradually expanded its field of action, and in the 1970s moved to block sale authorizations for certain organochlorine pesticides, including Aldrin and Dieldrin, on the grounds of alleged large-scale fraud that took place in some product risk assessments (Gillespie, Eva, and Johnston, 1979). Ralph Nader's Center for Study of Responsive Law, another key actor involved in the movement for tighter regulations on chemical products in the United States, raised similar criticisms at that time. In 1972, it published a well-researched and widely read report entitled *Sowing the Wind: Food Safety and the Chemical Harvest*, which took a critical look at industry influence on food and pesticide regulations. The report uses the term "conflicts of interest" to indicate a lack of neutrality in the laboratories hired by industry firms to conduct testing to secure authorization for their pesticides (Wellford, 1972, p. 351). It revealed that one of the leading laboratories that provided such services to chemical firms had submitted intentionally falsified toxicity data to public health authorities to hide internal organizational issues and to ensure client loyalty. This led to a lawsuit that lasted until 1983, as well as to congressional hearings that would play a central role in the development of EPA guidelines for producing and collecting data about pesticide toxicity (Jasanoff, 1990).

Throughout the 1980s, criticisms of corporate influence on the pesticide risk assessment process in the United States evolved in a context where the institutions in charge of regulating these products were growing weaker. The presidencies of Ronald Reagan and George H. W. Bush saw fewer resources invested in environmental protection (Fredrickson et al., 2018). The result was that social movements grew disenchanted with the idea that hazardous substances could be properly controlled by making risk assessment bodies stronger. While private research funding was on the rise,[1] these movements shifted their focus further upstream, to the production of the scientific data used in pesticide regulation, with the help of public health scientists. Several prominent figures got involved in organizations that opposed the negative environmental and health impacts of industrial activities. For example, Dr. Samuel Epstein, a researcher whose political importance has already been highlighted (Paehlke, 1981; Proctor, 1995), was directly involved in publicizing the dangers of pesticides. He served as an advisor to the Center for Study of Responsive Law for the above-mentioned *Sowing the Wind* report. More broadly, his own work was influential in drawing anti-pesticide activists' attention to the many dimensions of the COIs that influence pesticide regulation. Epstein used the concept of COI several times in his important and widely read work *The Politics of Cancer* (1978). In this book, he stressed the bias of USDA policies in favor of the interests of industrial agriculture organizations and denounced instances of fraud in laboratories involved in toxicological risk assessment. At the end of the 1970s, as part of a lawsuit, he obtained internal documents from asbestos-producing firms that provided him with a clearer understanding of firms' strategies with regard to science both within and beyond the asbestos industry (Epstein, 1978; 1979). In the years that followed, other documents revealed that these strategies were used with several toxic products. In the 1980s in particular, archives obtained during lawsuits against cigarette manufacturers[2] allowed journalists, activists, and researchers in public health[3] and the social sciences to understand the details of these firms' strategies for influencing scientific data. Activists drew on these revelations to broaden their criticisms against the pesticide industry's influence on regulation. They increasingly used the concept of COI to denounce the multifaceted industry strategies to leverage pesticide regulation and the production of scientific data itself.

In the 1990s, this broader framing of industry influence on the regulation of toxic substances led to debates within the environmental and public health scientific community about the declaration of interest policies. Such policies, which started to be implemented in biomedical journals in the 1980s (see Hauray, Chapter 1), were gradually adopted in public health, environment, and occupational health and safety journals, before becoming standard for all scientific disciplines (Resnik, Konecny, and Kissling, 2017; Daou et al., 2018). One of the first journals in this field to implement a mandatory policy of disclosing financial COIs was the *American Journal of Industrial Medicine*, in 1994, at the time headed by Philip J. Landrigan, a researcher who had worked on childhood exposure to pesticides. In 2003, *Toxicological Sciences*, the journal of the Society of Toxicology, also decided to adopt a disclosure policy (Lehman-McKeeman and Peterson, 2003), followed in 2005 by the leading journal *Epidemiology*, which had long been hostile to COI declarations. The systematic adoption of disclosure policies helped environmental activists to intensify their criticisms of industry influence on toxic substance regulations in general, and pesticide regulation in particular. Indeed, it has provided them with information to substantiate, in books or reports, "the hypothesis of a pro-industry bias in pesticide risk assessment" (see, for example, Fagin and Lavelle, 1996; Melnick and Huff, 2004; Sass and Needleman, 2004).

The late importation and circulation of COIs as a campaigning issue in France

French agriculture started to use synthetic pesticides at almost the same time as the United States, during the decades immediately after the Second World War. Along with mechanization, greater field sizes and the use of synthetic fertilizers, these chemicals constituted one of the pillars of French agricultural development policies (Fourche, 2004). However, the denunciation of corporate influence and COIs in pesticide regulation only gained prominence within anti-pesticide activists' repertoire at the end of the 20th century.

The first wave of public interest in the harmful effects of pesticides came after the publication of *Printemps silencieux*, the French translation of *Silent Spring*, in 1963, one year after the original edition was published in the United States. Roger Heim, a prominent biologist, well-known in the media for criticizing the environmental damage of technological progress, wrote the book's preface. In the 1968 edition, he stressed the responsibilities of pesticide producers and regulators:

> We arrest gangsters, we shoot at hold-up men, we guillotine assassins, we execute despots – or alleged despots – but who will jail the public poisoners who distribute every day the products that synthetic chemistry provides for their profit and their recklessness?
>
> (Heim, 1968)

This quote, however, does not accurately capture the controversies that surrounded the book's publication. These controversies focused essentially on whether or not the book's analysis on the dangerousness of pesticides was well-founded. On these grounds, *Printemps silencieux*'s conclusions on the dangers of DDT were attacked by researchers from the National Institute of Agricultural Research (INRA), France's leading agronomic research institution, as well as by representatives of the French Ministry of Agriculture, who were in charge of authorizing pesticides for sale (Fourche, 2004; Jas, 2007). The media also heavily discussed the book and received it with skepticism, "revealing the overwhelming trust in science to be found in the press at that time" (Trespeuch-Berthelot, 2015). Conversely, the book received a more enthusiastic reception among several activists' organizations, although interest in pesticides in general, and especially in industry influence on pesticide regulation, remained peripheral among these organizations. For instance, the French organizations promoting organic farming, very active in the 1960s, focused much more on the issues of land access policies or on the impact of the widespread diffusion of mineral fertilizers on soils than on the use of pesticides (Pessis, 2019). In the 1970s, a large "farmer-laborer" union movement was created to denounce the consequences of the so-called modernization policies promoted by the state and the majority farmers' union. This movement criticized the social consequences of industrialized agriculture and its dependence on pesticides. However, for this movement, the impact of pesticides on health and the environment, and industry influence on their regulation, were rarely considered a full-fledged issue. Instead, they were considered as one of the many examples of industrial capitalism's nefarious grip on agriculture and of farmers' growing dependence on technological progress (Martin, 2005; 2015; Pessis, 2019).

French activist organizations were not completely unaware of the US works and campaigns denouncing the influence of industry on pesticide regulation. They circulated among some of the environmental organizations that emerged in France in the 1960s and 1970s. For example, the newspaper *La Gueule ouverte*, which played an important role in facilitating the emergence of a left-wing libertarian environmental movement in France between 1972 and 1980 (Vrignon, 2015), mentioned one of Ralph Nader's lectures in its first issue. Nader's work was also known to the nascent French consumer movements (Lepiller, 2012, pp. 359–360). However, it was not until the late 1990s that the agrochemical industry's influence on pesticide regulation became central in the framing of opposition to pesticides.

At that time, several environmental health organizations, sometimes focused mainly on the fight against pesticides, began to dedicate important resources to denouncing the agrochemical industries' leverage on risk assessment agencies and on the production of scientific data on pesticide hazards. Several books that have highlighted and encouraged this shift in the protest repertoires of pesticide opponents have been published since then by NGO directors, scientists, journalists, and national political figures (see Box 10.1). Some achieved a great deal of commercial success and were accompanied by documentary films or television programs.

These books and their success indicate changing attitudes toward science and technology. Indeed, the groups that were most involved in denouncing pesticides in the 1970s mostly fought against techno-scientific progress in general, and its grip on farming practices (Bécot and Pessis, 2014). In contrast, the organizations that have been working on pesticides since the 1990s often express their faith in science's ability to provide objective risk assessments, as long as it is purged of the biases created by COIs between institutions and researchers on one side, and industry firms on the other. These books also illustrate the influence of US activists on French protest movements. In fact, most of the French authors mentioned above (see Box 10.1) cite US publications, including journalistic and activist writings about industry

Box 10.1   List of French books criticizing industry influence on pesticide regulation

1998: *Des lobbies contre la santé* ('Lobbies Against Public Health'), by Roger Lenglet and Bernard Topuz

1999: *La France toxique: Santé-environnement: Les risques cachés* ('Toxic France: Health and the Environment: The Hidden Risks'), by André Aschieri and Roger Lenglet

2004: *Quand les abeilles meurent, les jours sont comptés. Un scandale* ('When the bees die, our days are numbered. A public scandal'), by Philippe de Villiers

2005: *Alertes santé: Experts et citoyens face aux intérêts privés* ('Health Warnings: Experts and Citizens vs. Private Interests'), by André Cicolella and Dorothée Benoit Browaeys

2005: *Les empoisonneurs. Enquête sur ces polluants et produits qui nous tuent à petit feu* ('The Poisoners. A look at the pollutants and products that are killing us little by little'), by Vincent Nouzille

2007: *Pesticides, révélations sur un scandale français* ('Pesticides: Revelations of a French Scandal'), by François Veillerette and Fabrice Nicolino

2007: *Chronique d'un empoisonnement annoncé: Le scandale du chlordécone aux Antilles françaises, 1972–2002* ('Planned Poisoning: The Chlordecone Scandal in the French West Indies'), by Louis Boutrin and Raphaël Confiant

2008: *Le monde selon Monsanto. De la dioxine aux OGM, une multinationale qui vous veut du bien* ('The World According to Monsanto: From Dioxin to GMOs, a Multi-national that Wishes You Well'), by Marie-Monique Robin

2011: *Notre poison quotidien. La responsabilité de l'industrie chimique dans l'épidémie des maladies chroniques* ('Our Daily Poison: The Chemical Industry's Responsibility for the Chronic Illness Epidemic'), by Marie-Monique Robin

2012: *Tous cobayes! OGM, pesticides, produits chimiques* ('All Guinea Pigs! GMOs, Pesticides, and Chemical Products'), by Gilles-Eric Séralini and Abin Michel

2013: *La Fabrique du mensonge. Comment les industriels manipulent la science et nous mettent en danger* ('Manufacturing a Lie: How Industry Firms Manipulate Science and Put Us in Danger'), by Stéphane Foucart

2013: *Toxique Planète. Le scandale invisible des maladies chroniques* ('Toxic Planet: The Invisible Scandal of Chronic Illnesses'), by André Cicolella

2014: *La science asservie. Santé publique: Les collusions mortifères entre industriels et chercheurs* ('Science in Chains. Public Health: The Deadly Collusion Between Industry and Science'), by Annie Thébaud-Mony

2015: *Intoxication: Perturbateurs endocriniens, lobbyistes et eurocrates: Une bataille d'influence contre la santé* ('Intoxication: Endocrine Disruptors, Lobbyists, and Eurocrats: A Battle Between Influence and Public Health'), by Stéphane Horel

2019: *Et le monde devint silencieux* ('And the World Fell Silent'), by Stéphane Foucart

2019: *Le crime est presque parfait* ('The Almost Perfect Crime'), by Fabrice Nicolino

strategies to influence public health policy, beyond the sole issue of pesticide risks. In particular, they very often cite Robert Proctor's work on the tobacco industry (2011), David Michaels' work on chemical firms (2007), and the work by Naomie Oreskes and Erik Conway on energy producers (2010). They also sometimes directly discuss their personal relationships with scientists who are speaking out against the COIs that bias industry regulation in the United States.[4] Beyond such personal connections between French and US activists, major changes in the institutional and social context of French activism have supported this re-framing of the dangers of pesticides as an issue of industry influence and COIs.

A changing institutional and social context: Explaining the success of COIs as a protest repertoire

Putting the French situation into perspective with the US one, we identified three interrelated dynamics that have contributed to the rise of COIs as a prominent issue in the mobilizations against pesticides in France. These dynamics have involved pesticide regulation institutions, the media, and the field of environmental activism.

The institutionalization of risk assessment

In the United States, anti-pesticide organizations' focus on COIs was closely related to institutional changes in pesticide regulation. The new administrative bodies and regulatory assessment procedures put into place in the 1960s and 1970s to respond to concerns about the threats these substances posed to health and the environment created new expectations among social movements. They triggered a fresh round of activism, inclined to resort to legal action and attentive to the industry's influence on the regulation of toxic products. A similar phenomenon was observed in France, but 30 years later.

French pesticide policies have historically been the responsibility of the Ministry of Agriculture. For decades, it was in charge of assessing and managing all of these products' environmental and health risks and was able to fulfill this task following its own rules and procedures. Starting in the 1980s, however, the ministry's monopoly on these issues was called into question. As the creation of the European single market launched a first stage in the harmonization of pesticide risk assessments among its Member States, national-level authorities found themselves with less room for maneuver. Adopted in 1991, Council Directive 91/414/EEC formalized the common rules that all Member States must follow when considering authorization for pesticide sale requests. At the end of the 1990s, after a series of sanitary scandals, new public health and safety administrative bodies were created to shape risk assessment policies, further eroding the Ministry of Agriculture's monopoly and autonomy over pesticide regulation. In 1998, the French Food

Safety Agency (AFSSA) was created in France, followed four years later by the European Food Safety Authority (EFSA) at the European Union (EU) level (Demortain, 2009). Pesticides gradually came under the purview of these "new technocratic bureaucracies" (Benamouzig and Besançon, 2007). In France, this change was supported in particular by beekeepers' organizations, who claimed that neonicotinoid pesticides posed a serious threat to domestic honeybees. They focused particular attention on the Ministry of Agriculture's ComTox ("Commission on Toxics"), which had been responsible for pesticide risk assessments in France since 1943. In the 1970s, this commission had formed a "bee group", in charge of creating a "bee label" required for the authorization of pesticides to be applied during foraging periods. The commission, however, included interests that would be subject to any new pesticide regulations, with industry firms and the consultants handling their authorization requests allowed to participate.[5] This participation was regularly criticized by beekeeper unions and their political allies. The comtox credibility collapse led to its dissolution in 2006, with its pesticide risk assessment responsibility transferred to the AFSSA (Jouzel and Prete, 2017; Jouzel 2019).

Just as in the United States in the 1970s, such an institutional dynamic had several important consequences on anti-pesticide activism. By creating specific risk assessment agencies, lawmakers sought to protect themselves from accusations of COI (Boudia and Demortain, 2014). However, in many ways, the creation of these new agencies had the opposite effect. Indeed, it generated expectations among social movements and activist organizations in terms of the independence and transparency of the pesticide regulation process. The formalization of pesticide assessment rules, concerning either the nature of scientific information to be taken into account or to what extent industry firms could participate in the process, gave them levers to criticize industry influence on pesticide regulation. The work of Corporate Europe Observatory (CEO) illustrates this link between institutional transformations and activism. This NGO was founded in 1999 to scrutinize the influence of corporations on European public policy. Starting in the 2010s, it launched several campaigns and investigations that specifically looked at COIs in pesticide regulation. These investigations posit that the EU agencies do not respect the rules of transparency and independence they purport to uphold. These rules not only created expectations among the NGO activists but also helped them to access information. For instance, Stéphane Horel, a French journalist who worked with CEO, describes in detail in her works how she used transparency procedures to access European institutions' administrative files on pesticides and other toxic substances (Horel, 2015). In 2011, CEO launched an initiative to analyze COIs at the EFSA. More recently, CEO partnered with the NGO Pesticides Actions Network (PAN) Europe to uncover upstream industry influence on the tools and protocols that are used to conduct regulatory science (PAN Europe, 2018).

This denunciation of industry influence on pesticide regulation by CEO and other activist organizations received heavy press coverage in France. This increased publicity can be explained by the long-term changes in the press and the media that indirectly encouraged activists to invest time and resources in exploring the issue of COIs.

From activist journalism to investigative journalism

In the United States, environmental investigative journalism developed in the 1970s, and was readily critical of the chemical industry (Friedman et al., 1996; Friedman, 2015). Stories about plant protection industry firms committing fraud on their commercial authorization requests became a regular feature of investigative journalism, both in activist newspapers with limited circulation (such as *Mother Jones*, published by the Center for Investigative Reporting) and in national publications. In France, it was only over the course of the next two decades, with the environment becoming a regular topic in the media (Comby, 2009) and investigative journalism beginning to develop (Marchetti, 2002), especially in the public health field (Marchetti, 2010), that a similar journalistic treatment of information about industrial pollution emerged. Several journalists progressively covered this issue through the lens of COIs and the bias they introduce into risk assessment procedures. They highlighted that these are long-standing problems, and that scandals have significant moral, legal, and political ramifications. This treatment aligned with the prevailing ethos in professional journalism, allowing the journalists using it to base their criticisms on scientific authority, as well as helping them to not appear too close to environmental activist groups. It was also a way for journalists to set themselves apart in an increasingly competitive information market.

During the first decade of the 21st century, the issue of industry influence on pesticide regulation was initially taken up by independent journalists of a more investigatory bent, who tracked down COIs among scientists and administrators in charge of assessing these products' risks (Jouzel and Prete, 2016). More recently, this issue has begun to appear regularly in some mainstream newspapers. The way that the newspaper *Le Monde* has handled information about pesticides is a particularly interesting illustration of this shift. As the leading daily general-interest newspaper in France, *Le Monde* began to cover environmental issues in the 1970s, publishing its first dedicated "Environment" section in 1972. Up through the end of the 1990s, as in other national daily papers, coverage of these issues was intermittent,[6] peripheral, and handled by journalists who were often personally aligned with political ecology and environmental activist groups (Comby, 2009). In the 2000s, under the direction of editor-in-chief Éric Fottorino, this coverage intensified. The "Planet" and "Science" departments beefed up their staff and hired new generalist and scientific journalists. While their colleagues in more prestigious and established departments (International, Politics) sometimes suspected them of being political ecology "activists", they offered "critical expertise", combining a "refusal of political journalism with the ability to offer critique based on their technical knowledge of the issues at hand" (Neveu, 1999, p. 40), leading to more regular coverage of environmental issues. Stéphane Foucart was one of the journalists recruited during this period. He had a background in science and science journalism. Upon joining *Le Monde* in 2000 he initially covered technology, but later joined what would become the "Planet" department in 2009. Once in this department, he published several papers on the controversies surrounding climate change, the effects of neonicotinoids, and endocrine disruptors. While he did not specifically look at issues of COI in his early career, he came to write more and more on the topic as he became aware of industry firms' strategies for manipulating science. Many of his articles and books explore this theme, based on the work of French and US researchers, NGOs, and his own investigations. Foucart has published several articles about the impact of pesticides on health and the environment, where he questions the validity of regulatory agencies' toxicity tests. In 2018, along with Stéphane Horel, he received the European Press Prize's Investigative Reporting Award for a series of articles they wrote together using internal Monsanto documents obtained as part of a glyphosate lawsuit that was brought in California after the International Agency for Research on Cancer (IARC) classified the substance as a carcinogen in 2015. His work has been an important driver for communicating and legitimizing criticisms of pesticide regulation based on COIs in the French media. It has contributed to establishing a new way of discussing certain agricultural issues, which is not purely political or sector-based (as one might see in the "Agriculture" section of newspapers), but rather is based on a "scientific" point of view that goes beyond popularizing science and expressing scientific concepts in layman's terms.

The professionalization of environmental health organizations

In the United States, the coalitions of activists and scientists dedicated to environmental health protection that formed in the 1970s played a central role in placing industry influence on pesticide regulation in the spotlight. Similar coalitions emerged in France, but later. From the 1980s onward, French environmental organizations became more professional and invested their resources heavily in protest actions based on technical expertise (Ollitrault, 2001). Throughout the 2000s, a new sector formed in the non-profit activism field, made up of organizations that devoted resources and technical expertise to denouncing the harmful effects of environmental pollution on human health. Despite their diverse backgrounds, these organizations had something in common: they brought together activists who had a strong scientific social capital (researchers, doctors, science teachers).

They would base their claims on this capital, casting themselves as "whistleblowers" and drawing on the authority of science to condemn industry influence on the regulation of hazardous substances (Guilleux, 2015).

Within this sector, organizations have specialized in pesticides and played a prominent role. This was notably the case for the Mouvement pour la défense et le respect des générations futures (Movement for the Defense and Respect of Future Generations), founded by teacher and Greenpeace activist François Veillerette in 1996, and renamed Générations futures in 2011 (Jouzel and Prete, 2015). Its repertoire of contention includes science-based arguments and criticisms of COIs in the regulation and sale of pesticides. Over the last 20 years, Veillerette's editorial activity and the organization's alliances and campaigns have made it a force to be reckoned with. In 2002, with support from NGO PAN Europe (of which he became the administrator in 2003), he published *Pesticides: le piège se referme*, which popularized a lengthy review of toxicological and ecotoxicological literature. He followed this five years later with *Pesticides: révélations sur un scandale français*, co-written with Fabrice Nicolino, an environmental activist journalist who has written several books over the course of his career on the devastating effect of industrialized agriculture on the planet. This second book, which begins with the quote from Roger Heim's preface cited above, was the first fully documented critique of industry influence on pesticide regulation in France. It describes this influence at many levels: the personal relationships between industry firms and some representatives from the public authorities; the pressure from the Ministry of Agriculture and from industry lobbyists on expert agencies; and the financial ties between some scientists and industry firms. After selling tens of thousands of copies, it firmly established pro-industry bias in pesticide risk assessment as a serious issue for French organizations fighting against these products. Today, Générations futures continues to promote this issue, drawing on the work of journalists, activist organizations, and public health researchers, such as Annie Thébaud-Mony and André Cicolella. It also advocates for better procedures that would limit industry influence on pesticide regulation, as well as these companies' ability to "manufacture doubt".

Conclusion

This chapter describes three related dynamics – the institutionalization of risk assessment, the development of investigative environmental journalism, and the professionalization of environmental health advocacy organizations – that contributed to establishing the issue of industry influence as a central element of the protest repertoire of the US and French activists engaged in the fight against pesticides. For them, COI is a central concept that includes not only interpersonal financial relations between public agents and industries, but more broadly the corporate leverage on public expertise and decision covering different forms (manipulation of science, revolving doors, and so on). The concept is instrumental in connecting disparate phenomena, bringing to light various "incidents" or "scandals", and revealing recurring malpractices and repeat offenders. It helps these activists to generalize their criticisms of pesticide regulation and link them to other products (genetically modified organisms, endocrine disruptors, and so on), revealing the systemic nature of industry leverage on the expertise and scientific data used in formal risk assessment.

The critical discourse surrounding COIs is part of a particular historical process that began in the United States. We thus shed light, more generally, on how protest movements and the institutionalization of pesticide risk assessment are intertwined. New risk assessment procedures and expert agencies were created to manage pesticides and to respond to criticisms of COIs, just as in other sectors. The outcome of these institutional changes, however, was quite different than expected. They did not put an end to the denunciation of COIs. Instead, they encouraged activist organizations to shift their target further upstream in the risk assessment process, and to focus on the production of scientific data itself. What happened in France echoed what happened in the United States decades earlier: as risk assessment procedures became more formalized, they only created expectations of neutrality that were never met, to the disappointment of pesticide opponents. This chapter stresses that these expectations are largely based on the idea that risk assessment should be informed by "robust" and "pure" science. By condemning COIs and industry pressure on the production of scientific knowledge about pesticides' hazards, those who oppose their use are calling, more or less explicitly, for more science and expertise to guarantee that the environment and exposed populations will be protected. Over time, one may wonder whether or not this framing might disconnect the critiques of pesticides from a more radical condemnation of the hold of the ideology of technological progress over farmers' knowledge and practices.

Notes

1. The Bayh-Dole Act was passed in 1980, allowing universities to retain intellectual property rights to any innovations they develop using public research money. The law led to a boom in public–private partnerships, sparking a debate about the consequences this could ultimately have for researchers' independence.
2. Cipollone vs. Liggett (1988) was the first case to provide significant access to industry documents subpoenaed by the courts.
3. For example, Stanton Glantz, a researcher at the University of California. Sometimes called the "Ralph Nader of tobacco", Glantz has published several articles and has worked to make internal industry documents publicly available.
4. For example, influential journalist and activist Marie-Monique Robin describes how Devra Davis's work on industry influence inspired her own investigations. See https://blog.m2rfilms.com/la-fabrique-du-doute/#_ftn1 (last accessed December 23, 2020).

5. Of the 44 members of the Commission named in 2001 to serve in its penultimate term (of 3 years), there were 8 former industry representatives who had become consultants or directors of learned societies. It should be noted that this openness to economic interests went beyond industry representatives. For instance, the ComTox "bee group" was mostly made up of researchers who were also beekeepers themselves.
6. In 1982, for example, *Le Monde* replaced its dedicated "Environment" journalist with an editor who was only assigned to cover these issues part-time (Bodt, 2014).

References

Aschieri, A and Lenglet, R (1999) *La France toxique. Santé-environnement: les risques cachés*. Paris: La découverte.

Bécot, R and Pessis, C (2014) 'Improbables mais fécondes: les rencontres entre scientifiques critiques et syndicalistes dans les "années 1968"', *Mouvements*, 80(4), pp. 51–66.

Benamouzig, D and Besançon, J (2007) 'Les agences, alternatives administratives ou nouvelles bureaucraties techniques? Le cas des agences sanitaires', *Horizons stratégiques*, 3(1), pp. 10–24.

Bodt, J-M (2014) La 'cité écologique' dans l'espace public médiatique: trajectoires de controverses environnementales dans la presse généraliste française. PhD thesis, University of Toulouse II.

Bosso, CJ (1987) *Pesticides and politics. The life cycle of a public issue*. Pittsburgh: University of Pittsburgh Press.

Boudia, S and Demortain, D (2014) 'La production d'un instrument générique de gouvernement. Le "livre rouge" de l'analyse des risques', *Gouvernement et action publique*, 3(3), pp. 33–53.

Boudia, S and Jas, N (2014) *Powerless science? Science and politics in a toxic world*. New York: Berghahn Books.

Boutrin, L and Confiant, R (2007) *Chronique d'un empoisonnement annoncé: le scandale du chlordécone aux Antilles françaises, 1972–2002*. Paris: L'Harmattan.

Carson, R (1962) *Silent spring*. Cambridge: Houghton Mifflin Company.

Cicolella, A and Benoît-Browaeys, D (2005) *Alertes santé: experts et citoyens face aux intérêts privés*. Paris: Fayard.

Cicolella, A (2013) *Toxique planète. Le scandale invisible des maladies chroniques*. Paris: Le Seuil.

Comby, J-B (2009) 'Quand l'environnement devient "médiatique". Conditions et effets de l'institutionnalisation d'une spécialité journalistique', *Réseaux*, 157–158(5–6), pp. 157–190.

Daniel, P (2007) *Toxic drift: pesticides and health in the post-World War II south*. Baton Rouge: Louisiana State University Press.

Daou, KN, Hakoum, MB, Khamis, AM, Bou-Karroum, L, Ali, A, Habib, JR, Semaan, AT, Guyatt, G and Akl, EA (2018) 'Public health journals' requirements for authors to disclose funding and conflicts of interest: a cross-sectional study', *BMC Public Health*, 18(1), p. 533.

Demortain, D (2009) 'Standards of scientific advice. Risk analysis and the formation of the European food safety authority' in Weingart, P and Lentsch, J (eds.) *Scientific advice to policy making: international comparison*. Leverkusen: Verlag Barbara Budrich.

De Villiers, P (2004) *Quand les abeilles meurent, les jours de l'homme sont comptés*. Paris: Albin Michel.

Dunlap, TR (1981) *DDT: scientists, citizens, and public policy*. Princeton: Princeton University Press.

Epstein, S (1978) *The politics of cancer*. San Francisco: Sierra Club Books.

Epstein, S (1979) 'The politics of cancer', *Barrister*, 6, p. 11.

Fagin, D and Lavelle, M (1996) *Toxic deception. How the chemical industry manipulates science, bends the law and endangers your health*. New York: Carol Pub. Group.

Foucart, S (2013) *La fabrique du mensonge: comment les industriels manipulent la science et nous mettent en danger*. Paris: Editions Denoël.

Foucart, S (2019) *Et le monde devint silencieux. Comment l'agrochimie a détruit les insectes*. Paris: Le Seuil.

Fourche, R (2004) Contribution à l'histoire de la protection phytosanitaire dans l'agriculture française (1880–1970). PhD thesis, University of Lyon 2.

Fredrickson, L, Sellers, C, Dillon, L, Ohayon, JL, Shapiro, N, Sullivan, M, Bocking, S, Brown, P, de la Rosa, V, Harrison, J, Johns, S, Kulik, K, Lave, R, Murphy, M, Piper, L, Richter, L and Wylie, S (2018) 'History of US presidential assaults on modern environmental health protection', *American Journal of Public Health*, 108(S2), pp. 95–103.

Friedman, SM, Villamil, K, Suriano, RA and Egolf, BP (1996) Alar and apples: newspapers, risk and media responsibility', *Public Understanding of Science*, 5(1), pp. 1–20.

Friedman, SM (2015) 'The changing face of environmental journalism in the United States' in Hansen, A and Cox, R (eds.) *The Routledge handbook of environment and communication*. Abingdon-on-Thames: Routledge.

Gillespie, B, Eva, D and Johnston, R (1979) 'Carcinogenic risk assessment in the United States and Great Britain: the case of Aldrin/Dieldrin', *Social Studies of Science*, 9(3), pp. 265–301.

Guilleux, C (2015) L'institutionnalisation de la santé environnementale en France. D'une approche globale homme/environnement à la sectorisation d'actions de santé publique. PhD thesis, University of Aix-Marseille.

Heim, R (1968) 'Préface' in Carson, R (ed.) *Le printemps silencieux*. Paris: Plon, pp. 9–19.

Horel, S (2015) *Intoxication: perturbateurs endocriniens, lobbyistes et eurocrates: une bataille d'influence contre la santé*. Paris: La Découverte.

Jas, N (2007) 'Public health and pesticide regulation in France before and after *Silent Spring*', *History and Technology*, 23(4), pp. 369–388.

Jasanoff, S (1990) *The fifth branch: science advisers as policymakers*. Cambridge: Harvard University Press.

Jouzel, JN (2019) *Pesticides, comment ignorer ce que l'on sait?* Paris: Presses de Sciences Po.

Jouzel, JN and Prete, G (2015) 'Mettre en mouvement les agriculteurs victimes des pesticides. Émergence et évolution d'une coalition improbable', *Politix*, 111(3), pp. 175–196.

Jouzel, JN and Prete, G (2016) 'Des journalistes qui font les victimes? Le traitement médiatique des maladies professionnelles liées aux pesticides', *Études rurales*, 198(2), pp. 155–170.

Jouzel, JN and Prete, G (2017) 'La normalisation des alertes sanitaires. Le traitement administratif des données sur l'exposition des agriculteurs aux pesticides', *Droit et Société*, 96(2), pp. 241–256.

Kroll, G (2001) 'The "silent springs" of Rachel Carson: mass media and the origins of modern environmentalism', *Public Understanding of Science*, 10(4), pp. 403–420.

Lehman-McKeeman, L and Peterson, RE (2003) 'Guidelines governing conflict of interest', *Toxicological Sciences*, 72(2), pp. 183–184.

Lepiller, O (2012) Critiques de l'alimentation industrielle et valorisations du naturel: sociologie historique d'une 'digestion' difficile (1968–2010). PhD thesis, University of Toulouse II.

Marchetti, D (2002) 'Le "journalisme d'investigation". Genèse et consecration d'une spécialité journalistique' in Garraud, P and Briquet, JL (eds.) *Juger la politique. entreprises et entrepreneurs critiques de la politique*. Rennes: Presses universitaires de Rennes, pp. 167–191.

Marchetti, D (2010) *Quand la santé devient médiatique. Les logiques de production de l'information dans la presse*. Grenoble: Presses universitaires de Grenoble.

Martin, J-P (2005) *Histoire de la nouvelle gauche paysanne*. Paris: La Découverte.

Martin, J-P (2015) 'Des paysans environnementalistes? Comment les paysans contestataires se sont emparés de la question écologique', *Écologie & politique*, 50(1), pp. 99–111.

Melnick, RL and Huff, J (2004) 'Testing toxic pesticides in humans: health risks with no health benefits', *Environmental Health Perspectives*, 112(8), pp. 459–461.

Michaels, D (2007) *Doubt is their product. How industry's assault on science threatens your health*. Oxford: Oxford University Press.

Neveu, E (1999) 'Médias, mouvements sociaux, espaces publics', *Réseaux*, 98(7), pp. 17–85.

Nicolino, F and Veillerette, F (2007) *Pesticides: révélations sur un scandale français*. Paris: Fayard.

Nicolino, F (2019) *Le crime est presque parfait: l'enquête choc sur les pesticides et le SDHI*. Paris: Les liens qui libèrent.

Nouzille, V (2005) *Les empoisonneurs: enquête sur ces polluants et produits qui nous tuent à petit feu*. Paris: Fayard.

Ollitrault, S (2001) 'Les écologistes français, des experts en action', *Revue française de science politique*, 51(1–2), pp. 105–130.

Oreskes, N and Conway, E (2010) *Merchants of doubt: how a handful of scientists obscured the truth on issues from tobacco smoke to global warming*. Berkeley: University of California Press.

Paehlke, R (1981) 'Environnementalisme et syndicalisme au Canada anglais et aux États-Unis', *Sociologie et sociétés*, 13(1), pp. 161–179.

PAN Europe (2018) *Industry writing its own rules*. Report, Pesticide Action Network Europe [online]. Available at: https://www.pan-europe.info/sites/pan-europe.info/files/public/resources/reports/industry-writings-its-own-rules-pdf.pdf   (Accessed: January 26, 2021).

Parascandola, M (2007) 'A turning point for conflicts of interest: the controversy over the national academy of sciences' first conflicts of interest disclosure policy', *Journal of Clinical Oncology*, 25(24), pp. 3774–3779.

Pessis, C (2019) Défendre la terre. Scientifiques critiques et mobilisations environnementales des années 1940 aux années 1970. PhD thesis, EHESS.

Proctor, RN (1995) *Cancer wars: how politics shapes what we know and don't know about cancer*. New York: Basic Books.

Proctor, RN (2011) *Golden holocaust. Origins of the cigarette catastrophe and the case for abolition*. Berkeley: University of California Press.

Resnik, DB, Konecny, B and Kissling, GE (2017) 'Conflict of interest and funding disclosure policies of environmental, occupational, and public health journals', *Journal of Occupational and Environmental Medicine*, 59(1), pp. 28–33.

Robin, M-M (2010) *Le monde selon Monsanto: de la dioxine aux OGM, une multinationale qui vous veut du bien*. Paris: La Découverte.

Robin, M-M (2013) *Notre poison quotidien: la responsabilité de l'industrie chimique dans l'épidémie des maladies chroniques*. Paris: La Découverte.

Sass, JB and Needleman, HL (2004) 'Industry testing of toxic pesticides on human subjects concluded "no effect", despite the evidence', *Environmental Health Perspectives*, 112(3), pp. 150–156.

Séralini, G-E (2013) *Tous cobayes! OGM, pesticides, produits chimiques*. Paris: Flammarion.

Thébaud-Mony, A (2014) *La science asservie. Santé publique: les collusions mortifères entre industriels et chercheurs*. Paris: La Découverte.

Trespeuch-Berthelot, A (2015) 'La réception des ouvrages d'alerte environnementale dans les médias français (1948–1973)', *Le temps des médias*, 25(2), pp. 104–119.

Van den Bosch, R (1978) *The pesticide conspiracy*. New York: Doubleday.

Vogel, SA (2012) *Is it safe? BPA and the struggle to define the safety of chemicals*. Berkeley: University of California Press.

Vrignon, A (2015) 'Journalistes et militants. Les périodiques écologistes dans les années 1970', *Le temps des médias*, 25(2), pp. 120–134.

Wellford, H (1972) *Sowing the wind: a report from Ralph Nader's Center for Study of Responsive law on food safety and the chemical harvest*. New York: Grossman Publishers.

Whorton, JC (1974) *Before Silent Spring: pesticides and public health in pre-DDT America*. Princeton: Princeton Legacy Library.

Chapter 11

Conflict of interest, capture, production of ignorance, and hegemony

Conceptualizing the influence of corporate interests on public health

Henri Boullier, Jean-Paul Gaudillière,
Boris Hauray and Emmanuel Henry

In 2003, UK citizens not only discovered that more than 50,000 children were taking antidepressants in the country (most notably selective serotonin reuptake inhibitors (SSRIs)), but also that these prescriptions were based on off-label use of drugs licensed for depressive illness in adults and that there were solid suspicions that they could cause suicide. Facing growing public and media attention about the use of antidepressants, the British Medicines and Healthcare Products Regulatory Agency (MHRA) decided, in May 2003, to set up an expert working group to review the efficacy and risks of these drugs. In June, it concluded that the reviewed data did not demonstrate the efficacy of paroxetine (the United Kingdom's largest-selling antidepressant) in treating depression in under-18s, and that children taking it were twice as likely to have suicidal thoughts or to harm themselves than those with similar mental health problems not taking it. The MHRA decided to contraindicate paroxetine for under-18s and, in December, it did the same for all the other SSRIs except one (fluoxetine) that had a formal pediatric marketing license in the United States. In June 2003, the US Food and Drug Administration (FDA) issued a statement recommending that paroxetine not be used in treating depression in children and adolescents and in 2004 issued a black box warning on all the other SSRIs.

Since the marketing of Prozac®, the new class of SSRI antidepressants has been a huge commercial success and the influence of the producing firms – most notably in the form of conflict of interest (COI) – was rapidly pointed out as the main offender in this long-lasting situation of overprescribing or issuing risky prescriptions. Following this controversy, researchers have indeed revealed the existence of COIs that have caused bias in clinical trials conducted on antidepressants and other psychoactive drugs. For example, a group of researchers conducted a systematic analysis of the clinical

10.4324/9781003161035-11

trial results published in the major psychiatry journals and concluded that "author conflict of interest appears to be prevalent among psychiatric clinical trials and to be associated with a greater likelihood of reporting a drug to be superior to placebo" (Perlis et al., 2005). An inquiry report ordered by the House of Commons (House of Commons Health Committee, 2005) indicated that it was perhaps not a coincidence if the committee that decided to ban the use of antidepressants in children was the first one that had no expert with links to the producing firms sitting on it (before that, these experts could participate as long as they disclosed their links of interest). More broadly, the field of psychiatry was particularly targeted by COI accusations in the years that followed. Lisa Cosgrove and her colleagues have, for example, shown that 56 percent of the panel members of the highly influential Diagnostic and Statistical Manual of Mental Disorders (DSM-IV) "had one or more financial associations with companies in the pharmaceutical industry" (Cosgrove et al., 2006).

However, other ways of conceptualizing the influence of industrial actors have also emerged from this antidepressants case. First of all, it was pointed that the "blind" prescription of antidepressants to children was the result of the pharmaceutical firms' lack of willingness to conduct (costly and risky) trials on this population. Instead, they had chosen to rely on the evidence they had managed to gather from adults and from direct communication with physicians through their medical sales representatives. This "production of ignorance" had an even darker side. In June 2004, the attorney general of the state of New York decided to pursue GlaxoSmithKline (GSK) because the company had hidden the results of some clinical trials that showed that paroxetine was ineffective in treating depression in children and adolescents. In March 2004, a GSK internal memo was disclosed. It stated, as concerns two trials that had failed to demonstrate any separation of paroxetine from placebo: "It would be commercially unacceptable to include a statement that efficacy had not been demonstrated, as this would undermine the profile of paroxetine" (Rennie, 2004). A group of researchers compared all the published and unpublished data on SSRIs and children and showed that the inclusion of the latter was undoubtedly changing the risk–benefit profile of the drugs (Whittington et al., 2004). Second, it is also possible to assert that the late response from regulatory agencies to the off-label prescribing of antidepressants falls within a more general permissive attitude of these organizations, i.e., their "regulatory capture". At that time, the MHRA had for several years been facing repeated criticism for being too close to the pharmaceutical industry: it was run by a former executive director of medical affairs at Merck, it was entirely funded by industry fees, and it promoted its incomparable speed in reviewing new drugs (Hauray, 2006). Third, other analysts would consider it necessary to understand this controversy within a broader context, that of the hegemonic position of the pharmaceutical industry. They would underline the role of industry in building a shared Western ideology on psychiatric problems, in disease mongering, and in the pharmaceuticalization of social problems, as well as draw attention to the broader consequences of the articulation of capitalism and health issues.

For several decades, the social sciences have directly participated in the critical analysis of corporate influence on public health and in the controversies it generates. In order to evaluate the relevance of COI, not as a social category[1] but as an analytical tool for the social sciences, this last chapter compares this notion to three dominant conceptualizations of corporate influence in the public health sector.[2] The notions of capture, production of ignorance, and hegemony have the same high degree of generality and are used in very different sectors (not just in medicine, but also in environmental health, food, chemicals, etc.). They analyze partially overlapping social phenomena and are sometimes used indiscriminately, but they have developed in distinct historical and intellectual contexts and convey different conceptions of the influence[3] of corporate interests. This chapter compares their foundations, presents the main studies attached to them, and details their benefits and drawbacks for the social sciences.

Trajectories and literature review

The case of antidepressants reminds us that the influence of economic actors on public health can be looked at through different analytical lenses. The notions of COI, capture, production of ignorance, and hegemony have emerged at different points in time and in different contexts, but in response to a common set of questions. Our objective here is to retrace the trajectory of each of them and present the main contributions through which they have been developed and refined.

Conflict of interest

The trajectory of the notion of COI and its use in academic literature have been already discussed in the introduction of this book and in Chapter 1. In this analytical comparison, we will only summarize its main features. The use of COI in its current meaning developed in the legal and political domain in the United States after the Second World War. It was used as a portmanteau word to designate the common purpose of seven different statutes dealing with the private activities and revenues of employees of the Federal Government, even if none of these legislations used this notion. Highly publicized controversies that had affected top officials of both the Truman and Eisenhower administrations, coupled with the desire to encourage and secure a growing involvement of experts and consultants in the public administration, fostered the adoption of the 1962 "Bribery, Graft and Conflicts of Interest Law". This created a special status for these experts: they would be authorized to have more financial interests than ordinary government employees as long as they disclosed them to an official, who would certify that they did not affect their public duty. Whereas COI had been particularly discussed in relation to the "military-industrial complex", it gained greater visibility in public health from the 1970s onward. While the consumerist movement developed, the weak implementation of COI regulation in regulatory agencies and in scientific committees was highlighted. Most of all, the 1980s saw the development – in relation to a nascent biotechnology field – of scientific entrepreneurship, and worries about the commercialization of academic research developed. COI, as a description of a problematic kind of influence and as a solution to it (disclosure), was thus imported from the administrative/political domain to scientific institutions: universities, research organizations, and academic journals. Evidence on the influence of big corporations – those from the tobacco or pharmaceutical industries – mounted in the late 1990s and early 2000s, and COI was increasingly used to designate a wide range of links between these corporations and experts/scientists (not only equity, but also funding, honoraria, and board participation). After several health scandals and controversies in the mid-2000s (most notably the Vioxx® crisis of 2004), the media and NGOs began to pay more attention to COI. Unveiling undeclared interests turned out to be a powerful "action repertoire" for criticizing public decisions or scientific/technical statements. In the 2010s, the COIs of "regular" health professionals (such as general practitioners and pharmacists), students, and patients' organizations also came under political scrutiny. This led to the creation (in 2010 in the United States and in 2011 in France, for example) of public "transparency databases" disclosing their links with health industries.

As the introduction of this book has underlined, academic research on COI (in relation to public health) has been mostly conducted within ethics, law, and philosophy and has focused on the legal and ethical implications of the notion. The most influential works falling more directly within the social sciences (Rodwin, 2011; Krimsky, 2019) have tended to consider COI as a concept that enables us to designate a tangible phenomenon: the impact of commercial incentives on the ethos of scientists/physicians. Their analyses focus on the legal and social context explaining these problematic influences and, along with a few other works (Parascandola, 2007; Lexchin and O'Donovan, 2010; Hauray, 2018), on the adoption of COI policies. These policies have generally been criticized for their permissiveness and limited effectiveness. Researchers in social psychology have even evoked a perverse effect of the development of COI disclosure procedures, which are considered to produce a form of "moral licensing" (Dana and Loewenstein, 2003). Very little work has focused on the implications of this increasing problematization of COIs within the health sector. Its impact on expert committees and on professional hierarchies has been underlined in the case of Alzheimer's medications (Dalgalarrondo and Hauray, 2020). But the rare works available have tended to relativize its importance by placing the issue of COIs in the lived experience and concrete activities of the actors concerned – doctors (Wadmann, 2014) or patients' organizations (Jones, 2008).

On the whole, social scientists have thus been suspicious about the notion and there has been little empirical research conducted on COI in the social studies of health/science/medicine (Abraham, 2010). Sergio Sismondo has indicated, for example, that the term COI "is well established and is best retained, but is misleading. The term suggests that researchers act inappropriately to further their own interests" (Sismondo, 2008, p. 1910). As a consequence, he has favored empirical research on more specific social mechanisms, like "ghostwriting" or the role played by "key opinion leaders", and has chosen hegemony as an analytical framework (Sismondo, 2018). We can understand this situation. On the one hand, the denunciation of COI, infused with a defense of Mertonian norms of science (disinterestedness, communalism), has clashed with the dominant programs in science and technology studies and in the sociology of health and medicine that have long pursued opposite objectives (a deconstruction of scientific authority and a plea for an increased involvement of "civil society" actors). On the other hand, the strong connection of the concept with the implementation of disclosure policies encouraged political sociologists to consider this notion as part of a neoliberal regulation, aiming at managing corporate influence instead of prohibiting it (Lexchin and O'Donovan, 2010; Hauray, 2018).

Capture

Like the notion of COI, that of "capture" also emerged in the 1950s, in a context of concerns over the fact that the functioning of US federal commissions and agencies, because of the technicality of the laws they implement or flaws in their design, could tend to favor the interests of the regulated industry. These concerns were linked to the growing involvement of the Federal Government in the economy, and the challenge of promoting the "public interest", with a specific focus on organizational issues rather than individual ones. The 1970s and 1980s could be said to represent the "golden age" of regulatory capture, when the notion became frequently used by economists – along with other social scientists – and journalists to analyze situations in which public regulatory bodies seemed "captured" by industry interests. In this period, the question of the health and environmental impact of toxic chemicals had become widely discussed and numerous reforms were adopted, such as the Clean Air Act (1970), the Clean Water Act (1972), and the Toxic Substances Control Act (1976). However, as the United States entered the Reagan era, conservative policies and decisions increased the worry that federal bodies were under the influence of large chemical companies and had become "captive". Controversies over the political appointees at the Environmental Protection Agency (EPA) and the impossible regulation of chemicals like formaldehyde and asbestos fueled such concerns.

In the early years, the hypothesis of "captured" federal bodies was mainly formulated in relation to trade, finance, transportation, and energy commissions (Huntington, 1952; Bernstein, 1955). In the 1950s, Marver H. Bernstein, who had previously worked for the government, embarked on a project to critically evaluate the role and functioning of seven agencies. He explored the idea of "captive" agencies by describing their life cycle as they go through four stages. The "gestation" stage usually ends with the passing of ambiguous statutes. In the "youthful" stage, an agency uses a lot of technical procedures and litigation to achieve its goals, a dynamic that benefits the industry. It then enters a "maturity" phase during which it becomes more and more attentive to the interest of the regulated industry. In the final, "old age" phase, it becomes "retrogressive, lethargic, sluggish", and "surrenders" – in other words, it ends up "captive".

Later on, the work of economist George Stigler progressively became the most cited on the notion (Stigler, 1971). Stigler had a different take on regulatory capture. He proposed considering that governments and industry operate in a regulatory marketplace. Governments supply products such as subsidies, control over competitive entry, the regulation of product substitutes or complements, and the fixing of prices. Obtaining some of these products can then be a way of taking them away from one's competitors and dominating the regulatory market. Although Stigler's work did not focus on health-related agencies, his general theory has inspired a great deal of research on the pathways to capture since the 1980s (Shapiro, 2012).

More recently, the academic uses of "capture" have become less frequent. As far as public health is concerned, Daniel Carpenter is one of the few scholars to have discussed the concept at length in the context of pharmaceutical regulation (Carpenter, 2010). His argument, however, is that the patterns of influence, and the power relationships at play in the context of American pharmaceutical regulation, are better explained by the politics of reputation than by those of capture (companies have arguably resisted, not participated, in the institution of the FDA; big firms are not systematically favored over their smaller competitors; etc.). The discussions that followed his work on this issue led to the publication of an edited volume in which the authors defend the provocative idea that capture is always both preventable and manageable (Carpenter and Moss, 2013).

Following different lines of research, the scholars who developed and used the notion of capture have identified a series of mechanisms that tend to lead to the maximization of industry benefits and the failure of agencies to protect the public. Over the years, they have identified four main pathways to capture. The first is that of "industry-oriented mandates" that, for instance, led the now-defunct Minerals Management Service to promote oil drilling in the Gulf rather than focus on safety or protection of the environment (Glicksman, 2010). The second is the existence of anti-regulatory administrators, like the ones appointed at the EPA by Reagan during the conservative revolution. These EPA administrators, who denied the car-cinogenicity of formaldehyde in the 1980s, inspired what was also called "staff capture" (Graham, Green, and Roberts, 1988), i.e. the capture of agencies through their employees. A third pathway to capture is the inten-tional scarcity of funding that slowed down the operation of the EPA, or slight increases that aimed at accelerating the marketing of new drugs by the FDA (Steinzor and Shapiro, 2006) – a tactic that has been used by the Reagan, Bush, and Trump administrations. Finally, a fourth pathway to capture could be described as rulemaking "ossification", in other words, an excess of rules and procedures that tends to slow down the functioning of agencies, which is for instance what has been happening in the regulation of industrial chemicals in the United States since the 1970s (McGarity, 1979; Boullier, 2019).

Production of ignorance

Research about the production of ignorance has grown significantly in the field of social sciences in recent years, notably with the publication of a col-lective volume intended to promote this type of research, via the neologism "agnotology" (Proctor and Schiebinger, 2008), and the recent publication of a handbook that confirmed the importance of this theme (Gross and McGoey, 2015). These studies differ from a representation of the progress of science that flows straight from ignorance to knowledge. It emphasizes the role of economic actors in the deliberate production of ignorance or at least in the slowing down of the production of potentially inconvenient knowl-edge and more globally in the shaping of scientific knowledge as a whole.

The most obvious way of examining companies' influence on the produc-tion of ignorance is to see it as stemming from a struggle against the emer-gence of new knowledge. The most well-known and widely documented case is the tobacco industry in the United States, and its efforts to weaken and cast doubt on the connection between cigarette smoke and lung cancer. The tobacco industry's litigation provided the opportunity to promote a great deal of research on this industry, which then served as a model to analyze strategies for producing false controversies (Proctor, 2011). Thus, several studies have been carried out on firms that try to downplay as much as possible the toxicity of products to which their employees are exposed. As a follow-up to their history of silicosis (Rosner and Markowitz, 1991), Gerald Markowitz and David Rosner's research on the lead and vinyl chlo-ride industries highlights these industrial strategies of opposing the pro-duction of scientific knowledge, with the aim of maintaining dangerous industrial activities (Markowitz and Rosner, 2002; see also other examples in Michaels, 2008; 2020). One other emblematic case is that of asbestos. In this case, the industrial investment was made very early and lasted a long time, spanning the entire 20th century (McCulloch and Tweedale, 2008).

This research shows the numerous cases where firms have refused to publish certain results, have encouraged research that promoted their own interests, or have concentrated research on subjects that did not directly challenge their economic interests or that directly financed scientists so that they would publicly criticize academic research that ran counter to their own interests. More broadly, this research shows also how scientists working with industry contribute to the creation of false controversies, notably on the question of global warming (Oreskes and Conway, 2010). Globally, these studies tend to emphasize the individual and intentional nature of the production of ignorance. They propose a highly political reading of the conflicts between, on the one hand, firms seeking to format scientific knowledge in order to minimize the negative consequences for their own interests and, on the other, government services or regulatory agencies, especially at the federal level, seeking to thwart these strategies in order to regulate dangerous activities.

Yet, although those works are important, they should not overshadow the more structural dimensions of the production of ignorance, especially the more discrete power plays in this regard. The notion of "undone science", as developed in several sociology of science studies, can facilitate such a change of perspective (Frickel et al., 2010). It highlights that, apart from the direct pressure exerted by industry, many other factors explain the unequal development of scientific knowledge, depending on the economic or social interests involved. Hence, talking of undone science means emphasizing the structural inequalities between, on the one hand, the groups that are mobilized to denounce a risk (workers, unions, or people living near a polluted area) and, on the other, the companies and industries that produce those dangers (Hess, 2016). These approaches, therefore, focus on the fact that the production of knowledge (and of ignorance) is strongly correlated with the resources of the actors likely to be interested in the results of the research. Thus, studies on toxins used in industry, which could be useful to the workers concerned, are not carried out due to a lack of interest by the employers and therefore to the lack of the necessary financial and human resources. By producing ignorance and undone science, these situations of strong inequality of resources between actors also facilitate non-decisions and public inaction (Henry, 2017).

Further complicating the picture of questions on the unequal development of knowledge, research has also questioned how administrations and regulatory agencies contribute to producing ignorance. They can do this by setting aside some knowledge to continue their regulatory activities, as has been shown in the case of drug regulation (McGoey, 2012) and more globally regarding knowledge that appears uncomfortable for decision-makers (Rayner, 2012). They may also focus on certain dimensions of problems that are beyond administrative apprehension in an attempt to make them more easily manageable, as has been shown in the management of pollution after Hurricane Katrina in New Orleans (Frickel and Edwards, 2014), or highlight how industry influences the way an issue is regulated by the administration

(Suryanarayanan and Kleinman, 2017). In the case of undone science and of organized or institutionalized ignorance, ignorance is not only the result of manipulation of science by industry but appears to be the result of social inequalities or institutional logics.

Hegemony

The concept of hegemony as a means of apprehending the ways in which capitalism (understood as a system of economic relationships centered on the maximizing of profit, the organization of industrial production, and the control of surplus value generated through salaried work) is deeply rooted in the 1960s and 1970s political and intellectual debates about Marxism, which led to renewed interest in the writings of Antonio Gramsci.

Gramsci introduced hegemony in his *Prison Notebooks*. Hegemony was thought of as a key notion to avoid any kind of economic reductionism, namely the reification of "capital" into a purely economic arrangement of production forces and production relationships whose existence or non-existence determine (in a strong and quasi-causal manner) the politics and culture of a given society. At stake was the mere possibility of radical political change in "backward" – weakly industrialized – countries like Russia or Italy where "feudalism" and peasantry still dominated the social landscape.

Hegemony is rooted in a historical reading of the social, rather than a structural one. It is not a given, but an achievement – something that is built and rebuilt through the whole dynamics of social interactions. For Gramsci, every really existing society is a terrain of competition between different classes and political economies. It can only survive if certain social groups achieve alliances and turn their peculiar interests into that of society at large. Hegemony is the result of this process through which "civil society" and its multiple bodies manage to produce a hierarchy of values, political aims, and economic practices providing for a relatively coherent exercise of power. At the center is therefore the ways in which the law and the state, as core political institutions, "rule" the contradictory nature of capital, i.e., the conflicts between workers and employers, those between various economic sectors, or the competition with other modes of production. Gramsci's approach thus granted strong autonomy and specificity to politics and culture, stressing the role of consensus and "common sense" in the mere existence of power. As an effect of political and intellectual work, hegemony also preserves the possibility of counter-hegemony, meaning, for Gramsci, the possibility for the working class to build its own vision of society and its own institutions.

Hegemony has gained some visibility in studies of science, technology, and medicine over the past ten years since the category has been increasingly used to analyze the changing relationships between research and markets, originating in the rise of biotechnology, on the one hand (Kleinman, 1998; Holloway, 2015; Salter, Zhou, and Datta, 2015), and with studies of pharmaceutical capitalism and its role in the production of knowledge on the other. Sismondo (2018) apprehends hegemony in a rather straightforward manner, i.e., as the domination of capitalistic firms in the making and diffusion of pharmaceutical knowledge. His core argument focuses on the industry-based system of knowledge legitimation and dissemination with its cortege of contract research organizations, ghostwriting, sales representatives, and collaborating key opinion leaders, which seeks to persuade physicians to act in alignment with the firms' interests. Industrial hegemony in the world of pharmacy is thus a form of medical common sense originating in the control of information. Sismondo thus echoes a significant body of historical and sociological work on the industry, its in-house research practices, its links to practitioners, and the development of "scientific marketing" (Greene, 2007; Greffion, 2014; Gaudillière; 2015; Gaudillière and Thoms, 2015; Ravelli, 2015).

Kaushik Sunder Rajan refers to Gramsci and hegemony in a more specific and theoretical way (Rajan, 2017). His recent book *Pharmocracy* explores the dynamics of pharmaceutical innovation, capital formation, and regulation in India, following two configurations of political conflicts over health and its appropriation: the mobilizations about the HPV vaccine and its adverse effects, and the denial of patent rights for Novartis's anticancer drug Gleevec® by Indian courts. Hegemony is central, as it makes it possible to understand the dynamics of capital in biomedicine beyond machinations or money greed:

> Acknowledging the power of the multinational pharmaceutical industry is important [...]. But pharmocracy is constituted in more complex ways than merely rational, strategic, or cynical action on the part of corporate actors. I argue that we must additionally understand the mechanisms by which health gets appropriated by capital, in order to instantiate forms of political economic value that are dictated by logics of capital; how these logics of capital materialize through regimes of governance; and how they are contested and rendered political.
>
> (Rajan, 2017, p. 7)

Four aspects of Gramsci's approach are then taken on board: (a) the dialectics between the "conjuncture" and the "organic" or between events and structures; (b) the political nature of hegemony and its roots in "common sense", which means that the question of value is not simply economical but entails multiple cultural and moral layers; (c) the "intellectual work" grounding hegemony as a process of pragmatic and highly contextual co-production of knowledge, value, and politics; and (d) "counter-hegemony" taking the form of public scandals, engagements with the law or economic competition, and revealing alternative forms of value-making. The case of Gleevec® and the contestation of intellectual property rights is especially enlightening as it sheds light on: (1) the tensions within the law and its practice: when India ratified the World Trade Organization agreement on Trade-Related Aspects of Intellectual Property Rights (TRIPS), it included a provision against the ever-greening of patents, which was used to deny Novartis IP rights; (2) the multiple political economies at stake and the involvement of different forms of capital: the existence of a strong Indian generic drug industry competing with Euro–American companies was decisive in the deployment of the case as a national issue; and (3) the multiple forms of values articulated and their respective political space: financial, philanthropic, constitutional, and postcolonial.

Diverging conceptualizations of influence

The notions of COI, capture, ignorance, and hegemony have all been used to designate a common set of issues regarding the relationship between science, industry, and the regulation of markets; all emphasizing the ability of powerful economic actors to shape science and the law as well as the ways in which professionals and consumers use commodities. These four lenses have shed light on different, complementary dimensions of industry influence. At the same time, they all suffer from their own limitations. In this section, we discuss the advantages and drawbacks of these four notions in order to document how they can help study the influence of corporate interests on public health.

Conflict of interest

The popularity of COI stems, we believe, from two main dynamics. On the one side, by pointing to the tensions between private and public interest, it can designate a wide range of problematic situations without assigning them to other concepts such as "bribery", "fraud", or "corruption", which have unequivocal moral meaning and are legally well-defined. It is a "thick concept" (Luebke, 1987) that articulates descriptive and normative dimensions and, as such, it is particularly well-suited to addressing ethical worries through the implementation of *soft* regulations. In the health sector, the reference to COI increased in response to the multifaceted strategies of corporate actors to steer the production of knowledge and public health decisions. But this development was directly linked to the enforcement by scientific organizations and public health officials of disclosure procedures, transparency policies that fundamentally allowed the continuation of the problematic interactions under consideration. On the other side, COI refers to an apparently simple psychological mechanism, which everyone has experienced. The archetypal representation of COI enacts two forces clashing in the definition of a person's behavior, a representation that allows the definition of thresholds in terms of amount (the implicit being that the amount will determine the strength of the bad force) or timeframe (the force will decrease with time). But the situations analyzed through the COI category are diverse. Some imply clear power relationships, through rewards (such as speaking fees, consultancies, the direct funding of organizations) or threats and conflicts *between* interests (when a researcher is forbidden to publish bad results from a financing firm). Others seem to involve mainly persuasion (when a researcher is enrolled in a promissory claim about a drug through a collaboration) or imply complex diachronic processes (as in revolving doors issues).

These characteristics can explain why the notion has not been used in the social sciences as much as in legal/ethical studies or in public health/medical research. As a descriptive tool, it is mainly cartographic: it points to the existence of a link but tells us nothing about the nature of the interaction or about the power relationships involved in it. Furthermore, it conveys a very individualistic understanding of these power relationships and can be considered unsuited to capture the structural dimension of corporate influence. From a more normative point of view, it refers to an ideal of objective knowledge and independent practices, which is at odds with the constructivist nature of the dominant programs in the social sciences of health, science, or medicine.

However, the notion also has important merits and benefits for the social sciences. First, by encapsulating diverse, individualistic, and sometimes evasive forms of influence, it mirrors the multiple and connected channels of influence that industries have cultivated with a growing intensity for several decades. COIs can thus be considered as traces of corporate strategies, even if the precise product of these strategies cannot be established. Second, in questioning scientists and health professionals' motives, it problematizes their "ethos" (Bourdieu, 1984) and the contradictory demands they receive (being "independent", but building public–private partnerships). It is thus a useful tool for grasping sociological ambivalence (Merton, 1976) in a rapidly evolving moral landscape. Finally, and from a more political point of view, for 30 years COI has been a major weapon of "counter-hegemony", widely used by professionals, watchdog organizations, or investigative journalists. By promoting their own approach to COI, the social sciences have the opportunity to directly participate in the public debate.

Capture

In the last few decades of its existence, the notion of capture has mainly been used to respond to overtly normative questions about whether and how regulatory agencies are influenced by industry. Much of the existing research can be described, on the one hand, as "assessments" detailing whether agencies are captured or not – a trend in which political scientists and legal scholars are the main contributors – and, on the other hand, as analyses that aim to model the behavior and rationale of federal agencies and companies, from a political economy perspective.

Through the different cases it has explored, this scholarship has managed to identify a series of mechanisms that lead to some degree of capture. However, as this literature has largely been based on case studies merely asking whether a specific agency, commission, or public organization is captive or not, many authors now agree on the limitations of the notion. They call for a number of displacements in the study of how capture is achieved but, in the end, they tend to propose more concepts to show how capture is never total and can always be managed. This is for instance the case of the recent refinements proposed by Carpenter and Moss. Instead of defining degrees of capture, such as "strong capture" (a case in which public interest is completely violated) and "weak capture" (when the overall functioning of the agency/policy is positive despite industry influence), they propose to reflect on "corrosive capture", when the captured policy process does not "produce more rent-enhancing regulation" but results in "less public interest-serving regulation, and (as a consequence) reduce[s] or eliminate[s] regulatory costs that fall on industry" (Carpenter and Moss, 2013, p. 16). Some rare studies have made the hypothesis that there was actual capture and consequently proposed a more systemic analysis, like those promoting the idea of "institutional corruption" (Rodwin, 2012; Lessig, 2013), but have never pushed the promise much further.

Another striking trait of this literature is that its focus on public bodies tends to take for granted that capture is necessarily the result of industry strategies. This can be explained by disciplinary differences, as the questions posed by administrative sciences and economics are mostly normative, with the objective to design a generic analytical framework to respond to the question: is a given agency or commission "captive"? However, this poses a problem of symmetry for other social sciences: the presence of industrial actors in administrative settings can be the result of institutional arrangements or of situations of structural asymmetries that can be specific to a given sector, like that of medicines, foodstuffs, or chemicals. The scholars involved in the study of ignorance have precisely managed to take on board these specificities and reintroduce some symmetry in the analysis.

Production of ignorance

As a whole, ignorance studies are characterized by a *focus on economic actors* and their links with scientific spaces. They analyze their relations, which range from the manipulation or targeted funding of some research to the observation of a more structural imbalance of resources leading to a specific structuring of knowledge and ignorance. Industry strategies involve for example the funding of scientists and research programs and, in some cases, putting pressure on researchers to not publish or to delay publishing some of their results. In several cases, however, the mechanisms used by corporate entities can also be described as "non-decision-making processes" (Bachrach and Baratz, 1962, p. 949): these situations do not refer to active interventions by industries, but to the simple fact that corporate entities are in a position to authorize or prevent a scientific study requiring their product or concerning their employees. In the fields of environmental or occupational health, the agreement of companies using hazardous products is necessary to obtain samples or have access to exposed personnel. However, a mere refusal or unwillingness to launch a study is enough to prevent the production of knowledge and therefore can lead to more structural mechanisms, which will be developed in the hegemony model.

Highlighting the hidden links between industry and the academic research community is not easy work and numerous studies in this field have used data obtained from legal proceedings in the United States and to a lesser extent in the United Kingdom. In France and continental Europe, these kinds of work are less developed due to greater difficulties in accessing industry documents. Most of these works focus on past situations as it is easier to work from a historical perspective than to conduct contemporary sociological work, because the issues are less problematic and the interests to protect are less central.

Research in terms of ignorance can reveal *structural and lasting links between industry and scientific research* highlighting contemporary transformations of research funding with the increasing role of private actors (Krimsky, 2004). It has also made it possible to move away from a representation of the scientific space as a field characterized by a linear increase of knowledge. Going beyond approaches that emphasized the weight of economic interests in knowledge production (Gibbons et al., 1994), this research underlines the specific structuring of knowledge and ignorance in different sectors. It also makes it possible to highlight areas sustainably affected by undone science. However, it tends to put forward a strategic or even conspiring reading of social relations and insufficiently takes into account the effects of ignorance on public decisions. It is thus largely based on an intentional reading of the production of ignorance and leaves aside questions relating to the acceptance of these inequalities and the way in which these untruths are imposed beyond an explanation based on these individual strategies.

Hegemony

Hegemony is a broad notion introduced to reflect upon the entire historical dynamics of capitalism and the complex, systemic, and dialectical relationship between the economic and the political.

One of its main benefits is the ability to reveal the structural features contributing to the multiple links between researchers, regulators, and industrialists that result in specific and individualized COIs. As a general approach of the "structural" that helps placing capital (rather than industrial production) and the construction of markets at the center, hegemony is a powerful instrument in investigating pharmaceutical capitalism at work, i.e., the collective construction of markets and the processes of regulation. In addition, hegemony draws attention to the role legal arrangements, political decisions, and professional values play in the legitimization of strategic options, like the framing of intellectual property rights, the financing of clinical trials, or the high priority granted to chemical innovation when clinicians reflect about the sources of medical progress. All these features, some more practical, others more ideological, participate in an indirect, diffuse, and multilayered system of influence, which contributes to the obviousness and the naturalness of industrial interests.

However, the broadness and the encompassing character of hegemony is its main limitation. The category can easily become an umbrella notion loosely used to signal – rather than analyze – the elusive and diffuse dimensions of power. As such, it can become a mere synonym of ideology and therefore loose most of its value for understanding specific processes involved in the invention, production, and therapeutic use of drugs.

Based on the existing literature on pharmaceuticals linking hegemony, knowledge, and politics, one may suggest that the notion can be most fruitfully used to explore two kinds of systemic features. The first one – and in this respect hegemony echoes the concept of undone science – is the critical role knowledge, along with its social and cultural meanings, plays in the dynamics of influence with a special interest in the diverging ways in which various forms of knowledge are practically appropriated by capital. The second one is the political nature of pharmaceutical hegemony, looking at the intellectual work grounding the pragmatic and highly contextual production of legal values and regulatory mechanisms, as well as their contestation, i.e., the existence of "counter-hegemony". The latter must be understood both as an internal as well as an external alternative to the dominating regimes of accumulation. This is for instance the case, and in resonance with the work of Kaushik Sunder Rajan, in India where the generics industry opposes patents without challenging the biomedical model of innovation while the Indian firms promoting Ayurveda remedies do exactly the opposite (Pordié and Gaudillière, 2014).

Synthesis and conclusion

In order to evaluate the relevance of COI, not as a social category but as an analytical tool for the social sciences, this chapter has compared this notion with the three dominant conceptualizations of corporate influence mobilized by the social sciences in the recent past. One may consider that these categories are simply complementary tools that highlight different aspects of the same phenomenon: processes that can be analyzed in terms of COI often participate in the construction of fields characterized by false controversies or undone science.

Table 11.1 shows that this is to some extent the case. It also reveals striking differences in the mere definition of the problems and the putative responses, with the consequence that the four categories do not simply complement each other but are also used in alternative ways. As we have seen, COI is a category widely used by the actors themselves and has become a critical tool in the law

Table 11.1 Four categories to explore influence, their analytical framing, and their uses

	Main focus of the analysis	Mechanism/means of influence	Political response
COI	Individual Material/financial link between industry and scientists/experts, and their effects	Psychological bias Financial transfers, multi-positioning	Solution: disclosure policies and transparency, restriction measures
Regulatory capture	Organizations Agencies/ commissions' biased structure and decision-making	Adaptation to market construction imperatives Lobbying, campaign contributions, revolving door, staff recruitment of agencies	Solution: independent staff and funding of agencies, procedural reforms
Ignorance	Field Industries' activity and their strategy to weigh on the (non-)production of knowledge	False controversies and undone science. Funding of research, withholding of internal results, PR campaigns	Solution: declassification of industry's internal documents, through trials, public database and whistleblowing.
Hegemony	Political economy Legal and cultural legitimation of capitalism and/or domination	Organization of the cultural, legal, and political system, circulation of knowledge/ideas	Solution: alternative institutions and markets (public), counter-hegemony, political coalition

and in drug regulation. However, it is not the sole notion granted with some utility by the actors: capture also counts among the tools pharmacists, medical experts, economists, or regulators employ when discussing the nature of corporate influence and the ways to reduce it. In addition, both COI and capture point to "local" patterns, meaning either the links individual scientists and experts maintain with industry, or the institutional behavior of specific regulatory bodies. In contrast, ignorance and hegemony are categories developed by social scientists, and both point to the general, structural nature of influence even if the former targets the mode of knowledge production and the latter the capitalistic organization of the economy.

The question then arises of how they can contribute to a better understanding of pervasive powers and the attempts to counter them. It seems to us that the most problematic category in this theoretical package is that of capture. Beyond its limitations of scope, capture operates on the basis of a fundamental dichotomy between public institutions and science on the one hand, and markets and private actors on the other, with the former being contaminated by the latter *post hoc* and in contradiction to the nature of public institutions and/or science. Capture thus romanticizes the mere existence of regulation and it is presumably not by chance that it has so far been associated with insiders' discourses or with investigations, which in the end conclude that capture fails or remains peripheral.

We, therefore, conclude that a comprehensive analysis of influence requires an articulation of COI, ignorance, and hegemony: COI both as a reflection of the multiple channels of influence the industry has developed and as a powerful means of making visible the double-bind of scientists, experts, and regulators; ignorance as a way of exploring the asymmetries and power gradients at stake in the production and non-production of knowledge and their effects in regulation; and hegemony as a reminder of the key role processes of market construction and the competition between diverse political economies play in the logic of influence. Bringing these three concepts together would make it possible to reformulate the question of power in science and regulation, in an area – that of public health issues – in which asymmetries and inequalities are particularly strong.

Notes

1. See Chapter 1.
2. The analyses developed in this chapter were presented during the "Pervasive Powers" conference held in Paris in June 2018. We would like to thank its organizers and attendees for their helpful insights and comments on the previous version of this text.
3. Without entering into philosophical debates about the concepts of power and influence, and their links (is influence a sub-kind of power relationship? Or is power a sub-kind of influence mechanism? Or are the two concepts complementary conceptualizations of asymmetrical relationships? – see in particular Zimmerling [2005] for an overview), we have decided to use the concept of influence in this chapter. In fact, the four notions we discuss focus on social dynamics that aim at affecting people's beliefs and knowledge about what is true/false or good/bad, more than on the capacity of a person or a group to impose his/her/its preferences on others that do not share them. But, as the content of this chapter will show, we do not understand influence as a concept delimiting individualistic or *soft* forms of power.

References

Abraham, J (2010) 'On the prohibition of conflicts of interest in pharmaceutical regulation: precautionary limits and permissive challenges. A commentary on Sismondo (66:9, 2008, 1909–14) and O'Donovan and Lexchin', *Social Science & Medicine*, 70(5), pp. 648–651.

Bachrach, P and Baratz, MS (1962) 'Two faces of power', *The American Political Science Review*, 56(4), pp. 947–952.

Bernstein, MH (1955) *Regulating business by independent commission.* Princeton: Princeton University Press.

Boullier, H (2019) *Toxiques légaux. Comment les firmes chimiques ont mis la main sur le contrôle de leurs produits.* Paris: La Découverte.

Bourdieu, P (1984) *Questions de sociologie.* Paris : Éditions de Minuit.

Carpenter, D (2010) *Reputation and power: organizational image and pharmaceutical regulation at the FDA.* Princeton: Princeton University Press.

Carpenter, D and Moss, DA (2013) *Preventing regulatory capture: special interest influence and how to limit it.* New York: Cambridge University Press.

Cosgrove, L, Krimsky, S, Vijayaraghavan, M and Schneider, L (2006) 'Financial ties between DSM-IV panel members and the pharmaceutical industry', *Psychotherapy and Psychosomatics*, 75(3), pp. 154–160.

Dalgalarrondo, S and Hauray, B (2020) 'Conflit d'intérêts et traitements anti-Alzheimer: de la construction à la contestation d'une promesse médicale', *Sciences sociales et santé*, 38(3), pp. 77–104.

Dana, J and Loewenstein, G (2003) 'A social science perspective on gifts to physicians from industry', *JAMA*, 290(2), pp. 252–255.

Frickel, S and Edwards, M (2014) 'Untangling ignorance in environmental risk assessment' in Boudia, S and Jas, N (eds.) *Powerless science? Science and politics in a toxic world.* The Environment in History: International Perspectives. Berghahn Books, pp. 215–233.

Frickel, S, et al. (2010) 'Undone science: charting social movement and civil society challenges to research agenda setting', *Science, Technology & Human Values*, 35(4), pp. 444–473.

Gaudillière, J-P (2015) 'Une manière industrielle de savoir', *Histoire des sciences et des savoirs – 3. Le siècle des technosciences.* Paris: Le Seuil, pp. 85–106.

Gaudillière, J-P and Thoms, U (eds.) (2015) *The development of scientific marketing in the twentieth century.* New York: Picketing & Chatto.

Gibbons, M et al. (1994) *The new production of knowledge: the dynamics of science and research in contemporary societies.* London: Sage Publications.

Glicksman, RL (2010) 'Regulatory blowout: how regulatory failures made the BP disaster possible, and how the system can be fixed to avoid a recurrence', *George Washington Law Faculty Publications & Other Works,* article 608.

Graham, JD, Green, LC and Roberts, MJ (1988) *In search of safety: chemicals and cancer risk.* Cambridge: Harvard University Press.

Greene, J (2007) *Prescribing by numbers: drugs and the definition of disease.* Baltimore: Johns Hopkins University Press.

Greffion, J (2014) Faire passer la pilule: visiteurs médicaux and entreprises pharmaceutiques face aux médecins (1905–2014). PhD thesis, EHESS.

Gross, M and McGoey, L (eds.) (2015) *Routledge international handbook of ignorance studies.* Abingdon; New York: Routledge.

Guha, R (1989) *The unquiet wood. Ecological change and peasant resistance in the Himalaya.* New Delhi: Oxford University Press.

Hauray, B (2006) *L'Europe du médicament. Politique - expertise - intérêts privés.* Paris: Presses de Sciences Po.

Hauray, B (2018) 'Dispositifs de transparence et régulation des conflits d'intérêts dans le secteur du médicament', *Revue française d'administration publique*, 165(1), pp. 49–61.

Henry, E (2017) *Ignorance scientifique et inaction publique. Les politiques de santé au travail.* Paris: Presses de Sciences Po.

Hess, DJ (2016) *Undone science. Social movements, mobilized publics, and industrial transitions.* Cambridge: MIT Press.

Holloway, KJ (2015) 'Normalizing complaint: scientists and the challenge of commercialization', *Science, Technology & Human Values*, 40(5), pp. 744–765.

House of Commons Health Committee (2005) *The influence of the pharmaceutical industry: fourth report of session 2004–2005.* London: The Stationery Office Ltd.

Huntington, SP (1952) 'The marasmus of the ICC: the commission, the railroads, and the public interest', *The Yale Law Journal*, 61(4), pp. 467–509.

Jones, K (2008) 'In whose interest? Relationships between health consumer groups and the pharmaceutical industry in the UK', *Sociology of Health & Illness*, 30(6), pp. 929–943.

Kleinman, DL (1998) 'Untangling context: understanding a university laboratory in the commercial world', *Science, Technology & Human Values*, 23(3), pp. 285–314.

Krimsky, S (2004) *Science in the private interest: has the lure of profits corrupted biomedical research?* Lanham: Rowman & Littlefield Publishers.

Krimsky, S (2019) *Conflicts of interest in science: how corporate-funded academic research can threaten public health.* New York: Hot Books.

Lessig, L (2013) '"Institutional corruption" defined', *The Journal of Law, Medicine & Ethics*, 41(3), pp. 553–555.

Lexchin, J and O'Donovan, O (2010) 'Prohibiting or "managing" conflict of interest? A review of policies and procedures in three European drug regulation agencies', *Social Science & Medicine*, 70(5), pp. 643–647.

Luebke, NR (1987) 'Conflict of interest as a moral category', *Business and Professional Ethics Journal*, 6(1), pp. 66–81.

Markowitz, GE and Rosner, D (2002) *Deceit and denial: the deadly politics of industrial pollution.* Berkeley: University of California Press.

McCulloch, J and Tweedale, G (2008) *Defending the indefensible: the global asbestos industry and its fight for survival.* New York: Oxford University Press.

McGarity, TO (1979) 'Substantive and procedural discretion in administrative resolution of science policy questions: regulating carcinogens in EPA and OSHA', *Georgia Law Review*, 67, p. 729.

McGoey, L (2012) 'The logic of strategic ignorance', *British Journal of Sociology*, 63(3), pp. 553–576.

Merton, RK (1976) *Sociological ambivalence and other essays.* New York: Free Press.

Michaels, D (2008) *Doubt is their product: how industry's assault on science threatens your health.* Oxford: Oxford University Press.

Michaels, D (2020) *The triumph of doubt. Dark money and the science of deception.* Oxford: Oxford University Press.

Oreskes, N and Conway, EM (2010) *Merchants of doubt: how a handful of scientists obscured the truth on issues from tobacco smoke to global warming.* New York: Bloomsbury Press.

Parascandola, M (2007) 'A turning point for conflicts of interest: the controversy over the national academy of sciences' first conflicts of interest disclosure policy', *Journal of Clinical Oncology*, 25(24), pp. 3774–3779.

Perlis, RH, et al. (2005) 'Industry sponsorship and financial conflict of interest in the reporting of clinical trials in psychiatry', *The American Journal of Psychiatry*, 162(10), pp. 1957–1960.

Pordié, L and Gaudillière, J-P (2014) 'The reformulation regime in drug discovery: revisiting poly-herbals and property rights in the Ayurvedic industry', *East Asian Science, Technology and Society*, 8(1), pp. 57–79.

Proctor, RN (1995) *Cancer wars: how politics shapes what we know and don't know about cancer*. New York: Basic Books.

Proctor, RN (2011) *Golden holocaust: origins of the cigarette catastrophe and the case for abolition*. Berkeley: University of California Press.

Proctor, RN and Schiebinger, LL (eds.) (2008) *Agnotology: the making and unmaking of ignorance*. Stanford: Stanford University Press.

Rajan, KS (2017) *Pharmocracy: value, politics, and knowledge in global biomedicine*. Durham: Duke University Press.

Ravelli, Q (2015) *La stratégie de la bactérie. Une enquête au coeur de l'industrie pharmaceutique*. Paris: Le Seuil.

Rayner, S (2012) 'Uncomfortable knowledge: the social construction of ignorance in science and environmental policy discourses', *Economy and Society*, 41(1), pp. 107–125.

Rennie, D (2004) 'Trial registration: a great idea switches from ignored to irresistible', *JAMA*, 292(11), pp. 1359–1362.

Rodwin, MAMA (2011) *Conflicts of interest and the future of medicine: the United States, France and Japan*. Oxford: Oxford University Press.

Rodwin, MA (2012) 'Conflicts of interest, institutional corruption, and pharma: an agenda for reform', *The Journal of Law, Medicine & Ethics*, 40(3), pp. 511–522.

Rosner, D and Markowitz, GE (1991) *Deadly dust: silicosis and the politics of occupational disease in twentieth-century America*. Princeton: Princeton University Press.

Salter, B, Zhou, Y and Datta, S (2015) 'Hegemony in the marketplace of biomedical innovation: consumer demand and stem cell science', *Social Science & Medicine*, 131, pp. 156–163.

Shapiro, SA (2012) 'Blowout: legal legacy of the Deepwater Horizon catastrophe. The complexity of regulatory capture: diagnosis, causality, and remediation', *Roger Williams University Law Review*, 17(1), article 11.

Sismondo, S (2008) 'How pharmaceutical industry funding affects trial outcomes: causal structures and responses', *Social Science & Medicine*, 66(9), pp. 1909–1914.

Sismondo, S (2018) *Ghost-managed medicine: Big Pharma's invisible hands*. Manchester: Mattering Press.

Steinzor, R and Shapiro, SA (2006) *The people's agents and the battle to protect the American public. Special interests, government, and threats to health, safety, and the environment*. Chicago: Chicago University Press.

Stigler, GJ (1971) 'The theory of economic regulation', *The Bell Journal of Economics and Management Science*, 2(1), pp. 3–21.

Suryanarayanan, S and Kleinman, DL (2017) *Vanishing bees: science, politics, and honeybee health*. Durham: Rutgers University Press.

Wadmann, S (2014) 'Physician–industry collaboration: conflicts of interest and the imputation of motive', *Social Studies of Science*, 44(4), pp. 531–554.

Whittington, CJ, et al. (2004) 'Selective serotonin reuptake inhibitors in childhood depression: systematic review of published versus unpublished data', *The Lancet*, 363(9418) pp. 1341–1345.

Zimmerling, R (2005) *Influence and power. Variations on a messy theme*. Dordrecht: Springer.

Postface

Conflict of interest, industry hegemony and key opinion leader management[1]

Sergio Sismondo

The insightful chapters in this volume led me to revisit and rethink an anecdote that I have related elsewhere, one that can speak to some issues around conflicts of interest. The setting was a small conference on "KOL management", mostly attended by medical science liaisons and marketers who work directly or indirectly for the pharmaceutical industry. The speaker, whom I'll call "Dr. Kessel" (all informants are anonymized here), was a very prominent psychiatrist who was at this conference as a representative key opinion leader (KOL). The pharmaceutical industry refers to people as KOLs when they can be engaged to help companies shape medical knowledge and educate physicians.

Kessel started by announcing his conflicts of interest: "In the past decade, I have been a consultant to the manufacturer of every compound that has been developed for the treatment of depression or the treatment of bipolar disorder, and some number of other compounds that haven't made it through the multi phases stages of development." He added a list of six pharmaceutical companies that paid him to give talks in the previous three years, and listed another four that had recently funded research projects.

If he had been giving a more concrete medical talk, Kessel would have made a very similar disclosure of conflicts, ostensibly to allow his audience to discount some of what he might have to say about the treatment, definition, or understanding of particular conditions. At the same time, the breadth of Kessel's conflicts might be taken as evidence that he has no particular biases: I have heard several people claim that in having relationships with many pharmaceutical companies they dilute their conflicts, and that they wouldn't trust anybody with only a few conflicts. In this setting, though, Kessel was stepping away from the practice of psychiatry, so his rote performance was not serving to arouse or allay medical suspicion in the usual way.

Disclosure did mark Kessel as a responsible medical researcher and physician, following the norms even when they are unimportant. When an assistant and I interviewed a sample of very highly paid US KOLs, interviewees routinely emphasized that they abide by norms of transparency. Here, for example, is Dr. Koch: "You have to be, I think, in a milieu where you respect

10.4324/9781003161035

that and don't ignore it. [You have to] work with people who have management oversight of the activity where they can, put the handcuffs on you, and make sure that there are limits that your institution is comfortable with." Or Dr. King: "I'm a big believer in transparency, so I don't have a problem with that. In fact on my own personal website, I've got a transparency statement on there where I tell [patients], 'you know I want to make you aware of the fact that I have relationships with a number of companies and I derive a significant amount of my income from these activities and here's how I choose which companies I work with and here's why I do this – here are the potential good and bad parts of that but I just wanted you to know I do think about these things because none of us is free from bias you know' ... and I fully recognize that these kinds of relationships and doing these kind of works certainly has an influence and I think it's naive to say, 'Oh no, this doesn't affect me.'" That said, all of these KOLs also insisted that the relationships did *not* affect them. I'll come back to this.

It is remarkable, as Hauray notes in the opening chapter of this volume, that "conflict of interest" is a relatively new way of parsing the costs and risks of medicine's interactions with commerce and industry. Though the concept has much earlier origins, the term only acquired its current meaning in the 1950s, and only gained prominence in medicine in the 1980s and decades following. But as the chapters here relate, medicine has taken up conflict of interest, even while conflicts appear to multiply. And thus interviewed KOLs were keen to describe their transparency.

But let's return to Dr. Kessel. Although he was introduced as having authored more than 500 publications and as being "one of the brightest stars in neuroscience", the disclosure of conflicts, with its blanket coverage of the companies with potential produces in his areas of expertise, amplified his KOL status. His sweeping statement boasted of his importance. The boast was effective there, for his pharmaceutical industry audience, but it also would have been effective for medical audiences, marking Kessel as a genuine "player" in the game, and not merely an onlooker or follower of medical research. Again, this is a theme echoed by other KOLs. For example, Dr. Katz says, "When you're asked to be the thought leader, that's a bull's-eye exactly where academics live. They want to be thought leaders."

The industry actually creates and anoints thought leaders and KOLs, because it gives them platforms and prominence. It creates opportunities for talks and publications. Working with pharmaceutical companies increases researchers' status and builds reputations. Thus conflicts of interest are also signs and vehicles of importance. It is no surprise, then, that, as Greffion and Michel document in this volume, some people think that it is challenging to find highly qualified experts who do not also have conflicts of interest – which poses serious problems for staffing a regulatory committee explicitly focused on transparency!

This connection is pushed even further in the context of new political economies of university–industry relations. In her contribution to this volume, Jeske describes how the current emphasis on translational medicine reconfigures boundaries so that conflicts of interest once viewed as problematic have become markers of success. Translational medicine demands links that form chains of engagement between academic research and practical application. It is almost impossible to engage in translational medicine without acquiring a few conflicts of interest. As David Blake, then Vice Dean of Medicine at Johns Hopkins University, was reported to have frequently said, "No conflict, no interest" (Birch and Cohn, 2001). Alternatively, we could understand translational medicine as forging new roles by bringing together formerly competing ones – competing roles are at the heart of conflict of interest, as Rodwin argues in his chapter here. But whether translational medicine can dissipate the conflict or merely paper it over remains to be seen. Indeed, it will depend on how medicine is understood, organized, and regulated.

Since I was first introduced to Rodwin's work (e.g., Rodwin, 2011), I have been impressed by the clarity of his analysis of the concept of conflict of interest and the kinds of situations to which it is usefully applied, and even more so by the creativity of his suggestions for preventing, regulating and remedying conflicts. In this volume, Rodwin focuses on conflicts as applied to physicians in their practices, and convincingly makes the case for the value of the concept. In the conditions for its success, though, we might also see its limits.

Boullier et al. suggest that the success of conflict of interest as a frame for understanding economic interests in medicine stems from two features. First, Boullier and colleagues insightfully observe that conflict of interest serves as a device for doing boundary work, demarcating commercially-driven activities from public interest-driven ones. Second, conflict of interest is linked to familiar psychological mechanisms that can lead people to act in support of their or outside interests, rather than in terms of their duties in the absence of those interests.

Drawing attention to the psychological element is valuable for extending analyses to situations in which it might be challenging to identify a strict conflict of interest, but in which we might also want to be wary of influence. In their recounting of the Mediator® case, Lellinger and Bonah here refer to claims that the Servier company "anaesthetized" many actors in the drug chain. This lovely term captures how conflicted actors can become unaware, as if drugged, of their conflicts. But it also might capture how subtle influence can create compliance.

Too much of an emphasis on psychology leads many people to think in terms of actual biases, and not formal structures. Rodwin defines conflict of interest in terms of conflicting roles; put slightly differently, we might analyze it in terms of a conflict between duties and interests. When rooted in psychology, though, the ultimate problem is bias. And as such, people with formal conflicts of interest deny that they would ever let interests displace duties. Every single one of my interviewed KOLs strongly implied or loudly insisted that they could be unbiased about the drugs about which they were paid to speak – even when they were handsomely paid. Moreover, identifying biases demands detailed knowledge, as Dr. Kiley states: "There isn't anybody other than a doctor who's going to be able to decide whether there is a conflict, because nobody else has the fund of knowledge to really understand what they're doing." So all KOLs can deny being biased, as Dr. Koch does when he says: "If I don't believe the data, I won't do it. If I don't think the agent on label has a real role or a real niche, if it's not one I'm supportive of, then I don't do it. If I feel the drug company is pushing a sales pitch more than a proper therapeutic use, I won't do it." Different KOLs maintained that the conflicts are "manageable" or can be "minimized", and this needs to be done because "potential positives outweigh the negatives".

I would suggest a third source of success that I think is connected to the two that Boullier and colleagues identify. Conflict of interest is part of accounts focused on individual human agency, in which many of the actors involved in the regulation of medicine, not least physicians and medical researchers, are enormously invested. When the psychological mechanisms are conscious – as when a physician decides to prescribe a product because they will profit from that prescription – agency is front and center. And even when the psychological mechanisms are unconscious, a latent agency has been displaced. In my research, I have been interested in those situations in which the individual agency of medical researchers, physicians, and others is relatively unimportant. In those circumstances, I think that we should turn to one or another of the other frameworks that Boullier et al. discuss: agnotology, capture, or hegemony.

I again return to Dr. Kessel. Somewhat after his disclosures, Kessel described how he had been somewhat discredited as a witness in a lawsuit against a pharmaceutical company. The plaintiff's lawyers had introduced into the proceedings an "individual management plan" for Kessel as a KOL; the lawyers had acquired the plan from the company through a legal discovery procedure. The plan included statements that "so-and-so will meet with him on such-and-such a date with this expected result, and then we'll invite him to do this". The individual KOL management plan challenged Kessel as a witness not just because it showed a conflict of interest, but because it appeared to show him as a tool of the company. He wasn't acting independently.

When I introduced Dr. Kessel above, I mentioned that I heard him speaking at a workshop on KOL management – indeed, the name of the conference included the phrase "KOL management". The term is common in the industry, though it is out of favor as one to be used in public. KOLs and the data they present are carefully managed. Some KOLs are indoctrinated into promotional plans and are trained to give pre-prepared slide shows; they are told that they cannot, because of potential legal liability, deviate from their scripts, and are then placed in specific prepared settings to give their presentations. Higher-level researcher KOLs are brought into a company's ambit through advisory boards and consultancies, their interactions with medical science liaisons are carefully planned, they make presentations with company slide sets, are perhaps given research funds for commercially valuable projects, and may author ghosted articles, which are themselves carefully managed. Good management impinges on KOLs' actual independence, though they may not always be aware of it.

We can see this clearly when KOLs serve as authors on "ghost-managed" (Sismondo, 2018) manuscripts that populate medical journals. Even when pharmaceutical industry trials appear to be led by academic or other actors, chances are that they are run by contract research organizations. In his chapter here, Gaudillière, drawing on documents describing Wyeth's interactions with the agency DesignWrite, coins the term "scientific marketing organization". Scientific marketing organizations like DesignWrite use – and sometimes even direct – the work of contract research organizations to shape medical science. Manuscripts for medical journal articles are most likely drafted by ghostwriters on outlines created by publication planners, and then shepherded through to publication by those planners, with limited opportunities for their academic and other independent authors to contribute. All of this constitutes the ghost-management of medical research.

The ghost-management of trials affords many opportunities to intervene on publications, to affect the published record, and thus to shape medical knowledge. Funding almost certainly affects the interpretation of data and the writing of articles – writing mostly not done by those articles' apparently independent authors. Internal company documents and presentations show that the companies are fully aware of the opportunities for spin (e.g., McHenry, 2010). Just as important, companies can design studies that are likely to produce favorable results, making careful choices of comparators, doses, experimental populations, surrogate endpoints, trial durations, and definitions. For example, in Merck's testing of its COX-2 inhibitor rofecoxib, it used most of these techniques to improve one or another of its published trials (Whitstock, 2018), shaping the science to sell drugs. Sometimes the influence becomes scientific misconduct, through the direct manipulation of data, the omission of adverse events, etc. On the basis of documents from litigation against Forest for misleading marketing of citalopram, Jureidini, Amsterdam, and McHenry (2016) establish that the ghost-management of the research allowed company employees to publish efficacy and safety conclusions that were quite inconsistent with what the trial data could support. To ensure that the negative data wouldn't be known, the company insisted on tight control over the drafting of the manuscript, again leaving KOL authors unable to contribute. Authors' conflict of interest is at best a side-issue.

Many trials are performed when drugs are already on the market, and some are designed primarily to introduce or habituate physicians and patients to products. Such trials would be designed to test an already-studied drug in a way known to be effective, affecting the shape of the medical literature. For example, an important trial of gabapentin was designed as a seeding trial: an internal document about the trial announced, "Some indicators of success include a 20% increase in new patients' starts in March and a 3% market share in new prescriptions" (quoted in Krumholz, Egilman, and Ross, 2011).

Industry trials are more cited than are non-industry trials (Gorry, 2015). The higher level of citation may be partly a result of the fact that pharmaceutical companies have much better resources for promoting their own trials than individual researchers have. For example, the companies employ thousands upon thousands of KOLs to give talks to physicians, using prepared slide shows, on recent clinical research.

In no part of such ghost-management of medical science is conflict of interest particularly relevant. Instead, companies act in their own interest, attempting to establish hegemony over segments of medical science and the practice of medicine. In such situations, KOLs are essentially employees of pharmaceutical companies. Because they occupy other roles as well, we can sometimes understand their actions in terms of conflicts of interest. However, when their agency is tightly circumscribed it is more useful to look at their places in pharmaceutical company plans and actions. The KOLs involved have been anesthetized.

Note

1. Many of the interviews quoted were conducted by Zdenka Chloubova. The discussion here improved through conversations with Khadija Coxon. Any mistakes or failings are the responsibility of the author.

References

Birch, DM and Cohn, G (2001) 'The changing creed of Hopkins science', *The Baltimore Sun*, 25 June. Available at: https://www.baltimoresun.com/news/bs-xpm-2001-06-25-0106250161-story.html (accessed February 17, 2021).

Gorry, P (2015) 'Medical literature imprinting by Pharma ghost writing: A scientometric evaluation', *ISSI Proceedings* 0650. Available at: https://www.issi-society.org/proceedings/issi_2015/0650.pdf (accessed February 17, 2021).

Jureidini, JN, Amsterdam, JD and McHenry, LB (2016) 'The citalopram CIT-MD-18 pediatric depression trial: deconstruction of medical ghostwriting, data mischaracterisation and academic malfeasance', *International Journal of Risk & Safety in Medicine*, 28(1), pp. 33–43.

Krumholz, SD, Egilman, DS and Ross, JS (2011) 'Study of neurontin: titrate to effect, profile of safety (STEPS) trial: a narrative account of a gabapentin seeding trial', *Archives of Internal Medicine*, 171(12), pp. 1100–1107.

McHenry, L (2010) 'Of sophists and spin-doctors: industry-sponsored ghostwriting and the crisis of academic medicine', *Mens Sana Mongraphs*, 8(1), pp. 129–145.

Rodwin, MA (2011) *Conflicts of interest and the future of medicine: the United States, France, and Japan*. Oxford: Oxford University Press.

Sismondo, S (2018) *Ghost-managed medicine: Big Pharma's invisible hands*. Manchester: Mattering Press.

Whitstock, M (2018) 'Manufacturing the truth: from designing clinical trials to publishing trial data', *Indian Journal of Medical Ethics*, 3, pp. 152–3.

Index

accountability 70, 73, 77, 148, 173, 203
Act: Bayh-Dole 9, 35, 49, 73, 214n1;
    Bribery, Graft and Conflicts of
    Interest 14, 34, 221; Clean Air (US) 223;
    Clean Water (US) 223; Federal
    Advisory Committee 14, 34; Freedom
    of Information 14; Physician Payments
    Sunshine 42–43, 50, 87, 150, 160, 187;
    Social Security Financing (France) 131;
    Toxic Substances Control 223
activism 12, 21, 209–212
administrative law 70
adverse: effects 174, 184, 189, 228
    see also side effect; events 50, 168, 243
AFSSA (French Food Safety Agency) 210
AFSSAPS (French medicines
    regulatory agency) 181, 184, 187,
    193, 196
Alzheimer's disease 43, 167, 173–174, 222
*American Journal of Industrial
    Medicine* 205
amphetamine 186
Angell, Marcia 3, 12, 63, 110
ANSES (French Agency for Food,
    Environmental, and Occupational
    Health and Safety) 201
ANSM (French Agency for the Safety
    of Drug) 87 see also AFSSAPS
anti-pesticide: activists 202, 205–206, 210,
    movement 202–203; organizations 209
antidepressant 1, 12, 42, 139, 170–171,
    219–221
asbestos 205, 223, 225
Astra-Zeneca 138, 142
Autain, François 188

Baselga, José 43–44
Bertrand, Xavier 150, 187

Bertrand Law (2011) 87, 98, 159, 158, 187, 194
bias 4, 16–17, 22, 39–42, 50, 62–63, 77, 80,
    109, 112–116, 119–124, 175, 201–213,
    219, 234, 239–242
biased: evaluation 166, 174; knowledge 16
bioethics 4 see also ethics
biomedical research see research
biotechnology 7, 9, 18, 32, 35, 36–39,
    49–50, 55, 59–61, 65n1, 74, 222, 227
black box warning 219
blind trust 129
blockbuster 41, 74
The British Medical Journal 38, 51, 160
bureaucratic 4, 11, 23, 44, 188, 210
Bush, George H.W.: administration 225;
    President 37, 204

cancer 7, 20, 43, 66n3, 159, 165–168,
    173–174, 205, 212, 225, 228
capital 9, 36, 54, 212–213, 227–229,
    232–233
capitalism 8, 46n6, 169, 176, 221, 227–228,
    232, 234
capture 1, 5, 15, 166, 197, 219–221, 223–225,
    229–231, 234–235, 242; corrosive 231;
    strong 231; weak 231
cardiologists 190–195
cardiovascular: disorders 165, 167; risks 173
Carson, Rachel 203
Cenestin® 173
Center for Study of Responsive Law 204–205
CEO (Corporate Europe Observatory)
    14–15, 74, 81, 210–211
chemical industry 165, 203–204, 208, 211
Chiche, Georges 189
chronic heart failure 139
Ciba-Geigy 171
citalopram 243

civil servants 33, 44, 149, 153
    see also government employee
clinical research see research
clinical trials 50, 110, 170
Clinton, Bill: administration 167
CNIL (French data protection agency)
    153, 155–156
CNOM (French National Medical
    Council) 190–191
Cochrane Library 149
Code of Conduct 70–71, 73–78, 81
cohort study 20, 165
COI (conflicts of interest): apparent 111;
    category of 10–13, 16–17, 21, 31–41,
    44–46, 165–167, 175, 229; concept of 31,
    181–182, 188–190, 195–196, 202, 205;
    definition of 130, 187; financial 4, 63,
    131; governance 52, 65; institutional
    106n14, 112, 119–120; laws 33–35;
    management 5, 69, 75, 113, 121; notion
    of 14, 130, 221, 223; (disclosure) policies
    5, 12, 37–41, 51–52, 61–64, 73–75,
    81, 222; potential 15, 111, 114, 120;
    prohibition 79; regulations 33, 43, 222
Collins, Francis 55
competing interest 49, 61–64, 76, 81
ComTox (Commission on Toxics) 210, 215
confidence 31, 70, 137, 188–190, 193
Congress (US) 15, 34, 43, 66n8, 166–167, 203
consultancy 37, 65, 74, 78, 93, 106n14, 239
consultant see consultancy
consumers: interests of 34 see also patient,
    interests
controversies 2–3, 10–13, 18, 21, 31–36,
    42, 49, 74, 131, 144n2, 160, 165–168,
    174–175, 201–203, 206, 212, 219–226,
    233–234
cooling off period 79, 82n8
corporate: influence 1–3, 6, 13, 16,
    20–21, 45, 51, 204–206, 221–223, 230,
    233–234; interests 1, 4–6, 14, 18, 60,
    201, 219–221, 229
corruption 14–17, 51, 159, 197–198, 229–231
Council of Europe 74
Council of State (Conseil d'État, France) 156
counter-hegemony 227, 230, 233–234
Covid-19 1–2, 22n1, 160
criminal trial 182–183, 196
crisis 7–13, 42, 46n19, 52, 151, 165–168,
    173–175, 182, 187–190, 203, 222
culture 10, 38, 55, 114, 188, 227
cultural 58, 228, 233–234

database 2, 5, 15, 20, 65n1, 90–92, **95**,
    98, 106n14, 147–161, 162n6, 162n20,
    176n11, **234**
DDT (dichlorodiphenyltrichloroethane)
    203–204, 206
declaration of interest 32, 36–39, 42,
    45, 73–76, 96, 117–119, 198, 205
    see also (COI) conflicts of interest
denunciation 12–13, 21, 74, 189, 202, 206,
    211, 214, 223
DES (Diethylstilbestrol) 11, 165
DesignWrite 20, 168–169, 172–173,
    176n5–10, 243
DGCCRF (French Directorate for
    Competition Policy, Consumer Affairs
    and Fraud Control) 132
disclosure 2–5, 12–17, 20, 37–38, 50–52,
    61–64, 88, 98, 116–117, 121–125,
    147–149, 152, 160–161, 166, 185–187,
    205, 222–223, 229, **234**, 239–240
distrust see mistrust
DNA 35–36, 46n5
Dollars for Docs 157 see also EurosForDocs
domination 9, 13, 175–176, 228, **234**
Door, Jean-Pierre 187–188
Drazen, Jeffrey 62–63
drug: chain 21, 181–182, 187–193, 196–198,
    241; companies 132–134, 137, 142–143,
    167–169; development 8, 55, 60, 169;
    market 8, 93, 129; regulation 226,
    234; regulatory agencies 14, 18, 44;
    withdrawal of 11, 74, 182–186, 199n1
DSM (Diagnostic and Statistical Manual
    of Mental Disorders) 220
Duramed 173

EDF (Environmental Defense Fund) 204
Eisenhower, Dwight D. 33; administration
    33, 221
EMA (European Medicines Agency) 5, 19,
    38, 43–44, 69–71, 73–81, 81n2, 82n14,
    82n15, 82n16, 82n17, 82n21, 88
environment 35, 50, 201–205, 207–209,
    211–214, 215n6
EPA (Environmental Protection Agency)
    11, 204, 223–225
Epidemiology (Journal) 205
estrogens 165–168
Etalab 148, 155–156
ethics 2–3, 18, 31–32, 66n3, 71–73,
    82n12, 87, 109–111, 116, 133, 222
    see also bioethics

European: (regulatory) agencies 5, 14–15, 70; Commission 2, 38, 72–73, 81, 149; Court of Justice 71; EU (European Union) 2–3, 69, 149, 210; Food Safety Authority (EFSA) 15, 201, 210; governance 73; law 69, 71, 77; Ombudsman 72, 75, 80, 82n8, 82n9, 82n17, 82n20; Parliament 72–75, 81n2, 82n11; Transparency Initiative 15
EurosForDocs 148, 157–160, 162n19 see also Dollars for Docs
executive branch 14
expert: committees 2, 11, 33–34, 43, 149, 222; profile of 87–88, 100; quality of 100
expertise 12, 16–20, 34–35, 44, 56–58, 70, 78, 81, 89–90, 100, 105n4, 123, 129, 158, 166, 175–176, 202, 212–214, 240

falsification 17, 44
FDA (US Food and Drug Administration) 2, 11, 34–35, 38, 44, 53, 57–58, 70, 74, 87, 165–167, 173–174, 219, 224–225
federal (US): agencies 53, 57–59, 66n8, 223, 230; bodies 223–224; advisory committees 34; Government 55, 221–223
fiduciaries 109–110
FIFRA (Federal Insecticide, Fungicide, and Rodenticide Act) 203–204
financial: interests 19, 33–34, 61, 75–79, 110–114, 116–123, 125n3, 129–131, 134–136, 162, 221; relationships 1–2, 5–6, 16, 37, 45, 121, 213; ties 37, 40–43, 109–111, 115–116, 119–120, 131, 147–150, 152, 157–159, 162n6, 166, 174, 213
Formindep 43, 87, 149, 156, 158–160
Foucart, Stéphane 208, 212
Frachon, Irène 159, 184–185, 189
France 2–3, 21, 32, 38, 41–43, 74, 87–89, 117, 131–134, 142, 143n1, 149–150, 157, 161, 181–187, 198, 199n8, 201–202, 206–214, 222, 232
fraud 3, 11–12, 15, 35–37, 45, 132, 151, 196–197, 204–205, 211, 229
funding effect 5

gabapentin 243
Gallup poll 173
Geigy 169–171
Genentech, 35–37
Générations futures 213
generic 133–134, 136–140, 142, 173, 231; companies 20, 131–133, 143; drugs 129–143, 144n2, 173, 229; medicines 20

Germany 129, 143
ghost management 4
ghostwriting 10, 174, 176n4, 223, 228
gifts 4, 50, 76, 81, 115, 117–118, 151, 160, 190
Gilbert, Walter 36
Gilead 1, 160, 162n22
Gleevec® 228
global governance 70 see also European, governance
globalization 70
glyphosate 201, 212
government employee 33–34, 115, 119, 222 see also public, servant and civil servants
GPs (general practitioners) 89, 101, 130–131, 134–135, 137, 140–143, 167, 171–172, 175, 195, 222
Grassley, Chuck: Senator 42
GSK (GlaxoSmithKline) 220
guidelines 36–38, 70, 73–74, 81, 138, 165, 173, 204

h-index 101–104, 106n16–18
Harvard University 36
HAS (French National Authority for Health) 43, 88–89, 96–98, 104, 135
health maintenance organizations 172
hegemony 5, 21–22, 176, 219–223, 227–230, 232–235, 239, 242–244
Heim, Roger 206, 213
Hermange, Marie-Thérèse 187–188
historian 3, 7, 167, 203
history 13, 44, 72, 167, 174–175, 201, 225
honoraria 37, 222
Horel, Stéphane 15, 208–212
hospitality 76, 118, 152
hospitals 10, 50, 89–90, 101, 105n8, 112–113, 140–142, 144n8, 151, 159, 184, 192–193
House of Commons (UK) 12, 220
HPV (Human Papilloma Virus) vaccine 159, 228
HRT (hormone replacement therapies) 13, 20, 42, 165–168, 172–173, 175, 176n4
hypercholesterolemia 139
hypertension 139, 184

IARC (International Agency for Research on Cancer) 212
ICH (International Council for Harmonisation of Technical Requirements for Pharmaceuticals for Human) 81n3
ICMJE (International Committee of Medical Journal Editors) 40, 44

ideology 214, 220, 233
IGAS (French Inspectorate General of
    Social Affairs) 182, 185–188, 199n2
impartiality 69, 76–79, 188, 197
    see also partiality
IMS (Intercontinental Marketing
    Services) 143n1, 170
independence 38, 46n16, 69, 72, 75–77,
    110, 147, 210, 214n1
independent judgment 110, 115, 125
India 228, 233
Industry Documents database (University
    of California San Francisco) 168
inequalities 141, 226–227, 232, 235
Inexium® 138, 142
influence 1–2, 10–14, 17, 20–22, 31–33,
    36–42, 45–46, 49–51, 65, 70, 78, 117,
    130, 134, 142–143, 149–152, 154, 159–161,
    166–167, 171–172, 176, 187–188, 196,
    198, 202–213, 214n4, 219–225, 227–235,
    240–241, 243; channels of 230, 235;
    corporate see corporate, influence; forms
    of 230; peddling 17, 181–182, 185, 190,
    196–198
information: circulation of 13;
    infrastructures 148, 161
INRA (French National Institute
    of Agricultural Research) 206
insurer 130, 136
integrity 1, 5, 14–16, 34–36, 50–51,
    69–71, 112
intellectual property rights 9, 50, 82n13,
    214n1, 228–229, 233
investigative (environmental) journalism
    21, 202, 211

JAMA (Journal of the American Medical
    Association) 37–40, 65n1
Johns Hopkins University 241
Journal of Translational Medicine 54, 57

Kennedy, John F.: President 34, 203
key opinion leaders (KOLs) 3, 10, 22, 171,
    176n4, 228, 239–243

The Lancet 12, 38, 41–42
lawyer 21, 31, 34, 42, 72, 109, 202, 242
LEEM (Les entreprises du médicament)
    148, 150–152, 162n7
legal studies 230
legitimacy 13, 38, 72, 96, 100–102, 104, 167
legitimation 56, 129, 228, **234**

litigation 72–73, 76, 224–225, 243
lobbying 1, 9–10, 14–17, 82n9, 149, 161,
    162n12, **234**

Manning, Bayless 34
market: shares 133, 171–172
marketing authorization 79, 174, 187, 202
Marxism 227
MCA (Medicines Control Agency) 39,
    46n13
media 1–3, 11–12, 17–18, 21, 32–37, 41,
    44–45, 131, 147, 159–160, 166, 181,
    185–187, 191–195, 198, 206, 209,
    211–212, 219, 222
Mediator® (benfluorex) 21, 42, 74, 98, 147,
    150–151, 159, 181–186, 190–198, 241
medical: journal 4–5, 12–13, 16, 32, 35–36,
    39–41, 44, 166, 190, 198, 243; students
    144n7, 147, 190–191, 198
medicalization 12, 168, 175
Merck 39–41, 62, 220, 243
mergers 7
MHRA (Medicines and Healthcare
    Products Regulatory Agency) 219–220
Ministry of Agriculture (France) 206,
    209–210, 213
Ministry of Health (France) 143n1,
    147–148, 150–151, 153–157, 161, 162n8,
    162n13, 162n15
mistrust 33, 137
mobilization 11–14, 16–18, 33, 151, 155,
    169, 175, 201
Le Monde (newspaper) 158–159, 185,
    211–212, 215n6
Mopral® 138
moral: judgement 6; licensing 52, 222
Mother Jones 211

Nader, Ralph 14, 204, 207, 214n3
NAS (National Academy of Sciences) 34
National Assembly (France) 182, 187–188
Nature (journal) 38, 49, 61, 65n1
Nature Biotechnology (journal) 49, 65n1
Nature Cell Biology (journal) 61
NCATS (National Center for Advancing
    Translational Sciences) 58
NEJM (New England Journal of Medicine)
    37, 40–42, 51, 62–64, 166
neoliberal 70, 161, 223
neuroscience 240
New York Times (journal) 2, 33, 43,
    46n4–10, 168, 174, 176n2

NGO (non-profit organization) 11–17, 38, 43–45, 72–74, 80–81, 149, 201, 207, 210, 212–213, 222
NHI (French national health insurance scheme) 131–143, 144n3, 144n6
Nicolino, Fabrice 208, 213
NIH (National Institutes of Health) 37, 46n9, 53, 55–61, 167
Nimitz Commission 33
No Free Lunch 87, 149
Nobel Prize 36, 62
norms 4, 46, 54, 112, 181, 187, 190, 223, 239
Novartis 133, 228–229
NWHN (US National Women's Health Network) 167

OECD (Organization for Economic Co-operation and Development) 15, 70, 74, 82n12, 110–111, 117, 125n2, 129, 145
off-label 42, 219; prescriptions 175, 181, 220
Official Repository of Generic Drugs (France) 132, 134–135
openness 160, 210, 215n5
opioids 1, 139
osteoporosis 165–168, 173–174

PAN (Pesticides Actions Network) Europe 210, 213
paroxetine 219–220
partiality 98 see also impartiality
patent 8–10, 20, 35–37, 59, 74, 82n17, 130, 136, 144n5, 228–229, 233
patient: group, association 3, 5, 43, 74, 105n4, 105n8, 147; interests 134–136, 190 see also consumers, interest
patient-physician relationship 122–123, 125, 190–191
pediatric 219
Perec, Georges 182, 190, 195, 198
personal interests 33–35, 109–111, 117
pesticide risk assessment 201, 204, 209–210, 213
pharmaceutical: companies, firms 2, 5, 8, 11, 12, 16, 20–22, 39–41, 44, 50, 60–62, 69, 75–79, 91–92, 111, 117–119, 129–133, 136–138, 143, 144n8, 148, 150–152, 155, 159, 193, 195, 220, 244; industry 1–3, 11, 16, 22, 37–46, 50, 75–77, 88, 91, 96, 100, 104, 105n4, 142, 151, 154, 157, 161, 165, 168, 190–197, 220–222, 228, 239–242; market 20; regulation 224; (sales) representatives 8, 80, 88, 151, 167–172, 190, 195, 215n5, 220, 228

pharmaceuticalization 13, 169, 221
pharmacist 19–20, 89, 101, 109, 112, 129–143, 147, 170, 173–174, 184, 222, 234
placebo 46n12, 139, 220
Plavix® 137–138, 144n5
PLOS Medicine (journal) 168, 174
political economy 3, 6–7, 9–10, 41, 230, **234**
politicians 2, 11, 13, 33–35, 149, 161, 196
politicization 6, 10–13, 32, 44
power 12–13, 22, 35, 38–40, 44–45, 65, 66n3, 71, 76, 117, 125n3, 132, 139, 224, 226–230, 233–235
PPIs (proton pump inhibitors) 134, 138, 142
precautionary principle 71
Premarin® 168, 172–174, 176n6, 176n9, 176n10
Prempro® 167–168, 174, 176n3–10
prescribers 20, 135, 142–143, 172, 175, 198
prescribing 8, 21, 50, 110, 129, 131, 134–136, 138–141, 160, 173–175, 182, 190, 194, 220
prescription 4, 8, 19–20, 130–131, 134–135, 138–143, 159, 167, 170–173, 181, 190, 220, 242
Prescrire (journal) 149, 198
price 2, 8, 20, 43, 88, 132–135, 137–139, 142, 144n8 156, 166, 174, 224
problematization 3–5
production of ignorance 1, 21, 219–221, 225–226, 231–232
professional interest 129–131
profit 12–14, 31, 51, 59, 87, 112, 119, 140, 176, 206, 212, 227, 242
progestogens 168
ProPublica 15, 43
Prozac® 219
psychiatry 12, 43, 144n7, 220, 239
psychology 22, 222, 241
public: Citizen (organization) 14, 38; interest 13, 32, 37, 45, 73, 188, 206, 223, 229, 231, 241; servant 109–111, 113–114 see also government employee

R&D (research and development) 7, 9, 55–56, 59, 143, 169
raloxifene 174
Reagan, Ronald: administration 225; President 204, 223–224
Regards Citoyens 155–156, 158
regulation: regime of 176; soft 229
regulatory: agency 1–2, 5, 11, 14–16, 19, 31, 34, 38, 41, 41–44, 53, 73, 149, 166, 171, 181, 187, 212, 219–222, 226, 230; capture 5, 197, 220, 223, **234**

Relman, Arnold 37, 51, 64
repertoire 9, 206, 213; action 41–42, 45,
    222; protest 6, 201, 209, 213
representatives: drug 8, 167, 169, 172;
    medical 170; sales 190, 195, 220,
    228 see also pharmaceutical (sales)
    representatives
research: biomedical 10, 19, 32, 38, 41,
    49–54, 56–57, 59–60, 63–65, 66n4,
    66n7; clinical 3, 8–9 45, 50–55, 90,
    169–173, 194, 244; funding 39, 54, 205,
    232; medical 32, 51, 101, 230, 240, 243;
    translational see translational research
revolving door 3, 33, **234**
risk: assessment 21, 88, 201–202, 204–205,
    207–211, 213–214; reduction 168;
    society 12
risk–benefit: balance 138; profile 220
rofecoxib 243 see also Vioxx®
Rosenbaum, Lisa 4, 62–63, 112
Royal Society of Chemistry (UK) 62
royalties 112, 117–119

Sandoz 133
Sanofi-Aventis 137–138, 144n4
SBIR (Small Business Innovation
    Research) program 59, 66n8
scandal 37, 40, 44, 46n13, 208; Mediator®
    21, 42, 98, 147, 150–151, 181–182,
    185–186, 190–198
scandalization 6, 10, 12
science: financing of 5; misconduct in
    12, 36–37, 44, 243; undone 226–227,
    232–233, **234**
scientific: articles 4, 37, 39–41, 42–44,
    49, 52, 63, 65n1, 166, 172, 240, 243;
    entrepreneurship 12, 32, 35–36, 222; fraud
    3, 12, 35–37; knowledge 11, 18, 49, 110,
    214, 225–226; marketing 5, 8, 20, 137–138,
    165, 168–175, 228, 243; SMO (scientific
    marketing organization) 20, 168–169,
    172–174, 243; reputation 89–90, 104
secrecy 16
Senate (France) 87, 182, 187–189
SERMs (selective estrogen receptor
    modulators) 173–174
Servier (Laboratoires) 159, 181, 183–186,
    192, 196, 199n8, 241
side effects 12, 21, 137, 181–183, 195
    see also adverse, effects
social sciences 1–3, 7, 12, 18, 21, 72, 205,
    222, 225, 230–233
soft law 17, 69–73

Solomon, Jeff 172
speakers' bureau 172, 176n5
SSRIs (selective serotonin reuptake
    inhibitors) 219–220
statistics 32, 49, 63, **95**, 156
STS (science and technology studies) 11,
    51, 60, 64, 223
STTR (Small Business Technology
    Transfer) program 59, 66n8
studies of science 7, 227

technology transfer 58–59, 74
therapeutic: classes 8, 135, 170; interest 129
tobacco: industry 1, 209, 222, 225; papers 16
Tofranil® 170
Toxicological Sciences (journal) 205
trade secrets 150–152
tranquilizers 170
translational: medicine 18–19, 49, 52–58,
    60–65, 65n1, 66n4, 241; research 56–58
Transparence santé (database, France)
    16, 20, 90–92, **95**, 98, 105n7, 106n14,
    147–150, 153–161
transparency 3, 6, 13–20, 38, 42, 50–51,
    61–62, 69, 73–78, 87–88, 98, 115n147–152,
    154–161, 162n6, 187, 194, 198, 210,
    229, **234**, 239, 240; apparatus 13, 20;
    committee (France) 87–88, 105n4;
    data-driven 147; devices 17; industrial
    20, 147–148, 161; institutional 15, 148;
    movement 6; procedures 210; register
    15, 73, 149; studies 17, 148
Truman, Harry S.: administration 33, 221;
    President 33
Trump, Donald: administration 225;
    President 2
trust 4, 11, 13, 17, 31, 51, 76, 109–110,
    114, 115, 120–124, 147, 154, 161, 174,
    192–194, 206, 239
type 2 diabetes 139

the United Kingdom 39, 41, 46n13, 51,
    129, 143n1, 219, 232
the United States 2, 13, 32–34, 38–42,
    49–53, 73, 87, 112, 129, 143n1, 144n2,
    148–149, 166–168, 201–206, 209–214,
    219–223, 225, 232
university 2, 7, 14, 31–32, 35–37, 40, 43,
    49–51, 59, 74, 89–90, 105n8, 112, 121,
    214n1, 222; COI/disclosure policy 38,
    121, 159, 203, 240; financing 112
University of California 16, 35–36, 40,
    168, 214n3

USDA (US Department of Agriculture)
    202–205
US Senate 33, 43, 46n2
US Supreme Court 13, 33, 125

vaccines 1–2, 42, 159, 228
values 49–51, 60–65, 71, 143, 227–229,
    232–233
Veillerette, François 208, 213
VHDs (valvular heart diseases) 184, 192
Vioxx® 1, 12, 41–42, 147, 222

waivers 34, 116
Wakefield, Andrew 42

Waksman, Selman 62
watchdog organizations 1, 230
WHI (Women's Health Initiative) 20,
    165–168
whistleblowers 16, 31
WHO (World Health Organization) 42,
    74, 134, 183
World Trade Organization agreement
    on TRIPS (Trade-Related Aspects of
    Intellectual Property Rights) 74, 86,
    228–229
Wyeth 20, 167–169, 172–174, 176n5–10, 243

Yale University 36–37

For Product Safety Concerns and Information please contact our EU
representative GPSR@taylorandfrancis.com
Taylor & Francis Verlag GmbH, Kaufingerstraße 24, 80331 München, Germany

www.ingramcontent.com/pod-product-compliance
Lightning Source LLC
Chambersburg PA
CBHW060241220326
41598CB00027B/4003